# Algorithmic Selection and Interpretation of Diagnostic Tests

D1447303

1/27/15

To mark
good luck
9 cresery
re âro/um
your brother
Roicy

# Algorithmic Selection and Interpretation of Diagnostic Tests

R. Douglas Collins, M.D., F.A.C.P.
Diplomate, American Board of Internal Medicine
Diplomate, American Board of
Clinical Neurology
Consulting Neurologist and Internist
Lancaster Community Hospital
Lancaster, California

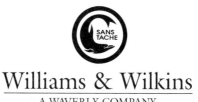

Williams & Wilkins
A WAVERLY COMPANY

BALTIMORE • PHILADELPHIA • LONDON • PARIS • BANGKOK
HONG KONG • MUNICH • SYDNEY • TOKYO • WROCLAW

Editor: Jonathan W. Pine, Jr
Managing Editor: Molly L. Mullen
Production Coordinator: Peter J. Carley
Project Editor: Ulita Lushnycky
Typesetter: Bi-Comp, Inc.
Printer/Binder: Transcontinental

*Printed in Canada*

**Library of Congress Cataloging-in-Publication
Data**

Collins, R. Douglas.
   Algorithmic selection and interpretation of
diagnostic tests / R. Douglas Collins.
      p.    cm.
   Includes bibliographical references.
   ISBN 0-683-30426-7
   1. Diagnosis, Laboratory—Handbooks, manuals,
etc.  2. Diagnosis, Radioscopic—Handbooks,
manuals, etc.  3. Medical protocols—Handbooks,
manuals, etc.  I. Title.
   [DNLM: 1. Diagnosis.  2. Algorithms.
3. Decision Support Techniques.  4. Diagnostic
Tests, Routine.    WB 141 C712a 1998]
   RB38.2.C64   1998
   616.07′5—dc21                 97-31730
                                     CIP

                                 98 99 00
          1 2 3 4 5 6 7 8 9 10

# Dedication

To Our Lord Jesus Christ

# Acknowledgments

I am indebted to Clayton Reynolds, M.D., F.A.C.P., who reviewed the book for accuracy and offered many valuable criticisms. My wife, Norie, gave up her time with me on two vacations to Florida so this book could be completed. Finally, Melissa Pelzer is gratefully acknowledged for typing the manuscript and assisting in laying out the algorithms.

# Preface

With the twentieth century has come an explosive expansion of the number of diagnostic tests, not just laboratory tests, but also radiographs and special diagnostic procedures such as ultrasonography and endoscopy. As a result, a need exists for a practical manual that will aid the clinician in the selection and interpretation of these tests in a cost-effective manner. *Algorithmic Selection and Interpretation of Diagnostic Tests* is designed to fulfill that need. With that in mind, the book has been divided into two useful sections.

Part I deals with the interpretation of diagnostic tests. Tests are arranged alphabetically with a discussion and often with an algorithm picturing the differential diagnosis of each test. Suggestions for additional tests to order to further nail down the diagnosis are displayed.

Part II, Section A deals with the selection of diagnostic tests for the workup of common symptoms and signs. The symptoms and signs are listed alphabetically. When confronted with a patient presenting with a certain symptom or sign, the clinician will have a handy list of tests to order in the diagnostic workup.

Finally, Part II, Section B provides the clinician with a quick reference to useful diagnostic tests to order in each disease. Many rare diseases are included in this section, along with more common disorders.

I hope that the clinician will find this book useful in both ordering and interpreting diagnostic tests in the office or hospital ward.

*Lancaster, California*                    R. Douglas Collins,
                                           M.D., F.A.C.P.

# INTRODUCTION

## HOW TO USE THIS BOOK

The diagnostic test comes back abnormal. Now what do you do? This quandary faces almost every clinician in this country on a daily basis. Knee deep in a busy medical practice, where do you turn for help? It is hard to get a quick answer from your local laboratory or library, and you do not want to bother a specialist or colleague.

This book was written to provide the answer. There are no chapters. Rather, the diagnostic tests are listed alphabetically so the clinician can immediately turn to the test to find out what an abnormal test result means. *Normal values* are supplied to allow the clinician to ascertain that the test is abnormal, and *additional tests* are listed that may be necessary to pin down the diagnosis. With this information at hand, the clinician can approach the problem accurately and efficiently.

Another common problem is the patient who presents with a certain symptom and sign. Where do you turn to find out what tests to order? This book provides the solution to that problem, in Part II, on diagnostic test selection. Here you will find a list of tests to order to work up each symptom and sign. Once again, these symptoms and signs are listed alphabetically for easy reference. Suppose you suspect a certain disease as an explanation of the patient's presenting symptom or sign but need a list of tests to order to confirm the diagnosis. Part II can provide the solution to that problem also. A second table provides a selection of tests to work up each disease. To make your choices cost-effective, the relative cost of each test is given in the section on test interpretation. Costs of tests are valued at low, medium, high, and very high. The actual cost varies by geographic area. The cost translates as follows:

Low: less than $100.00
Medium: $100.00 to $500.00
High: $500.00 to $1000.00
Very high: $1000.00 and above

In reviewing the charges of local hospitals and other resource material, I encountered a few surprises. For example, all but a few laboratory tests (such as parathyroid hormone, HLA typing, somatomedin C) were in the low cost range (under $100.00). Most radiographs were in the medium cost range. Ultrasonography was also usually in the medium price range, whereas radionucleotide scans were usually high in cost. Computed tomography was usually high in price, whereas magnetic resonance imaging procedures were very high.

# Contents

Preface                                                    vii
Introduction: How to Use This Book                         viii

Part I: Interpretation of Diagnostic Tests

Abdominal plain films                                        3
Acetone                                                      5
Acetylcholine receptor antibody test                        7
Acid phosphatase, blood                                     8
Acid phosphatase, vaginal                                  10
Adrenocorticotropic hormone (ACTH), plasma                 11
Adrenocorticotropic hormone (ACTH)
    infusion test                                          13
Albumin, serum                                             15
Aldolase                                                   17
Aldosterone, serum or urine                                18
Alkaline phosphatase                                       20
Allergy skin testing                                       24
Alpha$_1$-antitrypsin test                                 25
Alpha$_1$-fetoprotein                                      27
Amebiasis antibody tests                                   28
Amino acids                                                29
$\delta$-Aminolevulinic acid, urinary                      31
Ammonia                                                    32
Amniocentesis                                              33
Amylase, serum                                             34
Androstenedione                                            36
Angiography                                                38
Angiotensin I-converting enzyme                            41
Animal inoculation                                         42
Anion gap                                                  43
Ankle/brachial index                                       44
Antidiuretic hormone (ADH)                                 46
Anti-DNA antibody test                                     48
Anti-DNase-B                                               49
Antiglomerular basement membrane
    antibody titer                                         50
Antimitochondrial antibody test                            51
Antineutrophil cytoplasmic antigen
    antibodies (ANCA)                                      52
Antinuclear antibody test (ANA)                            53

| | |
|---|---|
| Antiparietal cell antibody | 55 |
| Antiplatelet antibody | 56 |
| Antisclerodermal antibody titer | 57 |
| Anti-Smith antibody titer | 58 |
| Antismooth muscle antibody test | 59 |
| Antisperm antibody test | 60 |
| Antistreptolysin O titer | 61 |
| Antithrombin III | 62 |
| Aortic sonography | 63 |
| Aortography | 64 |
| Arsenic, urine | 65 |
| Arthrography | 66 |
| Arthroscopy | 67 |
| Aspartate aminotransferase (AST) (SGOT) and Alanine aminotransferase (SGPT) | 68 |
| *Aspergillus* antibody titer | 70 |
| Audiometry, screening | 71 |
| Autohemolysis | 73 |
| Barium enema | 74 |
| Barr body analysis | 76 |
| Basophilic stippling | 77 |
| Basophils | 78 |
| Bence Jones protein, urine | 79 |
| Bernstein test | 80 |
| Bicarbonate | 81 |
| Bilirubin, serum | 83 |
| Bilirubin, urine | 86 |
| Biopsy | 87 |
| Blastomycosis antibody test | 88 |
| Blastomycosis skin test | 89 |
| Bleeding time | 90 |
| Blood cultures | 92 |
| Blood smear for morphology | 93 |
| Blood typing | 96 |
| Blood urea nitrogen (BUN) | 99 |
| Blood volume studies | 102 |
| Bone marrow examination | 104 |
| Bone marrow scan | 107 |
| Bone scan | 109 |
| Brain scan | 110 |
| Breast ultrasonography | 111 |
| Bronchography | 112 |
| Bronchoscopy | 113 |
| *Brucella* antibody | 114 |
| Brucellosis skin test | 115 |
| Calcitonin | 116 |

| | |
|---|---|
| Calcium | **118** |
| Calcium, urine, 24-hour | **121** |
| Cancer antigens | **123** |
| Capillary fragility test | **124** |
| Carbon dioxide | **126** |
| Carboxyhemoglobin | **128** |
| Carcinoembryonic antigen (CEA) | **129** |
| Cardiac catheterization and angiocardiography | **131** |
| Cardiac series | **133** |
| Carotene | **134** |
| Carotid duplex scan | **136** |
| Casts | **137** |
| CD4 and T-cell lymphocyte count | **139** |
| Cerebrospinal fluid (CSF) pressure | **140** |
| Chancroid skin test | **142** |
| Chest radiography | **143** |
| Chloride, blood | **150** |
| Cholecystography | **152** |
| Cholesterol | **154** |
| Chromosome analysis | **157** |
| Cisternography | **158** |
| *Clostridium difficile* toxin assay | **159** |
| Clot retraction | **160** |
| Coagulant factors | **162** |
| Coagulation time | **164** |
| *Coccidioides* antibody test | **166** |
| Coccidioidomycosis skin test | **167** |
| Cold agglutinins | **168** |
| Colonoscopy | **170** |
| Color, urine | **171** |
| Colposcopy | **173** |
| Complement C3 | **174** |
| Computed tomography, abdomen | **176** |
| Computed tomorophy, brain | **177** |
| Computed tomography, chest | **178** |
| Computed tomography, extremities and joints | **179** |
| Computed tomography, head | **180** |
| Computed tomography, neck | **181** |
| Computed tomography, pelvis | **182** |
| Computed tomography, spine | **183** |
| Coombs' test, direct and indirect | **184** |
| Copper and ceruloplasmin | **185** |
| Cortisol | **187** |
| C-peptide | **189** |
| C-reactive protein (CRP) | **191** |
| Creatine phosphokinase | **193** |

Creatinine 195
Creatinine clearance 197
Cryoglobulins 198
Cryptococcus antigen titer 199
Crystals, urine 200
Cultures of miscellaneous body fluids 201
Cutaneous immunofluorescence biopsy 207
Cyclic adenosine monophosphate (cAMP),
  renal 208
Cystine 209
Cystometric studies 210
Cystoscopy 211
Cytologic studies 212
Cytomegalovirus antibodies 217
Dehydroepiandrosterone sulfate (DHEA-S) 218
Dexamethasone suppression test 219
Digital subtraction angiography 221
Drug screen, serum and urine 222
Duodenal analysis 223
*Echinococcosis* stain test 224
Echocardiography 225
Echoencephalography 226
Electrocardiography 227
Electroencephalography 231
Electromyography 233
Endoscopic retrograde
  cholangiopancreatography 234
Eosinophil count 235
Epstein-Barr antibody test 236
Erythropoietin 238
Esophagogastroduodenoscopy 240
Estradiol, blood and urine 241
Estriol, blood 243
Estrogen and progesterone receptor proteins 244
Evoked potential studies 245
Exercise tolerance testing 246
Febrile agglutinins 247
Fern test 249
Ferritin 250
Ferrokinetic studies 252
Fetal hemoglobin in maternal blood 254
Fibrin split products 255
Fibrinogen 257
Fibrinolysis/euglobulin lysis time 258
Fishberg concentration test 260
Fluorescein angiography 261

Fluorescent treponemal antibody absorption
  test (FTA–ABS) ... 262
Folic acid ... 263
Follicle-stimulating hormone (FSH), blood
  and urine ... 265
Free thyroxine ($T_4$) ... 268
Free thyroxine index (FTI) ... 270
Free triiodothyronine ($T_3$) ... 271
Frei test ... 273
Fructosamine assay ... 274
Galactose-1-phosphate uridyl transferase ... 275
Gallbladder or hepatoiminodiacetic acid
  (HIDA) scan ... 276
Gallbladder ultrasonography ... 277
Gallium scan ... 278
Gastrin ... 279
Gastrointestinal bleeding scan ... 281
Gliadin antibody ... 282
Glucagon ... 283
Glucose, blood ... 285
Glucose, cerebrospinal fluid ... 287
Glucose, urine ... 289
Glucose tolerance test ... 291
Glucose-6-phosphate dehydrogenase (G6PD) ... 294
$\gamma$-Glutamyltransferase ... 296
Glycosylated hemoglobin ... 298
Growth hormone ... 299
Ham test ... 301
Haptoglobin ... 302
Heart shunt scan ... 304
Heavy metals ... 305
Heinz bodies ... 308
Hematocrit ... 309
Hematuria ... 311
Hemoglobin ... 313
Hemoglobin, Bart's ... 315
Hemoglobin electrophoresis ... 316
Hemoglobin F ... 318
Hepatitis panel ... 319
Histiocyte smear, blood ... 321
Histoplasmosis antibody test ... 322
Histoplasmosis skin test ... 323
HIV antibody tests ... 324
HLA testing ... 325
Holter monitoring ... 326
Homogentisic acid, urine ... 327

Homovanillic acid, urine 328
Hydrogen breath analysis 329
5-Hydroxyindoleacetic acid (5-HIAA) 330
Hydroxyproline, urine 331
Hysterosalpingography 333
Immunoelectrophoresis 334
Impedance phlebography 337
Insulin 338
Intravenous cholangiography 340
Intravenous pyelography 341
Iron, serum 343
Iron-binding capacity, total 345
17-Ketosteroids, 17-ketogenic steroids, urine 347
Lactic acid, arterial blood 349
Lactic acid dehydrogenase (LDH) 350
Lactic acid dehydrogenase (LDH),
    cerebrospinal fluid (CSF) 352
Lactic acid dehydrogenase (LDH) isozymes 354
Lactose tolerance 356
Laparoscopy 357
*Legionella* antibody 358
Leptospirosis antibody titer 359
Leucine aminopeptidase (LAP), blood, urine 360
Leukocyte alkaline phosphatase 362
Lipase 364
Lipoprotein electrophoresis 366
Liver scan 368
Liver ultrasonography 369
Long-acting thyroid stimulator (LATS) 370
Lyme disease antibody 371
Lymphangiography 372
Lysozyme, blood and urine 373
Magnesium 374
Magnetic resonance imaging, abdomen 376
Magnetic resonance imaging, brain 377
Magnetic resonance imaging, chest 378
Magnetic resonance imaging, joints 379
Magnetic resonance imaging, neck 380
Magnetic resonance imaging, pelvis 381
Magnetic resonance imaging, spine 382
Mammography 383
Mean corpuscular hemoglobin (MCH) 384
Mean corpuscular hemoglobin
    concentration (MCHC) 386
Mean corpuscular volume (MCV) 388
Melanin, urine 390

Mediastinoscopy 391
Methemoglobin 392
Metyrapone test 394
Minimum inhibitory concentration (MIC) 396
Monospot test 397
Mucopolysaccharide screen, urine 399
Mucoproteins 400
Myelin basic protein, cerebrospinal fluid 402
Myelography 403
Myoglobin, blood, urine 404
Nerve conduction studies 406
Nitrite test 408
Obstetric ultrasonography 409
Orbital and ocular ultrasonography 410
Osmolality, serum 411
Oval fat bodies and fatty casts 413
Oxygen, arterial 414
Pancreatic scan 416
Pancreatic ultrasonography 417
Paranasal sinus radiography 418
Parathyroid hormone 419
Parathyroid ultrasonography 421
Partial thromboplastin time (PTT) and
    activated partial thromboplastin time
    (APTT) 422
Pelvic ultrasonography 424
Pelvimetry 425
Peritoneal fluid analysis 426
pH 428
pH, urine 430
Pharyngeal smear 432
Phenylalanine, blood 433
Phonocardiography 434
Phosphorus 435
Platelet aggregation 438
Platelet antibodies 439
Platelet count 440
Pleural fluid analysis 442
Porphyrins, urine 444
Potassium 446
Potassium, urine 24-hour 448
Pregnancy test, blood and urine 450
Pregnanediol, urine 452
Pregnanetriol, urine 454
Prolactin 455
Prostate-specific antigen (PSA) 457

**Contents** **xvii**

| | |
|---|---|
| Protein, cerebrospinal fluid | **458** |
| Protein, urine | **460** |
| Protein electrophoresis | **462** |
| Protein electrophoresis, cerebrospinal fluid | **465** |
| Prothrombin consumption test (serum prothrombin time) | **466** |
| Prothrombin time | **468** |
| Pulmonary capillary wedge pressure | **470** |
| Pulmonary function studies | **471** |
| Pyruvate kinase | **479** |
| Radioactive iodine (RAI) fibrinogen venogram | **480** |
| Radioactive iodine (RAI) total body scan | **481** |
| Radioactive iodine (RAI) uptake and scan | **482** |
| Radioactive iodine (RAI) uptake stimulation test | **484** |
| Radioallergosorbent tests (RAST) | **485** |
| Red blood cell count (RBC) | **486** |
| Red cell casts | **488** |
| Red cell fragility | **490** |
| Red cell size distribution width (RDW) | **492** |
| Red cell survival time | **493** |
| Renal ultrasonography | **495** |
| Renin | **496** |
| Renogram | **498** |
| Residual volume, urine | **499** |
| Reticulocyte count | **500** |
| Retrograde pyelography | **502** |
| Retroperitoneal ultrasonography | **503** |
| Rheumatoid factor | **504** |
| Rocky Mountain spotted fever antibodies | **506** |
| Rubella antibody tests | **507** |
| Salivary gland scan | **508** |
| Schilling test | **509** |
| Sedimentation rate | **511** |
| Semen analysis | **513** |
| Shake test | **514** |
| Sickle cell test | **515** |
| Sigmoidoscopy and anoscopy | **516** |
| Sjögren's antibody test | **517** |
| Small bowel series | **518** |
| Smears and microscopic examination of body fluids | **519** |
| Sodium | **524** |
| Sodium, urine | **526** |
| Somatomedin C | **528** |

Specific gravity, urine 529
Spleen scan 531
Spleen ultrasonography 532
Sputum culture, routine 533
Stool analysis 535
Streptococcal antibody tests (ASO, ADB, streptozyme) 537
Sulfhemoglobin 538
Sweat test 539
Synovial fluid analysis 540
T and B lymphocytes 542
Technetium-99m resting heart scan 544
Teichoic acid antibody titer 545
Testosterone 546
Thallium gated equilibrium heart scan 548
Thallium stress scan 549
Therapeutic drug monitoring 550
Throat culture, routine 551
Thrombin time 553
Thyroglobulin 554
Thyroid antibodies 555
Thyroid ultrasonography 556
Thyroid-stimulating hormone (TSH)–sensitive assay 557
Thyrotropin-releasing hormone (TRH) stimulation test 559
Thyroxine-binding globulin (TBG) 561
TORCH test 563
Total protein 564
Total thyroxine ($T_4$) 566
Toxoplasmosis antibody tests 568
Toxoplasmosis skin test 569
Trichinella skin test 570
Triglyceride 571
Trypsin, stool 574
Tuberculin test 575
Tyrosine, urine 576
Upper gastrointestinal series and esophagogram 577
Uric acid 579
Uric acid, urine 581
Urinary bladder ultrasonography 583
Urine culture 584
Urobilinogen, stool 586
Urobilinogen, urine 588

Vanillylmandelic acid (VMA) and
   catecholamines                                   **590**
Venereal Disease Research Laboratory
   (VDRL) and rapid plasma reagin (RPR)      **591**
Venography                                        **592**
Ventilation-perfusion scan                   **593**
Viral isolation and antibody tests         **595**
Viscosity, blood                              **596**
Vitamin $B_{12}$                                    **598**
Vitamin D metabolites
   (25-hydroxycalciferol)                        **600**
Vitamins, miscellaneous                       **602**
White blood cell count (WBC), cerebrospinal
   fluid                                            **605**
White blood cell count (WBC), differential    **607**
White blood cell count (WBC), total         **609**
White blood cell count (WBC), urine        **611**
D-Xylose absorption                          **613**
Zinc protoporphyrins                        **614**

Part II: Diagnostic Test Selection

A.  Selection of Diagnostic Tests in the
    Workup of Symptoms and Signs       **617**
B.  Selection of Diagnostic Tests in the
    Workup of Diseases                 **662**

Bibliography                                **694**

# PART I

**INTERPRETATION OF
DIAGNOSTIC TESTS**

# ABDOMINAL PLAIN FILMS

Ask the following questions:

1. Is there increased air?
   a. Extraluminal: This may signify a ruptured peptic ulcer or other portion of the GI tract or a subphrenic abscess.
   b. Intraluminal: If it is in the small intestine, with air–fluid levels, it signifies intestinal obstruction; if it is in the large and small intestine, it indicates paralytic ileus. If it is in the large intestine alone, it is probably a normal finding but could result from obstruction.
2. Is there increased fluid?
   a. Extraluminal: Suspect ascites, blood from ruptured ectopic pregnancy, or abscess.
   b. Intraluminal: It may be due to bladder distension, distended intestine, ovarian cyst, or pancreatic cyst.
3. Are calcifications or other opacities present? Suspect gallstones, renal calculi, fecalith in the appendix, pancreatic calcifications, calcified blood vessels or lymph nodes, and foreign bodies.
4. Is a mass present? Suspect enlarged liver, kidney, spleen, uterus, or bladder or tumor.

## COST

Low.

## ADDITIONAL TESTS TO ORDER

CBC, chemistry panel, electrolytes, urinalysis, amylase and lipase, ultrasound of gallbladder, HIDA study, pregnancy test, IVP, CT scan of abdomen, peritoneoscopy, and surgical consult.

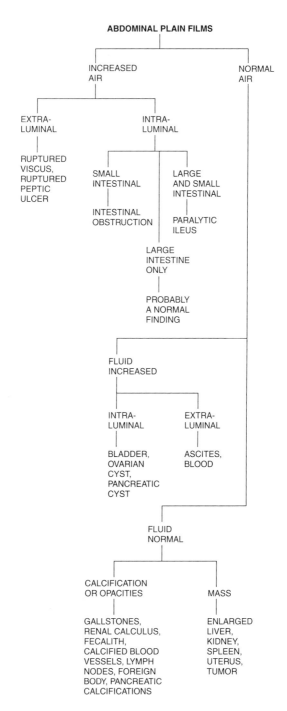

**ABDOMINAL PLAIN FILMS**

- INCREASED AIR
  - EXTRA-LUMINAL
    - RUPTURED VISCUS, RUPTURED PEPTIC ULCER
  - INTRA-LUMINAL
    - SMALL INTESTINAL
      - INTESTINAL OBSTRUCTION
    - LARGE AND SMALL INTESTINAL
      - PARALYTIC ILEUS
    - LARGE INTESTINE ONLY
      - PROBABLY A NORMAL FINDING
- NORMAL AIR
  - FLUID INCREASED
    - INTRA-LUMINAL
      - BLADDER, OVARIAN CYST, PANCREATIC CYST
    - EXTRA-LUMINAL
      - ASCITES, BLOOD
  - FLUID NORMAL
    - CALCIFICATION OR OPACITIES
      - GALLSTONES, RENAL CALCULUS, FECALITH, CALCIFIED BLOOD VESSELS, LYMPH NODES, FOREIGN BODY, PANCREATIC CALCIFICATIONS
    - MASS
      - ENLARGED LIVER, KIDNEY, SPLEEN, UTERUS, TUMOR

**4    Abdominal Plain Films**

# ACETONE

## POSITIVE

Acetone is increased in the plasma and urine in diabetic acidosis, drug effects, starvation, acute illnesses, prolonged vomiting, and febrile states. To differentiate this condition from diabetic acidosis, one should determine blood or urine glucose levels. To determine whether drugs are the cause, a thorough history of drug ingestion is necessary.

## NORMAL VALUES

Negative.

## COST

Low.

## ADDITIONAL TESTS TO ORDER

CBC, urinalysis, urine drug screen, chemistry panel, glucose tolerance test, serum electrolytes, arterial blood gas analysis, glycosylated hemoglobin, blood volume, osmolarity, and endocrinology consult.

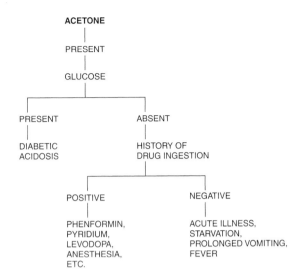

ACETONE
|
PRESENT
|
GLUCOSE
|
┌──────────────────────────┴──────────────────────────┐
PRESENT                                          ABSENT
|                                                |
DIABETIC                                         HISTORY OF
ACIDOSIS                                         DRUG INGESTION
                                    ┌────────────────────────┴────────────────────────┐
                                 POSITIVE                                          NEGATIVE
                                    |                                                |
                                 PHENFORMIN,                                      ACUTE ILLNESS,
                                 PYRIDIUM,                                        STARVATION,
                                 LEVODOPA,                                        PROLONGED VOMITING,
                                 ANESTHESIA,                                      FEVER
                                 ETC.

# ACETYLCHOLINE RECEPTOR ANTIBODY TEST

## INCREASED

In patients with myasthenia gravis.

## FALSE-POSITIVE RESULTS

Found in patients with amyotrophic lateral sclerosis treated with snake venom.

## NORMAL VALUES

$< 0.03$ nmol/L.

## COST

Low.

## ADDITIONAL TESTS TO ORDER

CBC, chemistry panel, muscle enzymes, Tensilon test, muscle biopsy, chest radiograph, and CT scan of mediastinum to look for thymoma. An antistriatal antibody titer also may indicate thymoma.

# ACID PHOSPHATASE, BLOOD

## INCREASED

Ask yourself the following questions:

1. Is the PSA increased? An increased PSA suggests that the acid phosphatase increase is due to a disorder of the prostate. If the PSA is not increased, suspect Gaucher's disease, liver disease, Niemann–Pick disease, or various hematologic disorders.
2. Is the alkaline phosphatase increased? An elevated alkaline phosphatase, along with a positive PSA, suggests prostatic carcinoma that has metastasized to the bone. If the alkaline phosphatase is not elevated, the prostatic carcinoma may be confined to the prostate; that is, of course, good news. An elevated alkaline phosphatase with a normal PSA suggests Gaucher's disease, Paget's disease, or osteogenic sarcoma. In these cases, the alkaline phosphatase is markedly increased.
3. Is the alkaline phosphatase decreased, with an increased acid phosphatase? This situation may be found in liver disease, early Gaucher's disease, and multiple myeloma.

## NORMAL VALUES

0.1–0/8 IU/L (varies with method).

## COST

Low.

## ADDITIONAL TESTS TO ORDER

CBC, PSA, chemistry panel, liver profile, skeletal survey, bone scan, and biopsy of the prostate.

**ACID PHOSPHATASE**

INCREASED

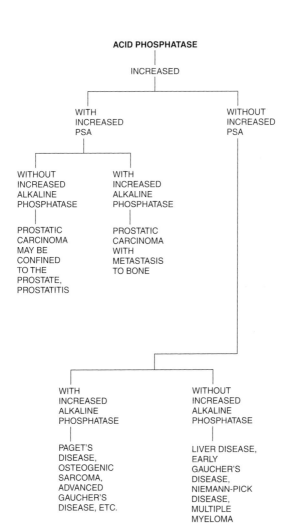

WITH INCREASED PSA

WITHOUT INCREASED PSA

WITHOUT INCREASED ALKALINE PHOSPHATASE

PROSTATIC CARCINOMA MAY BE CONFINED TO THE PROSTATE, PROSTATITIS

WITH INCREASED ALKALINE PHOSPHATASE

PROSTATIC CARCINOMA WITH METASTASIS TO BONE

WITH INCREASED ALKALINE PHOSPHATASE

PAGET'S DISEASE, OSTEOGENIC SARCOMA, ADVANCED GAUCHER'S DISEASE, ETC.

WITHOUT INCREASED ALKALINE PHOSPHATASE

LIVER DISEASE, EARLY GAUCHER'S DISEASE, NIEMANN-PICK DISEASE, MULTIPLE MYELOMA

# ACID PHOSPHATASE, VAGINAL

## INCREASED

An increased vaginal acid phosphatase indicates recent sexual intercourse. The acid phosphatase elevation may persist long after sperm are discernible.

## NORMAL VALUES

Less than 10 U/L.

## COST

Low.

## ADDITIONAL TESTS TO ORDER

A sperm count on vaginal fluid is also valuable in diagnosing recent sexual intercourse.

# ADRENOCORTICOTROPIC HORMONE (ACTH), PLASMA

## INCREASED

Ask the following questions:

1. Is the cortisol increased? If both the ACTH and cortisol are increased, suspect ACTH dependent Cushing's disease caused by basophilic adenoma of the pituitary or ectopic ACTH production.
2. Is the cortisol decreased? If the cortisol is decreased while the ACTH is increased, then suspect Addison's disease.

## DECREASED

Ask the following questions:

1. Is the cortisol decreased? This suggests pituitary insufficiency. A corticotropin-releasing hormone stimulation test can be done to confirm this diagnosis.
2. Is the cortisol increased? This suggests Cushing's syndrome resulting from adrenal neoplasm or hyperplasia. A dexamethasone suppression test (page 219) may be done to confirm the diagnosis.

## NORMAL VALUES

Morning specimen: 10–60 pg/mL.

## COST

Medium.

## ADDITIONAL TESTS TO ORDER

Serum cortisol, urinary free cortisol, ACTH infusion test, dexamethasone suppression test, metyrapone test, serial electrolytes, CT scan of the brain and abdomen, and endocrinology consult.

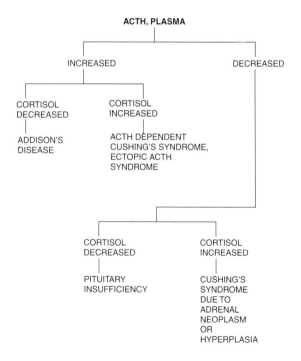

ACTH, PLASMA

INCREASED

CORTISOL DECREASED

ADDISON'S DISEASE

CORTISOL INCREASED

ACTH DEPENDENT CUSHING'S SYNDROME, ECTOPIC ACTH SYNDROME

DECREASED

CORTISOL DECREASED

PITUITARY INSUFFICIENCY

CORTISOL INCREASED

CUSHING'S SYNDROME DUE TO ADRENAL NEOPLASM OR HYPERPLASIA

# ADRENOCORTICOTROPIC HORMONE (ACTH) INFUSION TEST

## PROCEDURE

Administer 0.25 mg of Cortrosyn IM or IV (under 2 years old, 0.125 mg) and collect blood for baseline, 30-minute, and 60-minute determinations of plasma cortisol and aldosterone.
Ask the following questions:

1. Are both the cortisol and aldosterone increased? This response is normal.
2. Is the aldosterone increased alone? This indicates secondary adrenal insufficiency or hypopituitarism.
3. Do both the aldosterone and cortisol fail to increase? This response is typical in primary adrenal insufficiency.

## NORMAL VALUES

A greater than 10-$\mu$g/dL increase of cortisol and a 5-ng/dL increase of aldosterone after infusion of ACTH.

## COST

Medium.

## ADDITIONAL TESTS TO ORDER

Serial electrolytes, serum growth hormone, thyroid profile, serum estradiol or testosterone, serum KOH-progesterone after ACTH infusion, CT scan, or MRI of brain. Additional tests of adrenocortical function may be found on page 187.

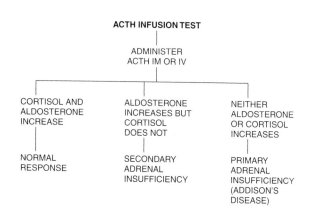

**ACTH INFUSION TEST**

ADMINISTER
ACTH IM OR IV

CORTISOL AND
ALDOSTERONE
INCREASE

ALDOSTERONE
INCREASES BUT
CORTISOL
DOES NOT

NEITHER
ALDOSTERONE
OR CORTISOL
INCREASES

NORMAL
RESPONSE

SECONDARY
ADRENAL
INSUFFICIENCY

PRIMARY
ADRENAL
INSUFFICIENCY
(ADDISON'S
DISEASE)

# ALBUMIN, SERUM

## DECREASED

Ask the following questions:

1. Are results of liver function tests abnormal? Abnormal liver function test results suggest that the low serum albumin is due to advanced liver disease such as alcoholic cirrhosis or postnecrotic cirrhosis.
2. Is the urine protein increased? This suggests nephrotic syndrome or chronic glomerulonephritis.
3. Is the blood volume increased? An increased blood volume suggests congestive heart failure or other causes of hemodilution. If the blood volume is normal, malnutrition, malabsorption, and other GI conditions should be considered, as well as third-degree burns and chronic dermatitis.

## INCREASED

An increased serum albumin is most likely the result of dehydration. Blood volume and electrolyte studies are useful in confirming this diagnosis.

## NORMAL VALUES

3.5–5.0 g/dL.

## COST

Low.

## ADDITIONAL TESTS TO ORDER

CBC, urinalysis, chemistry panel, liver function tests, protein electrophoresis, CT scan of abdomen, liver and renal biopsies, pulmonary function testing, echo-cardiography, chest radiograph, and D-xylose absorption testing.

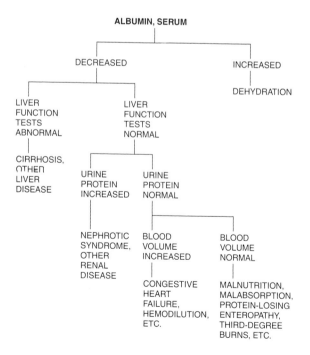

# ALDOLASE

## INCREASED

Serum or plasma aldolase is increased in most disorders of the skeletal muscles such as muscular dystrophy, polymyositis, viral myositis, and polymyalgia rheumatica. It is also increased in myocardial infarction, pancreatitis, thyroid disorders, renal disease, and various other disorders.

## NORMAL VALUES

Adults: 1–6 IU/L.
Children younger than 12 years: 2–12 IU/L, except in neonates 0–3 days old.

## COST

Low.

## ADDITIONAL TESTS TO ORDER

Serum enzymes (ALS, CPK, ALT, and LDH), chemistry panel, 24-hour urine creatine and creatinine, electromyography, muscle biopsy, and neurology consult.

# ALDOSTERONE, SERUM OR URINE

## INCREASED

Ask the following questions:

1. Is the plasma renin increased? If the plasma renin is increased, then secondary aldosteronism resulting from congestive heart failure, diuretic therapy, liver disease, or renal arteriosclerosis must be considered. Bartter's syndrome due to hyperplasia of the juxtaglomerular apparatus with increased renin output must also be considered. If the renin is decreased, then the patient probably has primary aldosteronism caused by adrenal adenoma, hyperplasia, or carcinoma.
2. What does the abdominal CT scan show? Bilateral adrenal masses suggest adrenocortical hyperplasia; a unilateral adrenal mass suggests carcinoma. A normal CT scan suggests adrenocortical adenoma, the most common cause of primary aldosteronism.

## DECREASED

The aldosterone level is decreased in Addison's disease, but so is the level of all adrenocortical steroids. However, a selective decrease in serum aldosterone is usually due to hyporeninemic hypoaldosteronism. Typically, these patients have renal failure.

## NORMAL VALUES

Supine: 3–10 ng/dL.
Upright: 5–30 ng/dL.

## COST

Medium.

## ADDITIONAL TESTS TO ORDER

Plasma renin, serial electrolytes, captopril inhibition test, 24-hour urine aldosterone, CT scan of abdomen, and exploratory surgery. Consult an endocrinologist.

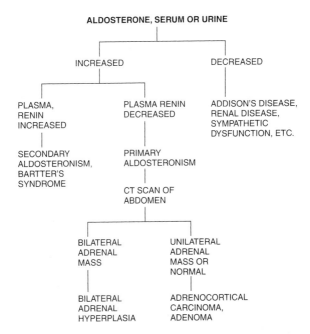

ALDOSTERONE, SERUM OR URINE

# ALKALINE PHOSPHATASE

## INCREASED

Ask the following questions:

1. Is a change in the serum calcium noted? If the serum calcium is increased, this may indicate primary hyperparathyroidism or bone metastasis. A PTH assay should be done to differentiate between these two conditions. If the calcium is decreased, the patient may have vitamin D deficiency or malabsorption syndrome or advanced renal disease. A serum phosphate determination distinguishes between these two groups.
2. Are the the results of liver function tests abnormal? Abnormalities of liver function tests should signify liver disease, obstructive jaundice, and liver metastasis (see page 83). However, these test results can be normal in patients with liver metastasis.
3. Another way to differentiate between liver and bone alkaline phosphatase is to do a 5'-nucleotidase or γ-glutamyltransferase level (Algorithm B). These values are increased in liver disease.

## DECREASED

Decreased alkaline phosphatase values are rarely found but may be associated with malnutrition, hypothyroidism, pernicious anemia, and hypophosphatasia.

## NORMAL VALUES

39–117 U/L.

## COST

Low.

## ADDITIONAL TESTS TO ORDER

CBC, sedimentation rate, urinalysis, chemistry panel, protein electrophoresis, liver profile, PTH assay, skeletal survey, bone scan, CT scan of abdomen, alkaline phosphatase isoenzymes, acid phosphatase, and PSA.

# ALKALINE PHOSPHATASE (ALGORITHM A)

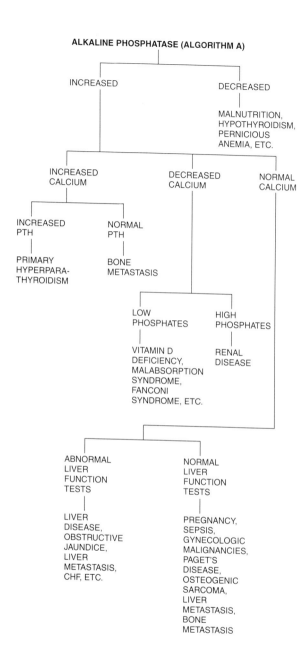

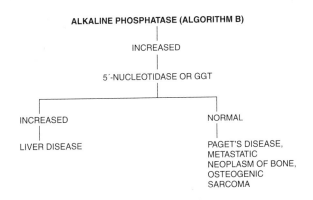

**ALKALINE PHOSPHATASE (ALGORITHM B)**

INCREASED

5´-NUCLEOTIDASE OR GGT

INCREASED

LIVER DISEASE

NORMAL

PAGET'S DISEASE,
METASTATIC
NEOPLASM OF BONE,
OSTEOGENIC
SARCOMA

# ALLERGY SKIN TESTING

## DEFINITION

Allergy skin testing is performed to detect a person's sensitivity to various substances, including dust, pollen, animal dander, drugs, and food. Allergy to trees, grass, ragweed, bee venom, and fungi may be determined. The cause of hay fever, asthma, and allergic skin disease may be diagnosed. The testing may be done by a patch test, scratch test, or intradermal injection of the allergen. Patch tests are helpful in diagnosing contact dermatitis.

## POSITIVE

Positive results are often obtained to house dust, pollen, animal dander, molds, foods, and drugs. Many false-positive results occur, as well as some false-negatives.

## NORMAL VALUES

No reaction.

## COST

Medium to high.

## ADDITIONAL TESTS TO ORDER

CBC, eosinophil count, RAST, serum IgE, nasal or sputum smear for eosinophils, therapeutic trial, pulmonary function tests, elimination diet, and consultation with an allergist.

# ALPHA$_1$-ANTITRYPSIN TEST

## INCREASED

This may occur in infectious diseases, particularly hepatitis, malignant diseases such as carcinoma of the cervix or lymphomas, and in conditions associated with increased plasma levels of estrogen or other steroids, such as pregnancy and contraceptive or steroid therapy.

## DECREASED

Ask the following question:
Is it associated with a low serum albumin? In this case, look for nephrotic syndrome, protein-losing enteropathy, and burns. When it is not associated with a low serum albumin, look for congenital deficiency, acute pancreatitis, or respiratory distress syndrome.

## NORMAL VALUES

150–350 mg/dL.

## COST

Low.

## ADDITIONAL TESTS TO ORDER

Serum protein electrophoresis, CBC, chemistry panel, chest radiograph, and pulmonary function tests.

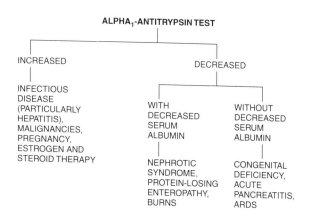

ALPHA₁-ANTITRYPSIN TEST

INCREASED

INFECTIOUS
DISEASE
(PARTICULARLY
HEPATITIS),
MALIGNANCIES,
PREGNANCY,
ESTROGEN AND
STEROID THERAPY

DECREASED

WITH
DECREASED
SERUM
ALBUMIN

NEPHROTIC
SYNDROME,
PROTEIN-LOSING
ENTEROPATHY,
BURNS

WITHOUT
DECREASED
SERUM
ALBUMIN

CONGENITAL
DEFICIENCY,
ACUTE
PANCREATITIS,
ARDS

# ALPHA$_1$-FETOPROTEIN

## INCREASED

The level is increased in the blood in hepatocellular carcinoma, embryonic gonadal teratoblastomas of the testicle, some ovarian tumors, neonatal hepatitis, lymphomas, and renal disease. It is most useful in the diagnosis of hepatocellular carcinoma, in which it is often markedly elevated. A normal level in newborns with jaundice helps to distinguish biliary atresia from neonatal hepatitis. An elevated maternal alpha-fetoprotein may indicate a fetal anomaly.

## NORMAL VALUES

< 25 ng/mL.

## COST

Low.

## ADDITIONAL TESTS TO ORDER

CBC, liver profile, urine for hCG, liver or testicular ultrasonography, and CT scans of the abdomen and pelvis.

# AMEBIASIS ANTIBODY TESTS

## POSITIVE

These tests are positive in infections caused by *Entamoeba histolytica*. Enzyme immunoassay is most sensitive, and specific IgM antibodies are a better marker of active disease. The indirect hemagglutination test identifies patients with liver abscess or invasive intestinal disease. False-positive results occur in carriers of the disease. False-negatives occur in immunocompromised hosts.

## NORMAL VALUES

Negative.

## COST

Low.

## ADDITIONAL TESTS TO ORDER

Sedimentation rate, stool for ova and parasites, barium enema, liver function tests, colonoscopy and biopsy, liver scan, CT scan of abdomen, and consultation with a parasitologist or infectious disease specialist.

# AMINO ACIDS

## INCREASED

Ask the following questions:

1. Is the increase of amino acids found in the urine only, or is it found in both the blood and urine? An increase of amino acids in the urine only suggests secondary aminoaciduria resulting from a renal defect such as may occur in Wilson's disease, lead poisoning, or Fanconi's syndrome. If the increase is in the blood and urine, an inborn error of metabolism is likely.
2. Is the aminoaciduria isolated to one to three amino acids, or are several amino acids involved? Isolated aminoaciduria occurs in phenylketonuria, alkaptonuria, homocystinuria, and cystinuria. The secondary aminoacidurias, such as Wilson's disease and Fanconi's syndrome, as well as a few primary aminoacidurias, such as maple syrup urine disease and Hartnup's disease, are associated with a generalized amino acid increase in the blood or urine.

## NORMAL VALUES

Negative qualitative or screening tests in blood and urine.

## COST

Medium.

## ADDITIONAL TESTS TO ORDER

Urinalysis, 24-hour urine quantitative tests for specific amino acids, blood and urine glucose, skeletal survey, blood lead levels, Guthrie test, and serum copper, and ceruloplasmin.

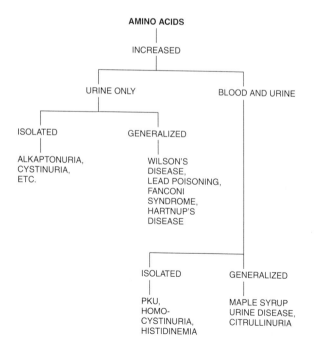

# δ-AMINOLEVULINIC ACID, URINARY

## INCREASED

This substance is increased most frequently in the urine in acute intermittent porphyria. However, lead poisoning and other types of porphyria, with the exception of porphyria erythropoietica, may cause an increase in urinary δ-aminolevulinic acid. Some increase may also occur in hereditary tyrosinemia, diabetic acidosis, and the third trimester of pregnancy.

## NORMAL VALUES

1.3–7 mg/24-hour urine specimen.

## COST

Low to medium.

## ADDITIONAL TESTS TO ORDER

CBC, liver profile, urine for uroporphyrins I and II and urine porphobilinogen, liver biopsy, nerve conduction velocity studies, and abdominal CT scan.

# AMMONIA

## INCREASED

Ammonia is increased in hepatic encephalopathy, and that is the most common reason to order this test. It is also increased in Reye's syndrome, liver bypass, GI bleeding, inherited metabolic disorders, systemic illnesses, and urinary tract abnormalities.

## NORMAL VALUES

The range varies with age from 65–105 $\mu$mol/L in the newborn to 5–50 in adults. Consult the laboratory where the test is performed.

## COST

Low.

## ADDITIONAL TESTS TO ORDER

CBC, sedimentation rate, chemistry panel, urinalysis, liver profile, CT scan of abdomen, liver biopsy, and consultation with a hepatologist.

# AMNIOCENTESIS

## ABNORMAL

The amniotic fluid is used to detect chromosomal abnormalities in Down's syndrome, hemophilia, muscular dystrophy, Lesch–Nyhan syndrome, Fabry's disease, ocular albinism, and other rare conditions. It is also abnormal in hemolytic disease of the newborn and may be used to evaluate fetal lung maturity.

## COST

Medium.

## INDICATIONS

1. Mother over 35 years old.
2. Previous child with neural tube defect (e.g., meningocele), chromosome anomaly, or known carrier of an inherited metabolic disorder.
3. Elevated maternal alpha-fetoprotein level.
4. Family history of a sex-linked recessive disease.

# AMYLASE, SERUM

## INCREASED

Ask the following questions:

1. Is the serum lipase increased? An increase of both the serum amylase and lipase makes pancreatitis likely. However, the elevation of both these enzymes may occur in biliary tract disease, intestinal obstruction, and other abdominal conditions.
2. What is the amylase clearance or urine amylase? If these values are decreased, the patient may have macroamylasemia. If they are increased, the patient could still have pancreatitis, primary or secondary to other abdominal conditions.
3. What does the isoamylaic electrophoresis show? This study identifies salivary amylase and confirms macroamylasemia.

## NORMAL VALUES

60–160 U/dL (Somogyi).

## COST

Low.

## ADDITIONAL TESTS TO ORDER

CBC, urinalysis, chemistry panel, serum lipase, urine amylase, flat plate of abdomen, chest radiograph, ECG, stool for occult blood, peritoneal tap, gastroenterology consult, surgical consult, laparoscopy, and exploratory laparotomy.

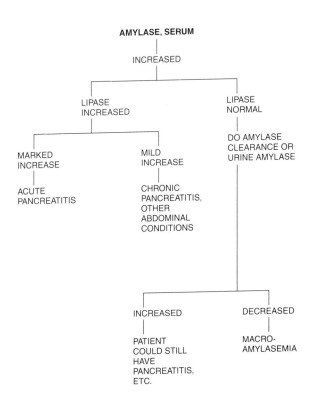

**AMYLASE, SERUM**

| |
INCREASED

LIPASE INCREASED — LIPASE NORMAL

**LIPASE INCREASED**

MARKED INCREASE — MILD INCREASE

MARKED INCREASE → ACUTE PANCREATITIS

MILD INCREASE → CHRONIC PANCREATITIS, OTHER ABDOMINAL CONDITIONS

**LIPASE NORMAL**

DO AMYLASE CLEARANCE OR URINE AMYLASE

INCREASED — DECREASED

INCREASED → PATIENT COULD STILL HAVE PANCREATITIS, ETC.

DECREASED → MACRO-AMYLASEMIA

# ANDROSTENEDIONE

## INCREASED

Ask the following questions:

1. What is the plasma ACTH? If this is increased, the patient may have a basophilic adenoma or ectopic ACTH-producing tumor.
2. What is the serum estradiol? If this is increased, the patient may have an ovarian tumor or ovarian stromal hyperplasia.
3. If the foregoing tests are normal, look for Stein–Leventhal syndrome or adrenal hyperplasia or tumors.

## NORMAL VALUES

Adult males: 75–205 ng/dL.
Adult females: 85–275 ng/dL.
Newborns: 20–290 ng/dL.

## COST

Low to medium.

## ADDITIONAL TESTS TO ORDER

Serum cortisol, serum testosterone and free testosterone, DHEA-S, CT scan of abdomen, pelvic ultrasonography, gynecology consult, and endocrinology consult.

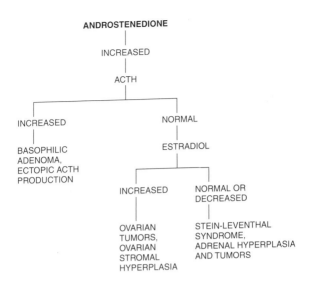

**ANDROSTENEDIONE**
|
INCREASED
|
ACTH

INCREASED
|
BASOPHILIC
ADENOMA,
ECTOPIC ACTH
PRODUCTION

NORMAL
|
ESTRADIOL

INCREASED
|
OVARIAN
TUMORS,
OVARIAN
STROMAL
HYPERPLASIA

NORMAL OR
DECREASED
|
STEIN-LEVENTHAL
SYNDROME,
ADRENAL HYPERPLASIA
AND TUMORS

# ANGIOGRAPHY

## INDICATIONS

1. *Cerebral angiography:* Indicated in *obstructive lesions,* particularly carotid stenosis, vertebral basilar artery insufficiency, thrombosis and embolism, *malformations* such as hemangiomas and A-V malformations, and *dilatation* such as occurs in congenital berry aneurysms. Its use in tumors, abscess, and hematoma has largely been replaced by MRI and CT scans.
2. *Coronary angiography:* Useful in assessing the cause and severity of coronary insufficiency (obstruction) resulting from stenosis, thrombosis, or atheromatous plaque. Occasionally helpful in *malformation* and *aneurysms* of the coronary arteries.
3. *Pulmonary angiography:* Standard in the diagnosis of pulmonary embolism.
4. *Renal angiography:* Useful in the diagnosis of renal artery stenosis, embolism, thrombosis, and fibromuscular dysplasia.
5. *Mesenteric arteriography:* Useful in diagnosis of mesenteric emboli and thrombosis in patients with abdominal angina or intestinal obstruction.
6. *Arteriography of the extremities:* Indicated when a proximal lesion (surgically correctable) is suspected as the cause of ischemia. It is useful in diagnosing Leriche's syndrome (see page 64).

## ADDITIONAL TESTS TO ORDER

Before ordering a *cerebral angiogram,* it may be wise to perform a carotid duplex scan, digital subtraction angiogram, CT scans, or MRI. Before ordering a *coronary angiogram,* it may be wise to do an exercise stress test or thallium scan. Pulmonary angiography is usually not done until a ventilation perfusion scan is performed. However, if a large embolism is suspected, angiography may be the procedure of choice.

*Renal angiography* is usually not performed until a hypertensive workup is completed, including 24-hour catecholamines, plasma renin and cortisol, and a hypertensive IVP or ultrasonography. Even when these tests fail to suggest renovascular hypertension, renal angiography may be worthwhile in young patients and in anyone who fails to respond to antihypertensive medication.

*Mesenteric angiography:* Appropriate testing to rule out other causes of abdominal pain (page 617) should be done before proceeding with this invasive procedure.

## COST

High to very high.

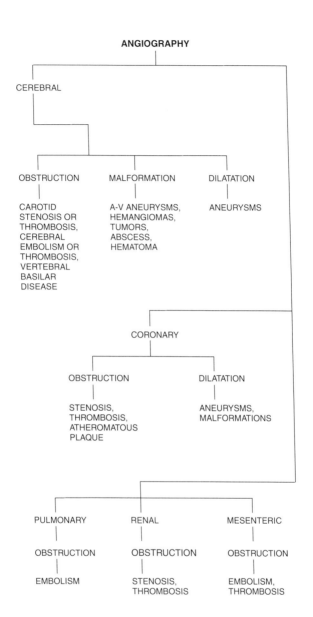

ANGIOGRAPHY

CEREBRAL

OBSTRUCTION

CAROTID
STENOSIS OR
THROMBOSIS,
CEREBRAL
EMBOLISM OR
THROMBOSIS,
VERTEBRAL
BASILAR
DISEASE

MALFORMATION

A-V ANEURYSMS,
HEMANGIOMAS,
TUMORS,
ABSCESS,
HEMATOMA

DILATATION

ANEURYSMS

CORONARY

OBSTRUCTION

STENOSIS,
THROMBOSIS,
ATHEROMATOUS
PLAQUE

DILATATION

ANEURYSMS,
MALFORMATIONS

PULMONARY

OBSTRUCTION

EMBOLISM

RENAL

OBSTRUCTION

STENOSIS,
THROMBOSIS

MESENTERIC

OBSTRUCTION

EMBOLISM,
THROMBOSIS

**40    Angiography**

# ANGIOTENSIN I–CONVERTING ENZYME

## INCREASED

The level of angiotensin I–converting enzyme may be increased in many lung conditions, but it is most consistently increased in *sarcoidosis,* especially in the advanced stages. A negative test in a patient suspected of having sarcoidosis is good evidence against the diagnosis. The test is usually negative in fungal or tuberculous lung diseases. It may also be elevated in nonpulmonary disorders such as cirrhosis, inflammatory bowel disease, diabetes, and hyperthyroidism.

## NORMAL VALUES

Variable, so the laboratory performing the test should be consulted.

## COST

Low.

## ADDITIONAL TESTS TO ORDER

CBC, sedimentation rate, chemistry panel, chest radiograph, tuberculin test, Kveim test, scalene node biopsy, sputum cultures, and guinea pig inoculation.

# ANIMAL INOCULATION

## INDICATIONS

This test is indicated in patients with suspected tuberculosis with negative smears and cultures, as well as in many other bacterial, spirochetal, and viral infections. It is useful in the diagnosis of anthrax, bubonic plague, glanders, leprosy, listeriosis, tetanus, tularemia, rat-bite fever, relapsing fever, Weil's disease, typhus fever, Colorado tick fever, cytomegalic inclusion disease, lymphogranuloma venereum, rabies, West Nile fever, yellow fever, coccidioidomycosis, histoplasmosis, Chagas' disease, kala-azar, toxoplasmosis, and trypanosomiasis. It is wise to consult the laboratory in any infectious disease case to see whether this test can be used in diagnosis.

## COST

Medium.

# ANION GAP

## INCREASED

The anion gap is increased in any case of metabolic acidosis associated with a foreign or intrinsic acid in the blood. Intrinsic acids may be increased in diabetic ketoacidosis (ketones), lactic acidosis, and renal failure (phosphates and sulfates). Foreign acids increase the anion gap in poisoning with ethylene glycol, salicylates, propyl alcohol, paraldehyde, and methyl alcohol.

## NORMAL VALUES

5–15 mmol/L. The anion gap may be calculated by the following formula:

anion gap = sodium − (chloride + bicarbonate)

Consequently, the normal anion gap would be:

140 - (102 + 26) or 12.

## COST

Low.

## ADDITIONAL TESTS TO ORDER

CBC, chemistry panel, serum electrolytes, arterial blood gases, serum ketones, serum phosphates, serum lactic acid, and urinalysis.

# ANKLE/BRACHIAL INDEX

## INDICATIONS

The test is indicated in suspected ischemia of the lower extremities, whether from obstruction of the terminal aorta (Leriche's syndrome), femoral artery atherosclerosis, embolism, or atherosclerosis of more peripheral arteries. It is done by taking the systolic pressure in the arms and legs, using a Doppler instrument. The index is calculated by dividing the systolic blood pressure from the leg by the systolic blood pressure from the arm.

## DECREASED

The ankle/brachial index is decreased in obstruction of the terminal aorta, femoral artery obstruction, and peripheral arteriosclerosis. Obstruction of the terminal aorta may be by atherosclerosis, embolism, thrombosis, and dissecting aneurysm. Obstruction of the femoral artery may result from similar disorders.

## NORMAL VALUES

0.96 or higher.

## MILD ISCHEMIA

0.85–0.95.

## MODERATE ISCHEMIA

0.84 and lower.

## SEVERE ISCHEMIA

0.50 and lower.

## COST

Low.

## ADDITIONAL TESTS TO ORDER

Lipid profile, ultrasonography, femoral angiography, and aortography.

# ANTIDIURETIC HORMONE (ADH)

## INCREASED

An increased ADH level is found in inappropriate ADH secretion as seen in porphyria, brain tumors, pneumonia, systemic neoplasms, congestive heart failure, and tuberculosis.

## DECREASED

A decreased level of antidiuretic hormone is found in pituitary diabetes insipidus. This may be due to pituitary adenomas, hypothalamic disorders, and idiopathic causes.

## NORMAL

The level of ADH is normal in renal diabetes insipidus and primary polydipsia.

## NORMAL VALUES

1–5 pg/mL.

## COST

Medium.

## ADDITIONAL TESTS TO ORDER

(Before and after ADH) water-deprivation stimulation test, serum and urine osmolality, 24-hour urine volume, serial electrolytes, CT scan of brain, other endocrine function studies, and water-loading suppression test.

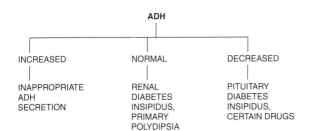

# ANTI-DNA ANTIBODY TEST

## INCREASED

This indicates active systemic lupus erythematosus. The higher the titer of anti-DNA antibody, the more active and intense the disease. Once the disease goes into remission, the titer decreases and may even disappear. Consequently, the anti-DNA antibody test is useful in following the disease. It is uncommon for the anti-DNA antibody test to be positive in other diseases.

## NORMAL VALUES

Consult the laboratory performing the test.

## COST

Low.

## ADDITIONAL TESTS TO ORDER

ANA, LE preparation, protein electrophoresis, CBC and chemistry panel, chest radiograph, ECG, renal biopsy, and skin biopsy.

# ANTI–DNASE-B

## INCREASED

An increased titer of this antibody is found after streptococcal infections such as pharyngitis and impetigo. It is a useful marker of glomerulonephritis secondary to these conditions.

## NORMAL VALUES

60–170 U (check normals for your local laboratory).

## COST

Low.

## ADDITIONAL TESTS TO ORDER

CBC, sedimentation rate, ASO titer, CRP, antihyaluronidase titer, chemistry panel, urinalysis, repeated titers, renal biopsy, nose and throat and skin cultures, ECG, and chest radiograph.

# ANTIGLOMERULAR BASEMENT MEMBRANE ANTIBODY TITER

## INCREASED

These antibodies are increased in Goodpasture's syndrome, tubulointerstitial nephritis, and other forms of anti-GBM glomerulonephritis.

## NORMAL VALUES

Negative.

## COST

Low to medium.

## ADDITIONAL TESTS TO ORDER

CBC, urinalysis, sedimentation rate, chemistry panel, serum complement, ANA, ASO titer, renal biopsy, and nephrology consult.

# ANTIMITOCHONDRIAL ANTIBODY TEST

## INCREASED

These antibodies are increased in disorders of the liver parenchyma, particularly *primary biliary cirrhosis* and is useful in diagnosing this disease. Titers higher than 1:160 are diagnostic of this disorder. Because these antibodies are rarely found in obstructive jaundice, they can be used to distinguish primary biliary cirrhosis from obstructive jaundice.

## NORMAL VALUES

Titer of 1:10 or below.

## COST

Low.

## ADDITIONAL TESTS TO ORDER

Rule out other causes of obstructive jaundice with ultrasonography, ERCP, and CT scan of the abdomen. A liver biopsy is useful in some cases, and this is best done during an exploratory laparotomy.

# ANTINEUTROPHIL CYTOPLASMIC ANTIGEN ANTIBODIES (ANCA)

## INCREASED

These antibodies are increased in autoimmune diseases, particularly those with vasculitis. More than 90% of patients with Wegener's granulomatosis have elevated titers, and it may be used to follow the course of the disease. The test is also positive in idiopathic crescentic glomerulonephritis, periarteritis nodosa, and non-syndrome vasculitis.

## NORMAL VALUES

None detected.

## COST

Low.

## ADDITIONAL TESTS TO ORDER

CBC, chemistry panel, sedimentation rate, ANA, anti-DNA, LE preparation, CT scan of brain and sinuses, cultures of exudates, and biopsy of lesions.

# ANTINUCLEAR ANTIBODY TEST (ANA)

## INCREASED

These antibodies are increased in collagen diseases, particularly systemic lupus erythematosus. The absence of a positive ANA almost completely rules out lupus erythematosus. Various fluorescent patterns are used to distinguish among the different collagen diseases (see Algorithm). Many drugs may cause a false-positive ANA.

## NORMAL VALUES

Lower than 1:40.

## COST

Low.

## ADDITIONAL TESTS TO ORDER

Repeat the test after withdrawing drugs. CBC, sedimentation rate, urinalysis, chemistry panel, anti-DNA, anti-Smith antibody test, VDRL, serum protein electrophoresis, LE preparation, chest radiograph, ECG, and skin, muscle, and renal biopsy.

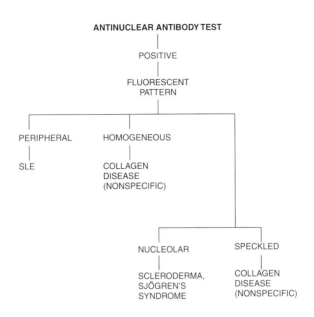

ANTINUCLEAR ANTIBODY TEST
|
POSITIVE
|
FLUORESCENT
PATTERN

PERIPHERAL    HOMOGENEOUS
|    |
SLE    COLLAGEN
DISEASE
(NONSPECIFIC)

NUCLEOLAR    SPECKLED
|    |
SCLERODERMA,    COLLAGEN
SJÖGREN'S    DISEASE
SYNDROME    (NONSPECIFIC)

# ANTIPARIETAL CELL ANTIBODY

## INCREASED

These antibodies are increased in autoimmune pernicious anemia. False-positive results occur in gastritis, gastric ulcer, and gastric carcinoma. These antibodies are also found in 2% of healthy children and up to 20% of the elderly.

## NORMAL VALUES

None detected.

## COST

Low to medium.

## ADDITIONAL TESTS TO ORDER

Serum $B_{12}$ and folic acid, Schilling test, upper GI series, gastric analysis, gastroscopy, and hematology consult.

# ANTIPLATELET ANTIBODY

## POSITIVE

A positive test for platelet antibodies is found in idiopathic thrombocytopenic purpura and is the principal reason for ordering this test. These antibodies are also found in some forms of drug-induced thrombocytopenia (e.g., quinidine, quinine, sulfa drugs). They are also found in pregnancy, autoimmune neonatal thrombocytopenic purpura, and post-transfusion purpura.

## NORMAL VALUES

Negative.

## COST

Medium.

## ADDITIONAL TESTS TO ORDER

CBC, platelet count, sedimentation rate, tourniquet test, coagulation profile, chemistry panel, platelet aggregation, platelet-associated IgG, and hematology consult.

# ANTISCLERODERMAL ANTIBODY TITER

## INCREASED

This antibody is increased in scleroderma. Because it is rarely found in other collagen diseases, it is almost specific for this disease.

## NORMAL VALUES

Negative.

## COST

Low.

## ADDITIONAL TESTS TO ORDER

ANA, nucleolar antibody titer, skin biopsy, chest radiograph, esophagoscopy and biopsy, and consultation with a rheumatologist.

# ANTI–SMITH
# ANTIBODY TITER

## POSITIVE

These antibodies appear in lupus erythematosus and are almost diagnostic of this disorder. This test is also useful in assessing the activity of the disease from time to time.

## NORMAL VALUES

Negative.

## COST

Low.

## ADDITIONAL TESTS TO ORDER

CBC, sedimentation rate, ANA, ds-DNA, chemistry panel, LE preparation, serum protein electrophoresis, renal biopsy, and rheumatology consult.

# ANTISMOOTH MUSCLE ANTIBODY TEST

## INCREASED

These antibodies are increased in chronic active hepatitis and primary biliary cirrhosis. Consequently, the test helps differentiate these two diseases from other liver disorders such as obstructive jaundice, viral hepatitis, and hepatoma.

## NORMAL VALUES

Negative.

## COST

Low.

## ADDITIONAL TESTS TO ORDER

Liver function tests, ANA, antimitochondrial antibody test, liver biopsy, CT scan, and gastroenterology consult.

# ANTISPERM ANTIBODY TEST

## INCREASED

A high titer of these antibodies in males is almost diagnostic of infertility. Mild to moderate titers are of uncertain diagnostic significance. Likewise, the sperm antibody titer in women is of uncertain importance. Antisperm antibodies in cervical mucus are more likely to be a cause of infertility.

## NORMAL VALUES

None detected.

## COST

Low.

## ADDITIONAL TESTS TO ORDER

Sperm count, testicular biopsy, cystoscopy, serum testosterone, serum FSH and LH, and CT scan of brain.

# ANTISTREPTOLYSIN O TITER

## INCREASED

These antibodies are increased in patients who have recently experienced a streptococcal infection such as streptococcal pharyngitis. The titer is also high in rheumatic fever (85–95%) and poststreptococcal glomerulonephritis. A rising titer is even more diagnostically significant.

## NORMAL VALUES

Less than 170 Todd U.

## COST

Low.

## ADDITIONAL TESTS TO ORDER

It is wise to order both an ASO titer and an anti-DNase titer in suspected streptococcal infections and their sequelae. CRP, sedimentation rate, ECG, and urinalysis may also be helpful. The tests should be repeated when doubt exists about the diagnosis.

# ANTITHROMBIN III

## DECREASED

This substance is decreased in patients with disseminated intravascular coagulation, familial antithrombin III deficiency, thrombophlebitis, deep vein thrombosis, postsurgical trauma, and various liver, kidney and neoplastic disorders (e.g., leukemia).

## NORMAL VALUES

17–30 mg/dL.

## COST

Medium.

## ADDITIONAL TESTS TO ORDER

CBC, sedimentation rate, chemistry panel, urinalysis, protein electrophoresis, bone marrow examination, coagulation profile, fibrin split products, fibrinogen levels, chest radiograph, ECG, and venography.

# AORTIC SONOGRAPHY

## INDICATIONS

This test is useful in both diagnosis and follow-up of abdominal aortic aneurysms to determine the optimal time for surgery. Most surgeons delay surgery until the aneurysms are 5 cm or more in diameter, but other factors must be taken into consideration. Consult a cardiovascular surgeon.

## COST

Medium.

## ADDITIONAL TESTS TO ORDER

Plain films of the abdomen, aortography, and CT scan of the abdomen.

# AORTOGRAPHY

## INDICATIONS

This test is useful in diagnosing aneurysms of the ascending and descending aorta and obstruction of the terminal aorta by saddle emboli or thrombosis.

## COST

High.

## ADDITIONAL TESTS TO ORDER

Plain films of the abdomen and chest, ultrasonography, and CT scans of the abdomen and thorax.

# ARSENIC, URINE

## INCREASED

Arsenic is increased in the urine in arsenic poisoning.

## NORMAL VALUES

Less than 20 $\mu$g/L. Patients with a high-seafood diet or industrial exposure may have higher values (up to 100–200 $\mu$g/L).

## COST

Low.

## ADDITIONAL TESTS TO ORDER

Repeat the urine test, arsenic on hair and toenail analysis, and nerve conduction velocity studies. Serum arsenic levels are not as accurate as urine determinations.

# ARTHROGRAPHY

## INDICATIONS

1. *Arthrography of the knee:* This examination is performed to diagnose a torn meniscus, torn cruciate ligaments, and other abnormalities of the knee joint, but it has become rare since the advent of MRI. Arthroscopy is also a useful test for diagnosing abnormalities of the knee joint.
2. *Arthrography of the shoulder joint:* This may be useful in diagnosing a ruptured rotator cuff or dislocation, but the MRI has largely replaced it.
3. *Arthrography of other joints:* This is rarely necessary but should be considered in difficult diagnostic cases.

## COST

Medium.

## ADDITIONAL TESTS TO ORDER

Plain radiographs, MRI of joint, bone scan, arthroscopy, synovial analysis, and orthopedic consult.

# ARTHROSCOPY

## INDICATIONS

The indications for arthroscopy are the same as for arthrography, but the test can be both diagnostic and therapeutic at the same time, especially when it is performed on the knee joint. It is useful in diagnosing a torn meniscus, torn cruciate ligament, various forms of arthritis, rotator cuff tears, chondromalacia, and loose fragments of cartilage and bone.

## COST

High.

## ADDITIONAL TESTS TO ORDER

Radiographs, MRI of joint, arthrography, bone scan, synovial fluid analysis, and orthopedic consult.

# ASPARTATE AMINOTRANSFERASE (AST) (SGOT) AND ALANINE AMINOTRANSFERASE (ALT) (SGPT)

## INCREASED

Ask the following questions:

1. Is the patient receiving heparin therapy? As many as 60% of patients taking heparin have an elevated ALT, and 27% have an elevated AST.
2. Are results of other liver function tests abnormal? This indicates that the elevated AST or ALT is due to liver disease. In acute viral hepatitis, these enzymes may be markedly elevated.
3. Is the CPK elevated? An elevated CPK most likely indicates either a myocardial infarction or muscle disease. For further differentiation of these conditions, see page 193.
4. Is the arm-to-tongue circulation time increased? This signifies congestive heart failure.
5. Is the serum amylase elevated? This signifies pancreatitis.

## NORMAL VALUES

AST: 0–35 U/L in adults; 20–65 U/L in infants.
ALT:7–35 U/L in adults; 6–62 U/L in infants.

## COST

Low.

## ADDITIONAL TESTS TO ORDER

CBC, serum amylase, chemistry panel, liver profile, urinalysis, CPK and CPK isoenzymes, LDH, serial ECGs, pulmonary function tests, chest radiograph, flat plate of abdomen, CT scan of abdomen, electromyography, liver biopsy, and muscle biopsy.

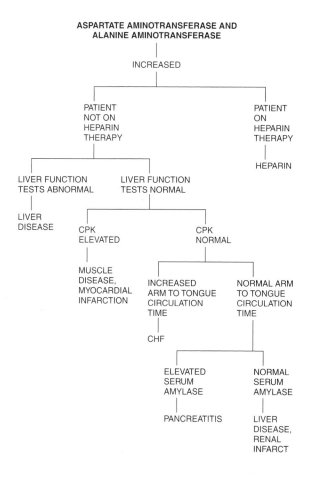

# *ASPERGILLUS* ANTIBODY TITER

## INCREASED

An increase in this antibody is found in *Aspergillus* infections (especially *A. fumigatus* and *A. flavus*). This type of infection is most often found in the immunocompromised host (e.g., leukemia). Antibodies to *A. fumigatus* antigens are also found in allergic bronchopulmonary aspergillosis.

## NORMAL VALUES

None detected.

## COST

Low.

## ADDITIONAL TESTS TO ORDER

CBC, chemistry panel, sedimentation rate, sputum culture, chest radiograph, serum IgE, eosinophil count, skin tests for aspergillus, and tomography for bronchiectasis.

# AUDIOMETRY, SCREENING

## DECREASED HEARING

Ask the following questions:

1. Is the loss unilateral or bilateral? Unilateral hearing loss suggests foreign body, wax, acute infectious otitis media, unilateral otosclerosis, traumatic ruptured eardrum, acoustic neuroma or other posterior fossa tumors, cholesteatoma, and unilateral Meniere's disease. Bilateral loss suggests congenital anomaly, bilateral serous otitis media, otosclerosis, and neural loss from traumatic, toxic, and metabolic causes. Multiple sclerosis and Meniere's disease are also more commonly bilateral.
2. Is the air-to-bone ratio (Rinne) 2:1 or 1:1? When the air-to-bone ratio is 1:1, a conductive loss is suspected, such as foreign body, otitis media, or otosclerosis, whereas a 2:1 air-to-bone hearing ratio suggests sensorineural loss due to traumatic, toxic, or metabolic conditions or tumor. Multiple sclerosis and Meniere's disease also cause neurosensory loss.

## NORMAL RANGE

Normal hearing means the subject is able to hear a sound of 20–25 dB intensity or less in all frequencies tested.

## COST

Low.

## ADDITIONAL TESTS TO ORDER

CBC, chemistry panel, sedimentation rate, VDRL, ANA, radiographs of skull, mastoid and petrous bones, CT scan of the brain, MRI, CSF examination, tympanometry, pure tone audiometry, speech audiometry, recruitment, Békésy audiometry, threshold tone decay, and consultation with an otologist or audiologist.

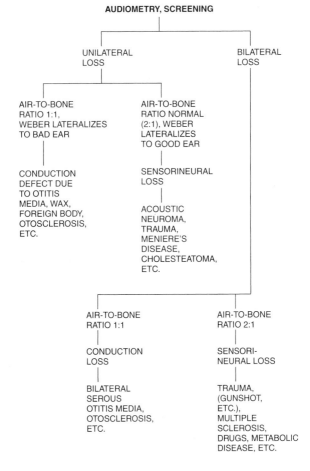

**AUDIOMETRY, SCREENING**

UNILATERAL LOSS

BILATERAL LOSS

AIR-TO-BONE RATIO 1:1, WEBER LATERALIZES TO BAD EAR

CONDUCTION DEFECT DUE TO OTITIS MEDIA, WAX, FOREIGN BODY, OTOSCLEROSIS, ETC.

AIR-TO-BONE RATIO NORMAL (2:1), WEBER LATERALIZES TO GOOD EAR

SENSORINEURAL LOSS

ACOUSTIC NEUROMA, TRAUMA, MENIERE'S DISEASE, CHOLESTEATOMA, ETC.

AIR-TO-BONE RATIO 1:1

CONDUCTION LOSS

BILATERAL SEROUS OTITIS MEDIA, OTOSCLEROSIS, ETC.

AIR-TO-BONE RATIO 2:1

SENSORI-NEURAL LOSS

TRAUMA, (GUNSHOT, ETC.), MULTIPLE SCLEROSIS, DRUGS, METABOLIC DISEASE, ETC.

# AUTOHEMOLYSIS

## INCREASED

Autohemolysis is increased in hereditary spherocytosis, G6PD deficiency, and pyruvate kinase deficiency. After the addition of glucose, the autohemolysis is significantly decreased in hereditary spherocytosis and G6PD deficiency, but not in pyruvate kinase deficiency and other congenital nonspherocytic hemolytic anemias.

## NORMAL VALUES

0.05−0.5% in 24 hours.

## COST

Low.

## ADDITIONAL TESTS TO ORDER

CBC, red cell fragility test, Coombs' test, serum haptoglobins, hemoglobin electrophoresis, red cell survival time, and hematology consult.

# BARIUM ENEMA

## INDICATIONS

Blood in the stool, a mass, chronic diarrhea, and persistent or recurrent abdominal pain are the most common symptoms to warrant this procedure.

## POSITIVE

The findings include *constriction* of the bowel, suggesting carcinoma, diverticulitis, and adhesions, *deformity* of the bowel as seen in volvulus, diverticula, colitis, amebiasis, intussusception, and fistulas, *dilatation* as seen in Hirschsprung's disease and toxic megacolon, and *filling defect* as seen in polyps, carcinoma, abscess, sarcoma, and impacted feces. A barium enema should not be ordered in toxic megacolon, and *water-soluble contrast* material should be used when intestinal obstruction or perforation is suspected. A double-contrast study with barium and air helps to diagnose polyps and early carcinoma.

## NORMAL VALUES

Normal size, shape, and position of the colon, with no filling defects, collections of barium, or obstruction.

## COST

Medium.

## ADDITIONAL TESTS TO ORDER

Stools for ova and parasites, stools for occult blood, stool culture, sigmoidoscopy, colonoscopy, CT scan of the abdomen and pelvis, peritoneoscopy and exploratory laparotomy, and consultation with a gastro-enterologist or abdominal surgeon.

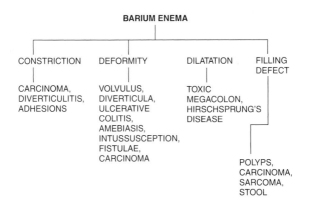

**BARIUM ENEMA**

| CONSTRICTION | DEFORMITY | DILATATION | FILLING DEFECT |
|---|---|---|---|
| CARCINOMA, DIVERTICULITIS, ADHESIONS | VOLVULUS, DIVERTICULA, ULCERATIVE COLITIS, AMEBIASIS, INTUSSUSCEPTION, FISTULAE, CARCINOMA | TOXIC MEGACOLON, HIRSCHSPRUNG'S DISEASE | POLYPS, CARCINOMA, SARCOMA, STOOL |

# BARR BODY ANALYSIS

## EXPLANATION OF TEST

Buccal or vaginal smears are prepared and stained with cresyl violet or similar dyes and are examined under the microscope. Normal female epithelial cells contain a dark-staining chromatin mass at the edge of the nucleus.

## NORMAL VALUES

Female: sex chromatin positive.
Male: sex chromatin negative.

## COST

Medium.

## ABNORMAL TESTS

In Turner's syndrome, the epithelial cells are negative for sex chromatin, whereas in Klinefelter's syndrome, the cells are sex chromatin positive (a Barr body is present). The Barr body analysis is useful in other less common chromosome disorders.

## ADDITIONAL TESTS TO ORDER

Chromosomal analysis, serum FSH and LH, estrogen, testosterone and progesterone.

# BASOPHILIC STIPPLING

## INTERPRETATION

This is found in red cells in lead poisoning. It may also be an indication of immaturity of the red cell (reticulocyte).

## NORMAL VALUES

Rare or absent on routine normal blood smears.

## COST

Low.

## ADDITIONAL TESTS TO ORDER

Blood lead level, urine porphyrins, radiographs of the long bones, reticulocyte count, bone marrow examination, and serum haptoglobins.

# BASOPHILS

## INCREASED

Basophils are increased in chronic myelogenous leukemia. They may also be increased in collagen disease, Hodgkin's disease, and allergic and toxic disorders.

## NORMAL VALUES

0–0.75%.

## COST

Low.

## ADDITIONAL TESTS TO ORDER

CBC, sedimentation rate, and bone marrow examination.

# BENCE JONES PROTEIN, URINE

## INTERPRETATION

The presence of Bence Jones protein in the urine usually indicates one of the following:

1. Multiple myeloma.
2. Macroglobulinemia.
3. Lymphocytic leukemia.
4. Lymphoma.

It can also be found in primary amyloidosis and rarely in benign monoclonal gammopathy.

## NORMAL RANGE

None detected.

## COST

Low.

## ADDITIONAL TESTS TO ORDER

CBC, sedimentation rate, serum protein electrophoresis and immunoelectrophoresis, radiographs of skull and long bones, bone scan, and bone marrow examination.

# BERNSTEIN TEST

## INDICATIONS

This test is used to differentiate between chest pain of cardiac origin and chest pain from esophagitis. A nasogastric tube is placed in the lower esophagus, and the esophagus is perfused first with normal saline and then with 0.1 N HCl.

## POSITIVE TEST

Esophagitis is indicated when the patient develops chest pain on perfusion with 0.1 N HCl only.

## COST

Low.

## ADDITIONAL TESTS TO ORDER

Upper GI series and esophagogram, esophagoscopy, and gastroenterology consult.

# BICARBONATE

## INCREASED

An *increased bicarbonate* is most likely due to *metabolic alkalosis,* which may be found in aldosteronism, vomiting, pyloric obstruction, diuretic use, and gastric suction. It may also be found in compensated respiratory acidosis found in pulmonary emphysema. To distinguish between these two groups of conditions, look at the pH. An increased pH signifies metabolic alkalosis, whereas a decreased pH signifies compensated respiratory acidosis.

## DECREASED

A decreased bicarbonate is most often associated with metabolic acidosis. This is found in diabetic acidosis, lactic acidosis, uremia, and chronic diarrhea. The bicarbonate is also reduced in compensated respiratory alkalosis. To distinguish between these two groups of conditions, look at the pH. If it is increased, the patient probably has compensated respiratory alkalosis. If it is decreased, the patient has metabolic acidosis.

## NORMAL VALUES

20–28 mEq/L.

## COST

Low.

## ADDITIONAL TESTS TO ORDER

CBC, urinalysis, chemistry panel, arterial blood gas analysis, serial electrolytes, serum and urine osmolality, blood volume, spirometry, chest radiograph, ECG, serum acetone, serum lactic acid, drug screen, anion gap, pulmonary consult, and endocrinology consult.

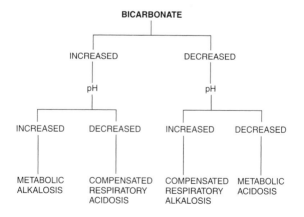

# BILIRUBIN, SERUM

## INCREASED

Ask yourself the following questions:

1. Is the direct or indirect bilirubin increased? (Algorithm A). If the increase in bilirubin is primarily direct, obstructive jaundice is the most likely diagnosis. If the increase in bilirubin is primarily indirect, a hemolytic anemia is the most likely diagnosis. If both the direct and indirect bilirubin are increased, primary liver disease (e.g., hepatitis or cirrhosis) is the most probable cause.
2. Is the alkaline phosphatase elevated? (Algorithm B). An increase in alkaline phosphatase points to liver disease or obstructive jaundice as the cause of an elevated bilirubin. A normal alkaline phosphatase suggests that the cause is hemolytic anemia, Gilbert's disease or Dubin–Johnson syndrome. The urine urobilinogen differentiates these disorders.
3. What is the serum transaminase (e.g., ALT)? An elevated serum transaminase points to liver disease, whereas a normal serum transaminase suggests that obstructive jaundice or hemolytic anemia is the cause of the increased bilirubin.

## NORMAL VALUES

Total: 0.3–1.2 mg/dL.
Direct: 0.1–0.4 mg/dL.
Indirect: 0.2–0.18 mg/dL.
Newborn: 1–12 mg/dL.

## COST

Low.

## ADDITIONAL TESTS TO ORDER

CBC, urinalysis, chemistry panel, hepatitis profile, Monospot test, blood smear, reticulocyte count, serum haptoglobin, bone marrow examination, gallbladder ultrasound, ERCP, percutaneous transhepatic cholangiography, abdominal CT scan, liver biopsy, and exploratory laparotomy. Consult a gastroenterologist.

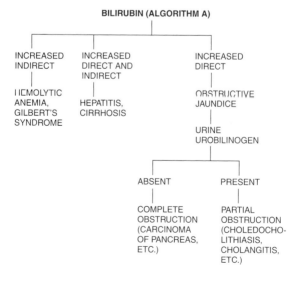

**BILIRUBIN (ALGORITHM A)**

INCREASED INDIRECT

I IEMOLYTIC ANEMIA, GILBERT'S SYNDROME

INCREASED DIRECT AND INDIRECT

HEPATITIS, CIRRHOSIS

INCREASED DIRECT

OBSTRUCTIVE JAUNDICE

URINE UROBILINOGEN

ABSENT

COMPLETE OBSTRUCTION (CARCINOMA OF PANCREAS, ETC.)

PRESENT

PARTIAL OBSTRUCTION (CHOLEDOCHO-LITHIASIS, CHOLANGITIS, ETC.)

**BILIRUBIN (ALGORITHM B)**

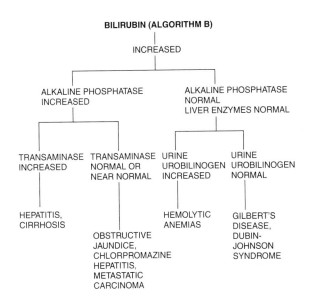

INCREASED

ALKALINE PHOSPHATASE
INCREASED

ALKALINE PHOSPHATASE
NORMAL
LIVER ENZYMES NORMAL

TRANSAMINASE
INCREASED

TRANSAMINASE
NORMAL OR
NEAR NORMAL

URINE
UROBILINOGEN
INCREASED

URINE
UROBILINOGEN
NORMAL

HEPATITIS,
CIRRHOSIS

OBSTRUCTIVE
JAUNDICE,
CHLORPROMAZINE
HEPATITIS,
METASTATIC
CARCINOMA

HEMOLYTIC
ANEMIAS

GILBERT'S
DISEASE,
DUBIN-
JOHNSON
SYNDROME

# BILIRUBIN, URINE

## POSITIVE

The presence of bilirubin in the urine should prompt one to check the *urine urobilinogen.* If it is *increased,* then the patient most likely has hepatitis or cirrhosis. Liver function tests further differentiate these conditions. If *no urobilinogen* is present in the urine, the patient probably has obstructive jaundice. Once again, the liver function tests have enormous diagnostic significance.

## NORMAL VALUES

Negative.

## COST

Low.

## ADDITIONAL TESTS TO ORDER

Liver function tests, ultrasonography, HIDA study, abdominal CT scan, and gastroenterology consult.

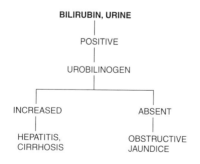

# BIOPSY

## INDICATIONS

Biopsy of various tissues is most commonly used to diagnose neoplasms, but it may also be useful to diagnose many inflammatory, toxic, and degenerative disorders. Listed here are some principal sites of biopsy and significant indications:

1. Bone: Neoplasm, osteomyelitis, congenital disorders.
2. Bone marrow: Aplastic anemia, leukemia, myelophthisic anemia, hemolytic anemia.
3. Brain: Alzheimer's disease, degenerative disease.
4. Colon: Neoplasms, ulcerative colitis, amebic colitis.
5. Endometrial: Neoplasm, dysfunctional uterine bleeding, infertility.
6. Esophageal: Neoplasm, esophagitis.
7. Gastric: Neoplasm, ulcer, pernicious anemia.
8. Liver: Neoplasm, anemia, hepatitis, cirrhosis, toxic disorders.
9. Lung: Neoplasm, pulmonary fibrosis, alveolar proteinosis.
10. Lymph node: Neoplasm, sarcoidosis, infectious diseases.
11. Muscle: Muscular dystrophy, collagen disease, trichinosis.
12. Ovary: Neoplasm, Turner's syndrome, Stein–Leventhal syndrome.
13. Prostate: Neoplasm.
14. Rectal: Neoplasm, ulcerative colitis, amyloidosis.
15. Renal: Neoplasm, collagen disease.
16. Small intestine: Malabsorption syndrome.
17. Skin: Neoplasm, collagen disease, dermatitis, infectious disease.
18. Synovial: Collagen disease.
19. Testicular: Infertility, neoplasm.
20. Thyroid: Neoplasm, thyroiditis.

## COST

Low to Medium.

# BLASTOMYCOSIS ANTIBODY TEST

## POSITIVE

This test is positive in blastomycosis infections. A rising titer is more definitive. The number of false-negative test results is significant.

## NORMAL VALUES

Negative.

## COST

Low.

## ADDITIONAL TESTS TO ORDER

Smear and culture of skin exudate and sputum, chest radiograph, skin test, and pulmonary consult.

# BLASTOMYCOSIS SKIN TEST

## POSITIVE

A positive response indicates present or past infection with *Blastomyces.* If a known case of blastomycosis converts from negative to positive, improvement can often be expected.

## NORMAL VALUES

Negative.

## COST

Low.

## ADDITIONAL TESTS TO ORDER

Chest radiograph, CBC, chemistry panel, sputum culture, culture of exudate from skin lesions, urine culture, KOH preparation of sputum or exudate, biopsy, and consultation with an infectious disease specialist or pulmonologist.

# BLEEDING TIME

## INCREASED

Ask the following questions:

1. Is the platelet count decreased? If the platelet count is decreased, consider thrombocytopenic purpura, lupus erythematosus, leukemia, or aplastic anemia. If not, consider Henoch–Schönlein purpura, thrombasthenia, vascular hemophilia, and scurvy.
2. What is the WBC? An increased WBC suggests leukemia. A decreased WBC suggests aplastic anemia and infiltrative disease of the bone marrow (myelophthisic anemia). A decrease can also be found in hypersplenism and aleukemic leukemia. A normal WBC with a decreased platelet count is typical of thrombocytopenic purpura.

## NORMAL VALUES

Duke: 1–5 minutes.
Ivy: 2–9.5 minutes.

## COST

Low.

## ADDITIONAL TESTS TO ORDER

CBC, sedimentation rate, urinalysis, chemistry panel, protein electrophoresis, coagulation profile, ANA, bone marrow examination, and hematology consult.

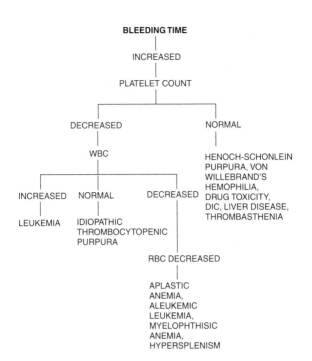

**BLEEDING TIME**
|
INCREASED
|
PLATELET COUNT

DECREASED — NORMAL

NORMAL:
HENOCH-SCHONLEIN
PURPURA, VON
WILLEBRAND'S
HEMOPHILIA,
DRUG TOXICITY,
DIC, LIVER DISEASE,
THROMBASTHENIA

WBC

INCREASED — NORMAL — DECREASED

INCREASED:
LEUKEMIA

NORMAL:
IDIOPATHIC
THROMBOCYTOPENIC
PURPURA

DECREASED:
RBC DECREASED

APLASTIC
ANEMIA,
ALEUKEMIC
LEUKEMIA,
MYELOPHTHISIC
ANEMIA,
HYPERSPLENISM

# BLOOD CULTURES

## INDICATIONS

Blood cultures are indicated any time a patient presents with a fever of unknown origin or is suspected of having bacterial endocarditis or septicemia.

## POSITIVE

The following organisms may be considered pathologic when found in the blood: *Staphylococcus aureus, Streptococcus pyogenes, Brucella* species, pneumococci, *Haemophilus influenzae, Neisseria meningitidis, Bacteroides* species, *Listeria monocytogenes, Francisella tularensis, Salmonella* species, coliform bacilli, malaria organisms, rickettsiae, trypanosomes, and filariae.

## NORMAL VALUES

Negative. However, *Staphylococcus epidermidis* and other skin flora may be found and are usually considered contamination.

## COST

Low.

## ADDITIONAL TESTS TO ORDER

CBC, urinalysis, chemistry panel, urine culture, culture of various body fluids, serologic tests, skin tests, chest radiograph, animal inoculation, sedimentation rate, ASO titer, CRP, febrile agglutinins, echocardiography, and consultation with an infectious disease specialist.

# BLOOD SMEAR FOR MORPHOLOGY

## RBC ABNORMALITIES

*Poikilocytosis* (variations and irregularities in shape): These are found in pernicious anemia, sickle cell anemia, hereditary spherocytosis, myeloid metaplasia, and other conditions.

*Anisocytosis* (variations in size): This may be microcytosis or macrocytosis. *Microcytosis* is typical of iron-deficiency anemia, spherocytic anemia, and thalassemia, whereas *macrocytosis* is typical of pernicious anemia, alcoholism, hypothyroidism, and folic acid deficiency.

*Normoblasts* (nucleated red cells): These are most often found in hemolytic anemia and infiltrative disease of the bone marrow.

*Target cells*: These are found in hemoglobin C disease, thalassemia, and sickle cell anemia.

*Sickle cells:* This is typical of sickle cell anemia.

*Elliptocytes:* These are oval RBCs found in hereditary elliptocytosis.

*Schistocytes:* These are broken red cells found in dissemination intravascular coagulation, among other disorders.

*Spherocytes:* These are spherical cells with no clear area in the center. They are found in congenital spherocytosis.

*Teardrop red cells:* These cells are associated with myeloid metaplasia.

## ABNORMAL CELLS

These are cells foreign to the blood, such as tumor cells, parasites, spirochetes, and histiocytes.

## WBC ABNORMALITIES

*Myelocytes, promyelocytes, myeloblasts:* These are large WBCs with big nuclei, often containing nucleoli. They are seen in leukemia and myeloid metaplasia.

*Lymphocytes, monocytes:* These are increased in infectious mononucleosis, monocytic leukemia, lymphatic leukemia, and plasma cell leukemia.

*Band cells:* This type of neutrophil is increased in infectious disease, in which their presence in large numbers is called a shift to the left.

## NORMAL VALUES

Abnormal cells are rarely present or present in insignificant numbers.

## COST

Low.

## ADDITIONAL TESTS TO ORDER

See page 105.

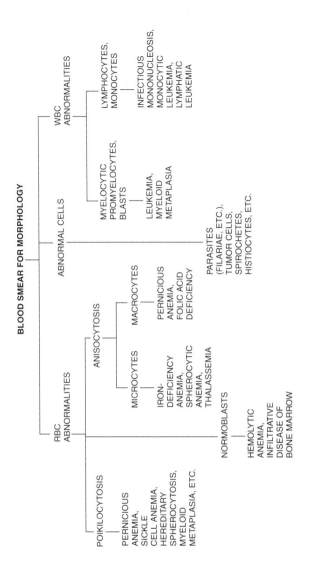

**BLOOD SMEAR FOR MORPHOLOGY**

BLOOD SMEAR FOR MORPHOLOGY

- RBC ABNORMALITIES
  - POIKILOCYTOSIS
    - PERNICIOUS ANEMIA, SICKLE CELL ANEMIA, HEREDITARY SPHEROCYTOSIS, MYELOID METAPLASIA, ETC.
  - ANISOCYTOSIS
    - MICROCYTES
      - IRON-DEFICIENCY ANEMIA, SPHEROCYTIC ANEMIA, THALASSEMIA
    - MACROCYTES
      - PERNICIOUS ANEMIA, FOLIC ACID DEFICIENCY
  - NORMOBLASTS
    - HEMOLYTIC ANEMIA, INFILTRATIVE DISEASE OF BONE MARROW
- ABNORMAL CELLS
  - MYELOCYTIC PROMYELOCYTES, BLASTS
    - LEUKEMIA, MYELOID METAPLASIA
  - PARASITES (FILARIAE, ETC.), TUMOR CELLS, SPIROCHETES, HISTIOCYTES, ETC.
- WBC ABNORMALITIES
  - LYMPHOCYTES, MONOCYTES
    - INFECTIOUS MONONUCLEOSIS, MONOCYTIC LEUKEMIA, LYMPHATIC LEUKEMIA

# BLOOD TYPING

## INDICATIONS

Diagnosis and prevention of transfusion reactions.

## PROCEDURE

1. Mix patient's blood cells with known antiserum (anti-A, anti-B and anti-AB):
   Group A: patient's cells react to anti-A and anti-AB.
   Group B: patient's cells react to anti-B and anti-AB.
   Group AB: patient's cells react to all three known antisera.
   Group O: patient's cells do not react to any of the known antisera.
2. Mix patient's cells with known Rho (D) antiserum:
   Rh+ = patient's cells react to anti-Rho.
   Rh− = patient's cells do not react to anti-Rho.
3. Mix patient's serum with known A, B, and AB red cells:
   Group A: reacts with B and AB red cells.
   Group B: reacts with A and AB red cells.
   Group AB: does not react at all.
   Group O: reacts with all three groups of known red cells.

The process is not complete until a cross match is done. The patient's blood cells are mixed with serum of the donor, and the patient's serum is mixed with the red cells of the donor. For the blood to be compatible, no reaction should occur.

## COST

Low.

## ADDITIONAL TESTS TO ORDER

Serum haptoglobins, CBC, chemistry panel, urinalysis for hemoglobin, serum heme albumin, direct and indirect Coombs test, blood culture, and IgA antibody titer.

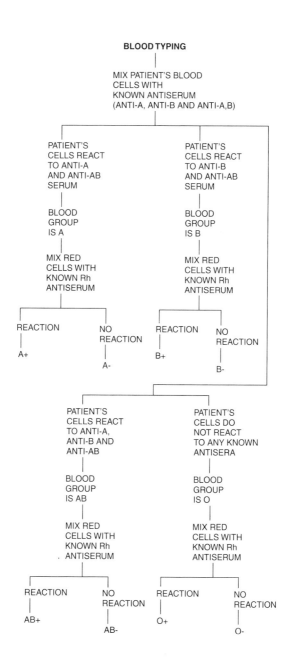

**BLOOD TYPING**

MIX PATIENT'S BLOOD CELLS WITH KNOWN ANTISERUM (ANTI-A, ANTI-B AND ANTI-A,B)

PATIENT'S CELLS REACT TO ANTI-A AND ANTI-AB SERUM

BLOOD GROUP IS A

MIX RED CELLS WITH KNOWN Rh ANTISERUM

REACTION — A+

NO REACTION — A-

PATIENT'S CELLS REACT TO ANTI-B AND ANTI-AB SERUM

BLOOD GROUP IS B

MIX RED CELLS WITH KNOWN Rh ANTISERUM

REACTION — B+

NO REACTION — B-

PATIENT'S CELLS REACT TO ANTI-A, ANTI-B AND ANTI-AB

BLOOD GROUP IS AB

MIX RED CELLS WITH KNOWN Rh ANTISERUM

REACTION — AB+

NO REACTION — AB-

PATIENT'S CELLS DO NOT REACT TO ANY KNOWN ANTISERA

BLOOD GROUP IS O

MIX RED CELLS WITH KNOWN Rh ANTISERUM

REACTION — O+

NO REACTION — O-

# BLOOD UREA NITROGEN (BUN)

## INCREASED

Ask the following questions:

1. What is the BUN/creatinine ratio (Algorithm A)? A BUN/creatinine ratio of 20:1 or more suggests prerenal azotemia as found in dehydration, shock, and numerous other conditions. A BUN/creatinine ratio of less than 10/1 suggests renal disease or obstructive uropathy. Consult a urologist to perform ultrasonography, retrograde pyelography, or cystoscopy to differentiate these two situations.
2. What is the serum osmolality (Algorithm B)? An increased serum osmolality suggests dehydration, diabetic acidosis, nonketotic diabetic coma, excessive protein intake, and starvation. A decreased serum osmolality suggests shock, congestive heart failure, pulmonary infarction, nephritis, and renal failure.
3. What is the urine osmolality? An increased urine osmolality coupled with a decreased serum osmolality suggests shock, congestive heart failure, or pulmonary infarction, whereas a normal or decreased urine osmolality with a decreased serum osmolality suggests nephritis or renal failure.

## DECREASED

A decreased BUN suggests cirrhosis, malnutrition, or malabsorption syndrome.

## NORMAL VALUES

10–15 mg/dL.

## COST

Low.

## ADDITIONAL TESTS TO ORDER

CBC, urinalysis, chemistry panel, liver function tests, sedimentation rate, serum and urine osmolality, plasma and urine acetone, arterial blood gas analysis, blood volume, spirometry, cystoscopy and retrograde pyelography, and nephrology and urology consult.

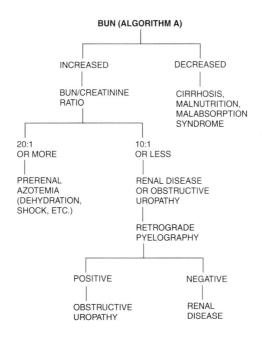

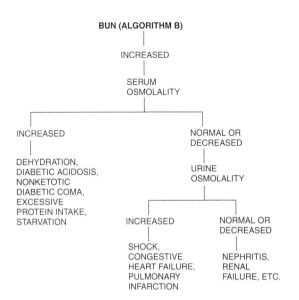

BUN (ALGORITHM B)
|
INCREASED
|
SERUM
OSMOLALITY
|
INCREASED — NORMAL OR DECREASED

INCREASED:
DEHYDRATION,
DIABETIC ACIDOSIS,
NONKETOTIC
DIABETIC COMA,
EXCESSIVE
PROTEIN INTAKE,
STARVATION

NORMAL OR DECREASED:
URINE
OSMOLALITY
|
INCREASED — NORMAL OR DECREASED

INCREASED:
SHOCK,
CONGESTIVE
HEART FAILURE,
PULMONARY
INFARCTION

NORMAL OR DECREASED:
NEPHRITIS,
RENAL
FAILURE, ETC.

**Blood Urea Nitrogen (BUN)    101**

# BLOOD VOLUME STUDIES

## TOTAL BLOOD VOLUME

### Increased

Blood volume is increased in polycythemia vera or after too vigorous administration of intravenous fluids. The blood volume is usually normal or decreased in secondary polycythemia.

### Decreased

Blood volume is decreased in acute hemorrhage (e.g., GI bleeding, uterine bleeding) and hypovolemic shock, whether from dehydration, diarrhea, vomiting, burns, or other causes.

## PLASMA VOLUME

This test is ordered to determine fluid-replacement therapy postoperatively and in burn and trauma cases.

## RED CELL VOLUME

This test is useful in acute GI hemorrhage, determination of red cell survival, and ferrokinetic studies.

## NORMAL VALUES

Total blood volume: 55–80 mL/kg.
Plasma volume: 30–45 mL/kg.
Red cell volume: 20–35 mL/kg.

## COST

Medium.

## ADDITIONAL TESTS TO ORDER

CBC, urinalysis, serum and urine osmolality, chemistry panel, total protein, chromium tagged red cell survival, arm-to-tongue circulation time, pulmonary capillary wedge pressure, chest radiograph, ECG, spot urine sodium, endoscopic procedures, surgical consult, and cardiology consult.

# BONE MARROW
# EXAMINATION

Ask the following questions:

1. Is the red blood cell series increased? An increase in this series suggests polycythemia vera, secondary polycythemia, hemolytic anemia, pernicious anemia, folic acid deficiency, and sideroblastic anemia. Blood loss may also produce these changes. To differentiate the disorders in this group further, look at the peripheral blood count. If the *RBC is increased,* then the patient has primary or secondary polycythemia. If the RBC is *decreased,* then the patient has hemolytic anemia, pernicious anemia, folic acid deficiency or sideroblastic anemia.

2. Is the red blood cell series decreased? A decrease in the red blood cell series in the bone marrow suggests leukemia, aplastic anemia, myelophthisic anemia, or myelofibrosis. Further distinction regarding this group can be achieved by looking at the WBC series. If the WBC series is increased, consider leukemia. If both the RBC and WBC series are decreased, consider aplastic anemia, myelophthisic anemia, or myelofibrosis.

3. Is the WBC series increased? An increase in the WBC series suggests leukemia or early myelofibrosis.

4. Is the WBC series decreased? This finding is typical of agranulocytosis, aplastic anemia, or advanced myelofibrosis. It is also noted in myelophthisic anemia. Further differentiation of the group of disorders is accomplished by examining the RBC and platelet series. If these are normal, the patient may have agranulocytosis or a viral disease. If these are decreased, look for aplastic anemia, myelofibrosis, or myelophthisic anemia.

5. Is the platelet series increased? This finding strongly suggests thrombocytopenic purpura or essential thrombocythemia. It is also found in myelofibrosis, but, of course, the WBC and RBC series are depressed in this disorder.

6. Is the platelet series decreased? This suggests aplastic anemia or myelophthisic anemia, but, of course, the RBC and WBC series are depressed.
7. Is the stainable iron in the bone marrow increased or decreased? Increased iron points to hemosiderosis, hemolytic anemia, or hemochromatosis. Decreased iron is found in iron-deficiency anemia and polycythemia vera.
8. Is there a dry tap? This suggests aplastic anemia and myelofibrosis.
9. Are there abnormal cells present? This would indicate metastatic neoplasm, Gaucher's disease, and other disorders.

## NORMAL VALUES

Myeloblasts: 0.3–5.0%.
Myelocytes: 5.0–19.0%.
Metamyelocytes: 17.5–33.7%.
Segmented granulocytes: 11–30%.
Normoblasts: 6–25%.
Megaloblasts: 0%.
Megakaryocytes: 0.0–3.0%.
M/E ratio: 2.1–6.1.

## COST

Medium.

## ADDITIONAL TESTS TO ORDER

CBC, platelet count, serum haptoglobins, serum iron and IBC, serum $B_{12}$ and folic acid, leukocyte alkaline phosphatase, coagulation profile, reticulocyte count, liver and spleen biopsy, and hematology consult.

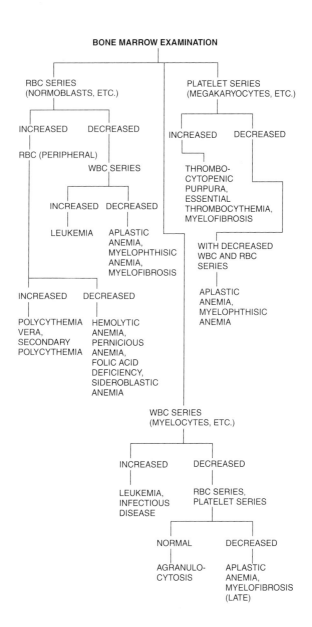

**BONE MARROW EXAMINATION**

RBC SERIES (NORMOBLASTS, ETC.)
- INCREASED
  - RBC (PERIPHERAL)
    - INCREASED
      - POLYCYTHEMIA VERA, SECONDARY POLYCYTHEMIA
    - DECREASED
      - HEMOLYTIC ANEMIA, PERNICIOUS ANEMIA, FOLIC ACID DEFICIENCY, SIDEROBLASTIC ANEMIA
- DECREASED
  - WBC SERIES
    - INCREASED
      - LEUKEMIA
    - DECREASED
      - APLASTIC ANEMIA, MYELOPHTHISIC ANEMIA, MYELOFIBROSIS

PLATELET SERIES (MEGAKARYOCYTES, ETC.)
- INCREASED
  - THROMBO-CYTOPENIC PURPURA, ESSENTIAL THROMBOCYTHEMIA, MYELOFIBROSIS
- DECREASED
  - WITH DECREASED WBC AND RBC SERIES
    - APLASTIC ANEMIA, MYELOPHTHISIC ANEMIA

WBC SERIES (MYELOCYTES, ETC.)
- INCREASED
  - LEUKEMIA, INFECTIOUS DISEASE
- DECREASED
  - RBC SERIES, PLATELET SERIES
    - NORMAL
      - AGRANULO-CYTOSIS
    - DECREASED
      - APLASTIC ANEMIA, MYELOFIBROSIS (LATE)

# BONE MARROW SCAN

## INCREASED ACTIVITY

Increased activity on a bone marrow scan is seen in myelogenous leukemia, polycythemia vera, and chronic hemolytic anemia.

## DECREASED ACTIVITY

Activity is decreased in bone marrow depression from radiation and chemotherapy, myelofibrosis, and aplastic anemia.

## NORMAL VALUES

Normal uptake and distribution.

## COST

Medium.

## ADDITIONAL TESTS TO ORDER

CBC, chemistry panel, sedimentation rate, serum haptoglobins, and bone marrow examination.

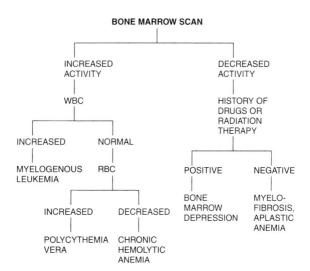

**BONE MARROW SCAN**

# BONE SCAN

## POSITIVE

Bone scans are positive in arthritis, osteomyelitis, fractures, benign and malignant bone tumors, metastases to bone, Paget's disease, osteochondrosis (e.g., Legg–Calvé–Perthes disease), and aseptic bone necrosis.

## NORMAL VALUES

Normal uptake.

## COST

Medium to high.

## ADDITIONAL TESTS TO ORDER

Skeletal survey, chemistry panel, sedimentation rate, acid phosphatase, PSA, bone biopsy, and orthopedic consult.

# BRAIN SCAN

## POSITIVE

The brain scan is positive in brain tumors, cerebro-vascular disease, subdural and epidural hematomas, aneurysms and arteriovenous malformations, and congenital malformations. The adequacy of carotid and cerebral blood flow can be assessed, and internal carotid artery thrombosis can be diagnosed.

## NORMAL VALUES

Homogeneous uptake and distribution of radioactive material and normal extracranial and intracranial blood flow.

## COST

High.

## ADDITIONAL TESTS TO ORDER

CT scan, MRI, carotid scan, EEG, spinal tap, and neurology consult.

# BREAST ULTRASONOGRAPHY

## POSITIVE

This test is positive in patients with cysts and benign and malignant tumors of the breast. It is most useful in differentiating benign cysts from solid tumors. It also can be used to guide the clinician in needle aspiration of a cyst.

## NORMAL VALUES

Symmetric echo pattern in both breasts.

## COST

High.

## ADDITIONAL TESTS TO ORDER

Mammography, xeroradiography, needle aspiration, surgical consult, and biopsy.

# BRONCHOGRAPHY

## POSITIVE

This test is positive in bronchiectasis, bronchial tumors, foreign bodies, and lung cysts and cavities. The principal reason for performing this test is to rule out bronchiectasis.

## NORMAL VALUES

Normal tracheobronchial tree without obstruction, dilatation, or filling defects.

## COST

Medium.

## ADDITIONAL TESTS TO ORDER

Sputum analysis and culture, 24-hour sputum volume, chest radiograph, bronchoscopy, CT scan of chest, and pulmonary consult.

# BRONCHOSCOPY

## POSITIVE

This test is used to diagnose bronchogenic carcinoma, bronchial adenomas, bronchitis, foreign bodies, bronchiectasis, tuberculosis, fungal disease, and abscess. Biopsies and specimens of bronchial washings are often taken.

## NORMAL VALUES

Normal-appearing mucosa, no dilatation or constriction of trachea or bronchi, no mass or foreign body present, and normal bronchial washings.

## COST

Medium.

## ADDITIONAL TESTS TO ORDER

CBC, sedimentation rate, chemistry panel, chest radiograph, sputum analysis, smear and culture, pulmonary function tests, arterial blood gas analysis, bronchography, CT scan of chest, biopsy, and pulmonary consult.

# *BRUCELLA* ANTIBODY

## INCREASED

This antibody is increased in *Brucella* infections except *B. canis.* False-positives occur after brucellergin skin test, *Yersinia, Salmonella,* and other infections.

## NORMAL VALUES

Less than 1:80 titer and no significant rise in titer.

## COST

Low.

## ADDITIONAL TESTS TO ORDER

CBC, sedimentation rate, chemistry panel, cultures of infected body fluids, guinea pig inoculation, and consultation with an infectious disease specialist.

# BRUCELLOSIS SKIN TEST

## POSITIVE

A positive result is an indication of both present or past infection with *Brucella* organisms. Because it may distort serologic tests for *Brucella,* it should not be done.

## NORMAL VALUES

Negative.

## COST

Low.

## ADDITIONAL TESTS TO ORDER

CBC, urinalysis, chemistry panel, febrile agglutinins, sedimentation rate, blood cultures, serologic tests, and consultation with an infectious disease specialist.

# CALCITONIN

## INCREASED

Increased calcitonin is most often due to *medullary carcinoma* and is the *principal indication* for ordering this test. However, it is also increased in chronic renal failure, pseudohypoparathyroidism, Zollinger–Ellison syndrome, pernicious anemia, carcinoma of breast, lung, and pancreas, thyroid C-cell hyperplasia, pregnancy, cirrhosis, and carcinoid syndrome. To differentiate chronic renal failure and pseudohypoparathyroidism from this group, order a serum calcium determination. This is decreased in these two disorders. To differentiate Zollinger–Ellison syndrome and pernicious anemia from this group, order a serum gastrin. Serum gastrin is elevated in these two disorders. Many other tests are available to differentiate other members of this group of disorders.

## NORMAL VALUES

0–30 pg/mL.

## COST

Low.

## ADDITIONAL TESTS TO ORDER

CBC, urinalysis, free $T_4$, chemistry panel, pregnancy test, urine 5-HIAA, chest radiograph, CT scan of abdomen, RAI uptake and scan, ultrasonography of thyroid, thyroid antibodies, needle biopsy of thyroid, and oncology consult.

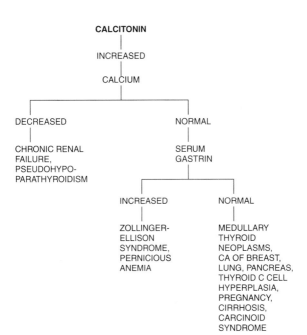

**CALCITONIN**

INCREASED

CALCIUM

DECREASED

CHRONIC RENAL
FAILURE,
PSEUDOHYPO-
PARATHYROIDISM

NORMAL

SERUM
GASTRIN

INCREASED

ZOLLINGER-
ELLISON
SYNDROME,
PERNICIOUS
ANEMIA

NORMAL

MEDULLARY
THYROID
NEOPLASMS,
CA OF BREAST,
LUNG, PANCREAS,
THYROID C CELL
HYPERPLASIA,
PREGNANCY,
CIRRHOSIS,
CARCINOID
SYNDROME

# CALCIUM

## INCREASED

Ask the following questions:

1. What is the phosphorus? An increased phosphorus with an increased calcium is associated with the milk-alkali syndrome and hypervitaminosis D. A decreased phosphorus and increased calcium is associated with hyperparathyroidism, metastatic neoplasm of the bone, Paget's disease, ectopic PTH secretion, multiple myeloma, and hyperproteinemia.
2. What is the alkaline phosphatase? An increased alkaline phosphatase with an increased calcium is associated with hyperparathyroidism, metastatic neoplasm of the bone, Paget's disease, and ectopic PTH production, but not with multiple myeloma or hyperproteinemia.

## DECREASED

Ask the following questions:

1. What is the phosphorus? If the phosphorus is increased, think of renal disease and hypoparathyroidism. If the phosphorus is decreased, think of malabsorption syndrome, rickets or osteomalacia, renal tubular acidosis, cirrhosis, nephrosis, and alkalosis.
2. What is the alkaline phosphatase? If the alkaline phosphatase is increased in the face of a decreased calcium and increased phosphorus, think of renal disease. If the alkaline phosphatase is increased with both a decreased calcium and phosphorus, consider malabsorption syndrome, rickets, osteomalacia, and renal tubular acidosis. A normal alkaline phosphatase with a decreased calcium and increased phosphorus is consistent with hypoparathyroidism.

## NORMAL VALUES

9–11 mg/L.

## COST

Low.

## ADDITIONAL TESTS TO ORDER

CBC, chemistry panel, 24-hour urine calcium, PTH assay, serum 25-COH vitamin D, free $T_4$, serum protein electrophoresis, skeletal survey, bone scan, D-xylose absorption test, serum 1,25-$(OH)^2$ vitamin D, and endocrinology consult.

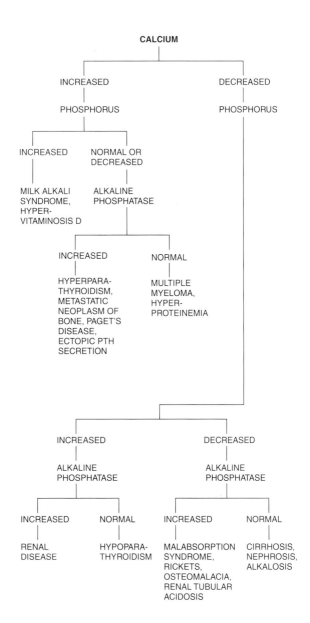

CALCIUM

INCREASED — PHOSPHORUS

INCREASED

MILK ALKALI
SYNDROME,
HYPER-
VITAMINOSIS D

NORMAL OR
DECREASED — ALKALINE
PHOSPHATASE

INCREASED

HYPERPARA-
THYROIDISM,
METASTATIC
NEOPLASM OF
BONE, PAGET'S
DISEASE,
ECTOPIC PTH
SECRETION

NORMAL

MULTIPLE
MYELOMA,
HYPER-
PROTEINEMIA

DECREASED — PHOSPHORUS

INCREASED — ALKALINE
PHOSPHATASE

INCREASED

RENAL
DISEASE

NORMAL

HYPOPARA-
THYROIDISM

DECREASED — ALKALINE
PHOSPHATASE

INCREASED

MALABSORPTION
SYNDROME,
RICKETS,
OSTEOMALACIA,
RENAL TUBULAR
ACIDOSIS

NORMAL

CIRRHOSIS,
NEPHROSIS,
ALKALOSIS

# CALCIUM, URINE 24-HOUR

## INCREASED

An increased 24-hour urine calcium is found in hyperparathyroidism, renal tubular acidosis, lymphoma, metastatic malignant disease, multiple myeloma, corticosteroid therapy, and sarcoidosis. To differentiate these conditions, a serum PTH assay is indicated. This value is increased in hyperparathyroidism and renal tubular acidosis, whereas it is normal in the other conditions.

## DECREASED

A decreased urine calcium is typical of hypoparathyroidism, vitamin D deficiency, malabsorption syndrome, pseudohypoparathyroidism, and familial benign hypercalcemia. To differentiate these conditions further, one should order a serum PTH assay. In primary hypoparathyroidism, the serum PTH is decreased or absent. In the other conditions, it is normal or increased.

## NORMAL VALUES

100–300 mg/24 hours.

## COST

Low.

## ADDITIONAL TESTS TO ORDER

CBC, urinalysis, chemistry panel, protein electrophoresis, survey of long bones, PTH assay, thyroid profile, lymph node biopsy, bone marrow examination, bone scan, ultrasonography of parathyroid glands, chest radiograph, and endocrinology consult.

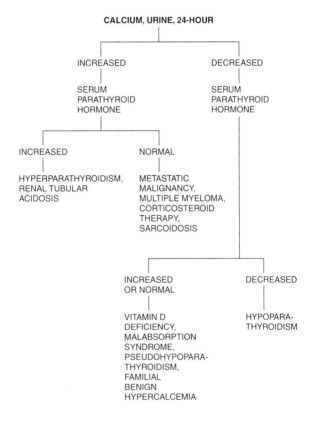

**CALCIUM, URINE, 24-HOUR**

INCREASED

SERUM PARATHYROID HORMONE

INCREASED

HYPERPARATHYROIDISM, RENAL TUBULAR ACIDOSIS

NORMAL

METASTATIC MALIGNANCY, MULTIPLE MYELOMA, CORTICOSTEROID THERAPY, SARCOIDOSIS

DECREASED

SERUM PARATHYROID HORMONE

INCREASED OR NORMAL

VITAMIN D DEFICIENCY, MALABSORPTION SYNDROME, PSEUDOHYPOPARA-THYROIDISM, FAMILIAL BENIGN HYPERCALCEMIA

DECREASED

HYPOPARA-THYROIDISM

# CANCER ANTIGENS

## CA-125

This is *positive* in carcinoma of the ovaries, especially the nonmucinous type. It may also be positive in early pregnancy, pelvic inflammatory disease, endometriosis, and other malignant diseases.

## CA-19-9

This test is positive in pancreatic and colonic carcinoma. Unfortunately, it is also positive in some cases of inflammation or neoplasm of almost any abdominal organ.

## CA-15-3

This test is positive in breast cancer 50–60% of the time. It may be used to follow the course of the disease. Unfortunately, it is also positive in neoplasms of other organs.

## NORMAL VALUES

Negative.

## COST

Low.

## ADDITIONAL TESTS TO ORDER

CEA, CBC, sedimentation rate, urinalysis, chemistry panel, pelvic ultrasound, CT scans, biopsy, endoscopy, cytology, and oncology consult.

# CAPILLARY FRAGILITY TEST

## INCREASED

Capillary fragility is increased in thrombocytopenic purpura, hypersplenism, allergic purpura, von Willebrand's disease, thrombasthenia, scurvy, and senile purpura. To differentiate these conditions, one should look further at the platelet count. It is decreased in idiopathic and secondary thrombocytopenic purpura (as in leukemia and aplastic anemia) and hypersplenism. It is normal in allergic purpura, von Willebrand's disease, thrombasthenia, and other causes of vascular purpura.

## NORMAL VALUES

Occasional petechiae: fewer than 10 petechiae in a 1-inch radius.

## COST

Low.

## ADDITIONAL TESTS TO ORDER

CBC, platelet count, blood smear, chemistry panel, coagulation profile, ANA, serum protein electrophoresis, bone marrow examination, and hematology consult.

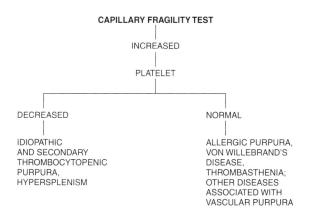

**CAPILLARY FRAGILITY TEST**
|
INCREASED
|
PLATELET

DECREASED

IDIOPATHIC
AND SECONDARY
THROMBOCYTOPENIC
PURPURA,
HYPERSPLENISM

NORMAL

ALLERGIC PURPURA,
VON WILLEBRAND'S
DISEASE,
THROMBASTHENIA;
OTHER DISEASES
ASSOCIATED WITH
VASCULAR PURPURA

# CARBON DIOXIDE

## INCREASED

The most likely cause of *increased* carbon dioxide is *respiratory acidosis.* This is seen most commonly in pulmonary emphysema, but it may also be found in asthma, pickwickian syndrome, kyphoscoliosis, central nervous system depression, and spinal cord trauma. Carbon dioxide is also *increased* in *compensated metabolic alkalosis* such as may be found in aldosteronism, pyloric obstruction, and the use of various diuretics. To distinguish between respiratory acidosis and compensated metabolic alkalosis, one should look at the pH. If it is near normal or increased, the patient has compensated metabolic alkalosis. It if is decreased, the patient has respiratory acidosis. In chronic respiratory acidosis, the pH may be only slightly decreased because the respiratory acidosis is compensated.

## DECREASED

The most likely cause of decreased carbon dioxide is respiratory alkalosis. This is seen most frequently in conditions associated with hyperventilation such as salicylate toxicity, congestive heart failure, shock, excessive mechanical ventilation, central nervous system disease, and hypermetabolic states. Carbon dioxide is also *decreased* in *compensated metabolic acidosis* such as may be found in diabetic ketoacidosis, chronic diarrhea whatever the cause, uremia, and lactic acidosis. To distinguish between these two groups of disorders, look at the pH. If the pH is *increased,* the patient has *respiratory alkalosis.* If it is *near normal* or *decreased*, the patient probably has *compensated metabolic acidosis*. In chronic respiratory alkalosis, the pH may be only slightly increased because the alkalosis is compensated.

## NORMAL VALUES

P$_{CO_2}$: 35–45 mm.

## COST

Low.

## ADDITIONAL TESTS TO ORDER

Arterial blood gas analysis, CBC, urinalysis, chemistry panel, blood volume, serum and urine osmolality, chest radiograph, drug screen, serial electrolytes, spirometry, plasma acetone, plasma lactic acid, anion gap, pulmonary consult, and endocrinology consult.

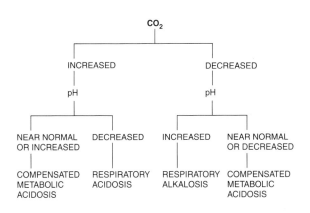

# CARBOXYHEMOGLOBIN

## INCREASED

Carbon monoxide poisoning from exposure to automobile exhaust, coal gas, and fires, for example.

## NORMAL VALUES

0–2.3% of hemoglobin (may be up to 15% in long-term cigarette smokers).

## COST

Low.

## ADDITIONAL TESTS TO ORDER

Arterial blood gas analysis, spirometry, and pulmonary and toxicology consult.

# CARCINOEMBRYONIC ANTIGEN (CEA)

## INCREASED

Ask the following questions:

1. What does the barium enema or colonoscopy show? If either of these is positive, the patient probably has carcinoma of the colon.
2. What does the CT scan of the abdomen and pelvis show? This test often reveals carcinoma of the pancreas, neuroblastoma, or carcinoma of the ovary.
3. If none of the foregoing tests is positive, consider cigarette smoking, inflammatory bowel disease, and malignant diseases of the prostate, bladder, breast, lung, bone, or blood as the possible cause.

The test may also be used to detect recurrence of colon cancer.

## NORMAL VALUES

0–2.5 ng/mL.

## COST

Low.

## ADDITIONAL TESTS TO ORDER

CBC, urinalysis, chemistry panel, liver function tests, stool for occult blood times three, sigmoidoscopy, laparoscopy, PSA, CA-125, abdominal ultrasonography, chest radiograph, bone scan, bone marrow examination, oncology consult, and gastroenterology consult.

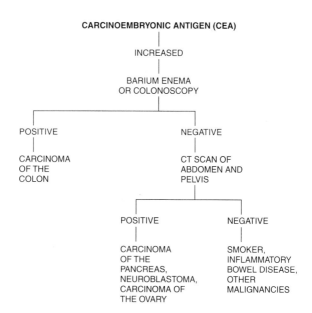

CARCINOEMBRYONIC ANTIGEN (CEA)
|
INCREASED
|
BARIUM ENEMA
OR COLONOSCOPY

POSITIVE — NEGATIVE

POSITIVE:
CARCINOMA
OF THE
COLON

NEGATIVE:
CT SCAN OF
ABDOMEN AND
PELVIS

POSITIVE — NEGATIVE

POSITIVE:
CARCINOMA
OF THE
PANCREAS,
NEUROBLASTOMA,
CARCINOMA OF
THE OVARY

NEGATIVE:
SMOKER,
INFLAMMATORY
BOWEL DISEASE,
OTHER
MALIGNANCIES

# CARDIAC CATHETERIZATION AND ANGIOCARDIOGRAPHY

## INDICATIONS

This test is performed primarily to diagnose congenital heart disease and valvular lesions caused by rheumatic fever. It may also be used to diagnose the various forms of myocardiopathy. Both left-heart and right-heart catheterization can be performed.

## POSITIVE RESULTS

This test is positive in atrial septal defects, ventricular septal defects, tetralogy of Fallot, transposition of great vessels, Ebstein abnormality, patent ductus arteriosus, coarctation of the aorta, pulmonic stenosis and insufficiency, aortic stenosis and insufficiency, subaortic stenosis, mitral stenosis and insufficiency, tricuspid stenosis and insufficiency, myocardiopathy, and pericarditis.

## NORMAL VALUES

Check with the local laboratory.

## COST

Very high.

## ADDITIONAL TESTS TO ORDER

CBC, urinalysis, sedimentation rate, chemistry panel, ANA, ASO titer, CRP, arterial blood gas analysis, chest radiograph, ECG, echocardiography, CT scans, and cardiac consult.

# CARDIAC SERIES

## DEFINITION

This is a series of four films of the chest, including a posteroanterior view, a lateral view, and both anterior oblique views. A barium swallow is coordinated with these views. This test is cost-effective.

## POSITIVE

This test shows cardiomegaly more clearly than a routine chest radiograph (see page 143). Left atrial enlargement, pericardial effusion, and left ventricular enlargement are easier to spot. Dilated pulmonary artery, and aortic and right atrial enlargement can also be diagnosed, but these diagnoses are more difficult. This test used to be routine in the workup of patients with congenital heart disease and chronic rheumatic valvulitis (e.g., mitral stenosis).

## NORMAL VALUES

Normal size, shape, and position of the heart on all views.

## COST

Medium.

## ADDITIONAL TESTS TO ORDER

ECG, echocardiography, CT scan of the chest, angiocardiography, cardiac catheterization, digital subtraction angiography, and cardiology consult.

# CAROTENE

## INCREASED

Carotene is increased in diabetes mellitus, myxedema, chronic nephritis, certain diets, hyperlipemia, and pregnancy. To differentiate these conditions further, one should order a blood glucose determination to rule out diabetes mellitus and a free $T_4$ to rule out myxedema.

## DECREASED

Carotene is decreased in liver disease, malabsorption syndrome, certain diets, and infection. To differentiate these conditions further, one should order liver function tests. These, of course, are abnormal in liver disease.

## NORMAL VALUES

60–300 $\mu$g/100 mL.

## COST

Low.

## ADDITIONAL TESTS TO ORDER

CBC, urinalysis, chemistry panel, liver function tests, free $T_4$, TSH, glucose tolerance test, D-xylose absorption, small bowel mucosal biopsy, mucosal biopsy, and gastroenterology consult.

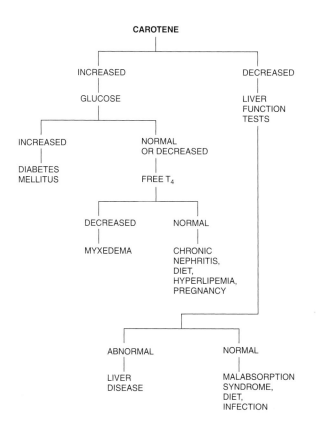

**CAROTENE**

├── INCREASED
│   └── GLUCOSE
│       ├── INCREASED
│       │   └── DIABETES MELLITUS
│       └── NORMAL OR DECREASED
│           └── FREE T$_4$
│               ├── DECREASED
│               │   └── MYXEDEMA
│               └── NORMAL
│                   └── CHRONIC NEPHRITIS, DIET, HYPERLIPEMIA, PREGNANCY
└── DECREASED
    └── LIVER FUNCTION TESTS
        ├── ABNORMAL
        │   └── LIVER DISEASE
        └── NORMAL
            └── MALABSORPTION SYNDROME, DIET, INFECTION

**Carotene**     135

# CAROTID DUPLEX SCAN

## POSITIVE

This test can detect stenosis and atherosclerotic plaques of the common and internal carotid arteries. Obstruction of greater than 70% may be an indication for carotid endarterectomy based on the clinical picture. Of course, surgery is not contemplated without confirmation by conventional angiography in most cases.

## NORMAL VALUES

Good flow through the carotid arteries and no evidence of plaques or obstruction on imaging.

## COST

Medium.

## ADDITIONAL TESTS TO ORDER

Digital subtraction angiography, brain scan and flow study, oculoplethysmography, carotid angiography, neurosurgical consult, and consultation with a vascular surgeon.

# CASTS

## RED CELL CASTS

These signify involvement of the glomerulus such as may occur in glomerulonephritis, collagen disease, subacute bacterial endocarditis, renal embolism, and lower nephron nephrosis.

## WHITE CELL CASTS

These usually signify pyelonephritis, but they are also found in interstitial nephritis, as in gentamicin toxicity.

## EPITHELIAL CASTS

These are found in amyloidosis, heavy metal poisoning and nephrosis.

## GRANULAR CASTS

These are found in acute tubular necrosis, glomerulonephritis, lead poisoning, and nephrosclerosis.

## HYALINE CASTS

Large numbers of these casts are found in the nephrotic syndrome, but they are also found in fever, stress, prolonged exercise, and cylindruria.

## NORMAL VALUES

Only occasional hyaline casts per low-power field.

## COST

Low.

## ADDITIONAL TESTS TO ORDER

CBC, urinalysis, sedimentation rate, Addis count, chemistry panel, ASO titer, ANA, serum complement, urine culture, 24-hour urine protein, IVP, cystoscopy, renal biopsy, and nephrology consult.

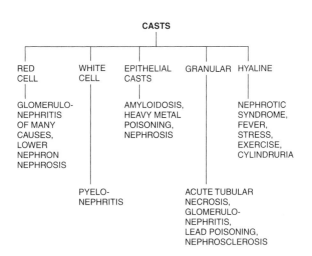

**CASTS**

| RED CELL | WHITE CELL | EPITHELIAL CASTS | GRANULAR | HYALINE |
|---|---|---|---|---|
| GLOMERULO-NEPHRITIS OF MANY CAUSES, LOWER NEPHRON NEPHROSIS | | AMYLOIDOSIS, HEAVY METAL POISONING, NEPHROSIS | | NEPHROTIC SYNDROME, FEVER, STRESS, EXERCISE, CYLINDRURIA |
| | PYELO-NEPHRITIS | | ACUTE TUBULAR NECROSIS, GLOMERULO-NEPHRITIS, LEAD POISONING, NEPHROSCLEROSIS | |

# CD4 AND T-CELL LYMPHOCYTE COUNT

## DECREASED

T-cell lymphocytes, particularly CD4, are decreased in AIDS and in rare patients with primary immune deficiency disorders (agammaglobulinemia). AIDS patients with CD4 counts below $200/\mu L$ should be placed on *Pneumocystis carinii* prophylaxis.

## NORMAL VALUES

$700-1100/\mu L$.

## COST

Medium.

## ADDITIONAL TESTS TO ORDER

HIV antibody titer (ELISA), CBC, differential count, sedimentation rate, blood smear, serum protein electrophoresis, serum protein immunoelectrophoresis, bone marrow, blood cultures, sputum culture, western blot test, oncology consult, and hematology consult.

# CEREBROSPINAL FLUID (CSF) PRESSURE

## INCREASED

Ask the following questions:

1. Is blood present in the spinal fluid? Increased pressure and bloody fluid suggest subarachnoid or cerebral hemorrhage. If the protein is elevated out of proportion to the amount of blood, consider a neoplasm.
2. Is the increase in WBCs significant? This finding, along with an increased pressure, suggests meningitis, encephalitis, or brain abscess.
3. Is the protein increased? This finding suggests brain tumor. An increased CSF pressure with normal protein and no increase in WBCs or RBCs suggests pseudotumor cerebri.

## DECREASED

If the CSF pressure is decreased, the patient may have a spinal cord tumor. One should then look for a spinal block by checking the response to jugular compression. A poor response is typical of subarachnoid block. The pressure is also decreased in dehydration and diabetic acidosis.

## NORMAL VALUES

75–150 mm $H_2O$ in lateral decubitus position.

## COST

Medium.

## ADDITIONAL TESTS TO ORDER

CBC, chemistry panel, urinalysis, CT scan or MRI of brain and spinal cord, lumbar puncture and spinal fluid analysis, myelography, radiographs of spine and skull, arteriography, and neurology or neurosurgical consult.

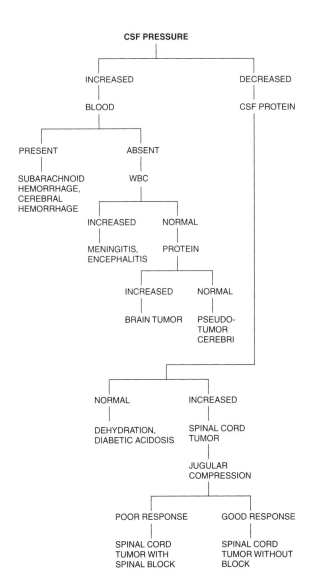

# CHANCROID SKIN TEST

## POSITIVE

A positive response to this test indicates that the patient has an active infection with *Haemophilus ducreyi* or has been infected in the past.

## NORMAL VALUES

Negative.

## COST

Low.

## ADDITIONAL TESTS TO ORDER

Smear or biopsy for Donovan bodies, culture with special media, VDRL and dark-field examination to rule out syphilis, and urology consult.

# CHEST RADIOGRAPHY

## LUNG ABNORMALITIES (ALGORITHM A)

1. Infiltrate:
   *Focal:* A focal infiltrate may be due to bacterial pneumonia, tuberculosis, fungal disease, atelectasis, sarcoidosis, Löffler's syndrome, neoplasm, pulmonary embolism, or Kerley's lines from mitral valve disease.
   *Diffuse:* Diffuse infiltrates may be due to bacterial pneumonia, miliary tuberculosis, fungal disease, pulmonary edema, aspiration pneumonia, and pneumoconiosis.
2. Cavity: A cavity may be due to tuberculosis, fungal disease, lung abscess, neoplasm, or a congenital cyst. Bullous emphysema may create a large cavity.
3. Increased air: Increased air in the pleura is due to pneumothorax, whereas increased alveolar air results from emphysema.
4. Fluid: Fluid in the pleural space may be due to tuberculosis, emphysema, traumatic hemorrhage, pulmonary embolism, and mesothelioma. It may also result from congestive heart failure. Fluid in the lung is caused by pulmonary edema.
5. The workup (Algorithm C):
   *Infiltrate:* When faced with a pulmonary infiltrate, one should order a sputum smear and routine culture. If there is a possibility of a pulmonary embolism, a ventilation perfusion scan should be obtained. If these tests are negative, then one should obtain cold agglutinins and culture for *Legionella.* If these results are negative, AFB smear and culture, culture for fungi, and skin tests for fungi and tuberculosis are indicated. When these results are also negative, it may be necessary to do guinea pig inoculation if tuberculosis is strongly suspected. Finally, a sputum cytology or needle biopsy of the lesion should be done to rule out a neoplasm.
   *Cavity:* The workup of a cavity is similar to the workup of an infiltrate. First, one should obtain a routine sputum smear and culture. If this is nega-

tive, a smear and culture for AFB and fungi are done, along with skin tests. When these tests are also negative, one should look for carcinoma of the lung or bullous emphysema.

*Bronchoscopy* is the next logical step in the workup of both infiltrates and cavities, both to look for intrabronchial lesions and to obtain bronchial washings for culture and cytology.

## ABNORMALITIES OF THE CARDIAC SILHOUETTE (ALGORITHM B)

1. Cardiac enlargement: Enlargement of the heart may be due to valvular disease, congestive heart failure, hypertensive cardiovascular disease, pericardial effusion, myocardiopathy, and cardiac aneurysms.
2. Straightening of the waste-line: This is seen in mitral valvular disease with an enlarged left atrium.
3. Small cardiac silhouette: This is seen in constrictive pericarditis.
4. Enlarged aorta: This is seen in aneurysms and atherosclerosis.
5. Leather bottle silhouette: This is seen in pericardial effusion.

## WORKUP OF PLEURAL EFFUSION (ALGORITHM D)

1. Large: With a large pleural effusion one may proceed with thoracentesis. If the fluid is a *transudate* one should consider congestive heart failure, Meigs' syndrome, pancreatitis, lupus erythematosus, ascites, and neoplasms as possibilities. If the fluid is *bloody,* one should consider pulmonary infarction, trauma, and mesothelioma as possibilities. If the fluid is an exudate, one should perform a routine culture. If the culture is positive, empyema and pneumonia are the likely causes. If the routine culture is negative, one should consider tuberculosis or fungal disease and order AFB and fungi smears, cultures, and skin tests.

2. Small: A small pleural effusion warrants the use of ultrasonography or CT scan to localize the effusion. Once this is done, the clinician may proceed with a thoracentesis, and the results are interpreted as a large pleural effusion.
3. Mediastinal abnormalities: These include an enlarged *thymus* (thymoma), *lymphadenopathy* due to Hodgkin's disease, sarcoidosis, and neoplasms, substernal thyroid, aneurysms, mediastinitis, esophageal diverticulum or neoplasm, and hiatal hernia.

## ABNORMALITIES OF THE THORACIC SPINE

These are discussed on page 382.
The clinician should consult standard radiology textbooks for further discussion of chest radiographic abnormalities.

## NORMAL VALUES

Normal size and shape and without abnormal radiopacity or radiolucency of the lung, heart, mediastinum, and spine.

## COST

Low.

## ADDITIONAL TESTS TO ORDER

CBC, urinalysis, sedimentation rate, chemistry panel, ECG, circulation time, sputum analysis and cultures, skin tests, sputum smear for eosinophils, ANA, CRP, CT scan of chest, bronchoscopy, bronchography, pulmonary function tests, needle biopsy, and pulmonary consult.

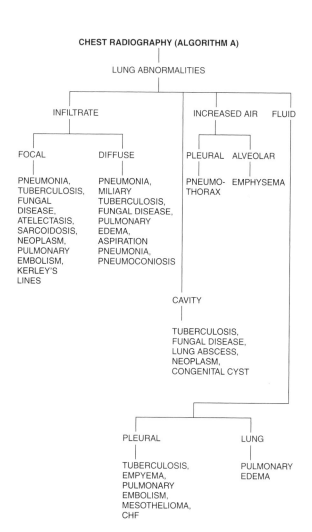

**CHEST RADIOGRAPHY (ALGORITHM A)**

LUNG ABNORMALITIES

INFILTRATE

INCREASED AIR    FLUID

FOCAL

PNEUMONIA,
TUBERCULOSIS,
FUNGAL
DISEASE,
ATELECTASIS,
SARCOIDOSIS,
NEOPLASM,
PULMONARY
EMBOLISM,
KERLEY'S
LINES

DIFFUSE

PNEUMONIA,
MILIARY
TUBERCULOSIS,
FUNGAL DISEASE,
PULMONARY
EDEMA,
ASPIRATION
PNEUMONIA,
PNEUMOCONIOSIS

PLEURAL    ALVEOLAR

PNEUMO-       EMPHYSEMA
THORAX

CAVITY

TUBERCULOSIS,
FUNGAL DISEASE,
LUNG ABSCESS,
NEOPLASM,
CONGENITAL CYST

PLEURAL

TUBERCULOSIS,
EMPYEMA,
PULMONARY
EMBOLISM,
MESOTHELIOMA,
CHF

LUNG

PULMONARY
EDEMA

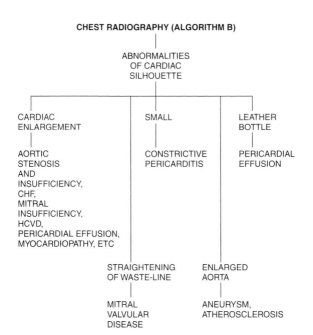

**CHEST RADIOGRAPHY (ALGORITHM B)**

ABNORMALITIES
OF CARDIAC
SILHOUETTE

CARDIAC
ENLARGEMENT

AORTIC
STENOSIS
AND
INSUFFICIENCY,
CHF,
MITRAL
INSUFFICIENCY,
HCVD,
PERICARDIAL EFFUSION,
MYOCARDIOPATHY, ETC

SMALL

CONSTRICTIVE
PERICARDITIS

LEATHER
BOTTLE

PERICARDIAL
EFFUSION

STRAIGHTENING
OF WASTE-LINE

MITRAL
VALVULAR
DISEASE

ENLARGED
AORTA

ANEURYSM,
ATHEROSCLEROSIS

**Chest Radiography   147**

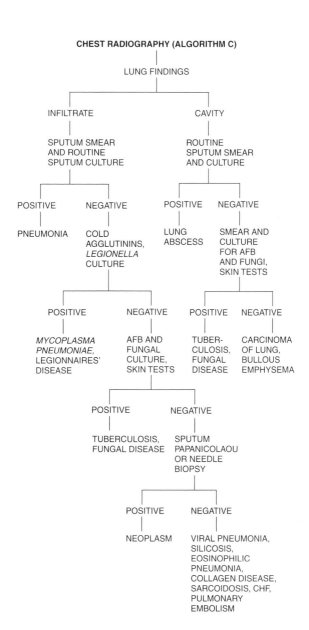

**CHEST RADIOGRAPHY (ALGORITHM C)**

LUNG FINDINGS

INFILTRATE — SPUTUM SMEAR AND ROUTINE SPUTUM CULTURE
- POSITIVE → PNEUMONIA
- NEGATIVE → COLD AGGLUTININS, *LEGIONELLA* CULTURE
  - POSITIVE → *MYCOPLASMA PNEUMONIAE*, LEGIONNAIRES' DISEASE
  - NEGATIVE → AFB AND FUNGAL CULTURE, SKIN TESTS
    - POSITIVE → TUBERCULOSIS, FUNGAL DISEASE
    - NEGATIVE → SPUTUM PAPANICOLAOU OR NEEDLE BIOPSY
      - POSITIVE → NEOPLASM
      - NEGATIVE → VIRAL PNEUMONIA, SILICOSIS, EOSINOPHILIC PNEUMONIA, COLLAGEN DISEASE, SARCOIDOSIS, CHF, PULMONARY EMBOLISM

CAVITY — ROUTINE SPUTUM SMEAR AND CULTURE
- POSITIVE → LUNG ABSCESS
- NEGATIVE → SMEAR AND CULTURE FOR AFB AND FUNGI, SKIN TESTS
  - POSITIVE → TUBERCULOSIS, FUNGAL DISEASE
  - NEGATIVE → CARCINOMA OF LUNG, BULLOUS EMPHYSEMA

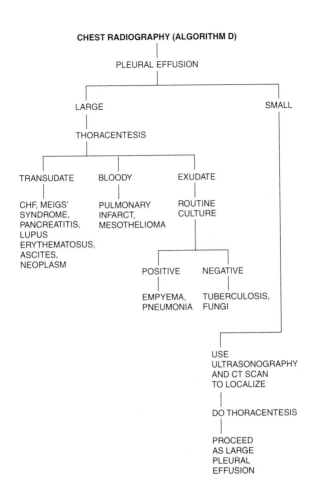

**CHEST RADIOGRAPHY (ALGORITHM D)**

PLEURAL EFFUSION

LARGE

SMALL

THORACENTESIS

TRANSUDATE

CHF, MEIGS'
SYNDROME,
PANCREATITIS,
LUPUS
ERYTHEMATOSUS,
ASCITES,
NEOPLASM

BLOODY

PULMONARY
INFARCT,
MESOTHELIOMA

EXUDATE

ROUTINE
CULTURE

POSITIVE

EMPYEMA,
PNEUMONIA

NEGATIVE

TUBERCULOSIS,
FUNGI

USE
ULTRASONOGRAPHY
AND CT SCAN
TO LOCALIZE

DO THORACENTESIS

PROCEED
AS LARGE
PLEURAL
EFFUSION

# CHLORIDE, BLOOD

## INCREASED

Ask the following questions:

1. What is the sodium? If both the chloride and sodium are increased, consider dehydration, diabetes insipidus, and hyperventilation syndrome as possible causes.
2. What is the bicarbonate? If the chloride is increased but the sodium and bicarbonate are decreased, consider nephritis, renal tubular acidosis, and diabetic acidosis as possible causes. An increased chloride with a normal bicarbonate, but a decreased sodium suggests Addison's disease.

## DECREASED

Ask the following questions:

1. What is the sodium? A decreased chloride with a decreased sodium suggests inappropriate ADH secretion, burns, diuretic use, diarrhea, and congestive heart failure. A decreased chloride with a normal or increased sodium suggests Cushing's syndrome, aldosteronism, pyloric obstruction, and infection.
2. What is the bicarbonate? The bicarbonate is increased in Cushing's syndrome, aldosteronism, and pyloric obstruction.

## NORMAL VALUES

95–105 mEq/L.

## COST

Low.

## ADDITIONAL TESTS TO ORDER

CBC, urinalysis, chemistry panel, sedimentation rate, serial electrolytes, blood volume, arterial blood gases, serum and urine osmolality, spot urine sodium, plasma renin, 24-hour urine aldosterone, plasma cortisol, plasma ADH, and endocrine consult.

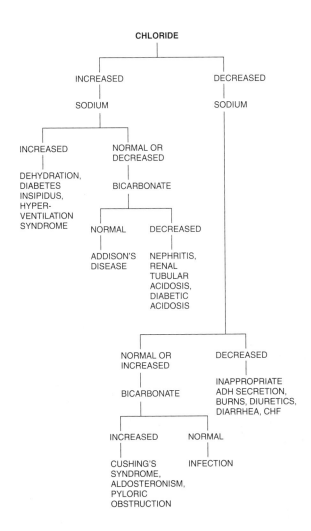

# CHOLECYSTOGRAPHY

## POSITIVE FINDINGS

1. Filling defects: These indicate gallstones, polyps, carcinoma, and congenital anomalies.
2. No evidence of gallbladder: This may be a sign of cholecystitis and cholelithiasis. *Repeat* the *study* with a double dose. If *gallstones* show up, one should obtain a *surgical consult.* If the gallbladder still fails to visualize, *ultrasonography* is indicated. If gallstones are found, a surgeon should be consulted. If not and the patient is asymptomatic, simple observation may suffice. If the patient is symptomatic, one should order transhepatic cholangiography or ERCP (endoscopic retrograde cholangiopancreatography).

## NORMAL VALUES

Good filling of gallbladder, normal size and shape; good response to fatty meal.

## COST

Medium.

## ADDITIONAL TESTS TO ORDER

CBC, urinalysis, chemistry panel, liver function tests, sedimentation rate, HIDA scan, gallbladder ultrasonography, transhepatic cholangiography, ERCP, duodenal analysis, CT scan of abdomen, upper GI series, gastroenterology consult, and surgical consult.

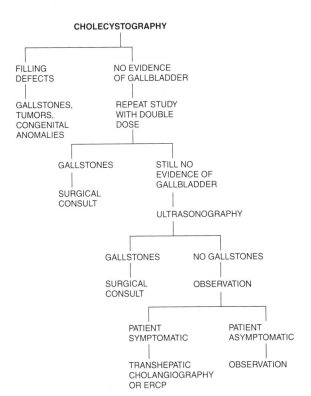

**CHOLECYSTOGRAPHY**

FILLING DEFECTS

GALLSTONES, TUMORS, CONGENITAL ANOMALIES

NO EVIDENCE OF GALLBLADDER

REPEAT STUDY WITH DOUBLE DOSE

GALLSTONES

SURGICAL CONSULT

STILL NO EVIDENCE OF GALLBLADDER

ULTRASONOGRAPHY

GALLSTONES

SURGICAL CONSULT

NO GALLSTONES

OBSERVATION

PATIENT SYMPTOMATIC

TRANSHEPATIC CHOLANGIOGRAPHY OR ERCP

PATIENT ASYMPTOMATIC

OBSERVATION

# CHOLESTEROL

## INCREASED

Ask the following questions (Algorithm A):

1. What is the serum albumin? A decreased serum albumin coupled with an increased cholesterol should prompt consideration of nephrosis, obstructive jaundice, and other liver disorders.
2. What is the free $T_4$? A decreased free $T_4$ with an increased cholesterol suggests myxedema.
3. What is the triglyceride? A marked increase in the triglyceride in association with an increased cholesterol is typical of type I and type II lipoproteinemia. A mild increase in triglyceride may be associated with a high cholesterol in types IIb, III, and IV lipoproteinemia, in diabetes, in atherosclerosis, in xanthomatosis, and in patients taking oral contraceptives.

## DECREASED

Ask the following questions (Algorithm A):

1. What is the free $T_4$? A high free $T_4$ coupled with a low cholesterol is found in hyperthyroidism.
2. What is the D-xylose absorption test? A low cholesterol with a decreased D-xylose absorption is found in malabsorption syndromes. If neither of the foregoing tests are positive, consider advanced cirrhosis or starvation as the cause. A look at the cholesterol esters helps in diagnosing cirrhosis because it is proportionately much lower than would be expected.

## DIFFERENTIATING THE LIPOPROTEINEMIAS (ALGORITHM B)

Cholesterol, triglyceride, and chylomicrons can be used to differentiate the various types of lipoproteinemias.

**154**

## Increased Cholesterol

Cholesterol is increased in type IIa, IIb, III, and V lipoproteinemia. To differentiate these further, one should look at the triglycerides. Triglyceride is increased in types IIb, III, and V. It is normal in type IIa. Further differentiation of types IIb, III, and V can be achieved by examining the chylomicrons (noted in the creamy layer of plasma refrigerated overnight). Chylomicrons are increased in type V but are normal in types IIb and III.

## Normal Cholesterol

Cholesterol is normal or near normal in types I and IV lipoproteinemia, whereas triglyceride is increased. To differentiate these two, one should order a chylomicron test as previously described. Chylomicrons are increased in type I but are normal in type IV lipoproteinemia.

## NORMAL VALUES

Total cholesterol: 125–200 mg/dL.
Cholesterol esters 60–75% of total cholesterol.

## COST

Low.

## ADDITIONAL TESTS TO ORDER

CBC, urinalysis, chemistry panel, overnight refrigeration of plasma, free T4, TSH, lipoprotein electrophoresis, liver function tests, renal function test, 24-hour urine protein, liver biopsy, renal biopsy, D-xylose absorption, and consultation with a metabolic disease specialist or endocrinologist.

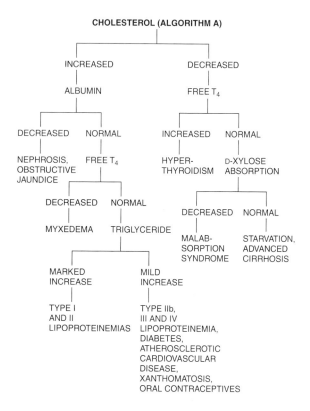

**CHOLESTEROL (ALGORITHM A)**

- INCREASED
  - ALBUMIN
    - DECREASED
      - NEPHROSIS, OBSTRUCTIVE JAUNDICE
    - NORMAL
      - FREE T₄
        - DECREASED
          - MYXEDEMA
        - NORMAL
          - TRIGLYCERIDE
            - MARKED INCREASE
              - TYPE I AND II LIPOPROTEINEMIAS
            - MILD INCREASE
              - TYPE IIb, III AND IV LIPOPROTEINEMIA, DIABETES, ATHEROSCLEROTIC CARDIOVASCULAR DISEASE, XANTHOMATOSIS, ORAL CONTRACEPTIVES
- DECREASED
  - FREE T₄
    - INCREASED
      - HYPER-THYROIDISM
    - NORMAL
      - D-XYLOSE ABSORPTION
        - DECREASED
          - MALAB-SORPTION SYNDROME
        - NORMAL
          - STARVATION, ADVANCED CIRRHOSIS

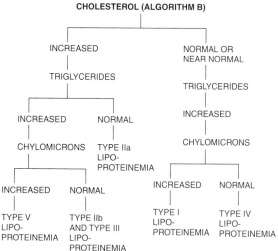

**CHOLESTEROL (ALGORITHM B)**

- INCREASED
  - TRIGLYCERIDES
    - INCREASED
      - CHYLOMICRONS
        - INCREASED
          - TYPE V LIPO-PROTEINEMIA
        - NORMAL
          - TYPE IIb AND TYPE III LIPO-PROTEINEMIA
    - NORMAL
      - TYPE IIa LIPO-PROTEINEMIA
- NORMAL OR NEAR NORMAL
  - TRIGLYCERIDES
    - INCREASED
      - CHYLOMICRONS
        - INCREASED
          - TYPE I LIPO-PROTEINEMIA
        - NORMAL
          - TYPE IV LIPO-PROTEINEMIA

# CHROMOSOME ANALYSIS

## POSITIVE RESULTS

1. Trisomy 21: Three No. 21 chromosomes are present. This is the most common form of Down's syndrome.
2. Translocation 21 trisomy: This is another form of Down's syndrome with extra chromosome 21 material becoming attached to chromosome 16.
3. Philadelphia chromosome: This is associated with chronic granulocytic leukemia.
4. XXY: This indicates an extra X chromosome and is associated with Klinefelter's syndrome or male hypogonadism.
5. A single X chromosome: This is associated with Turner's syndrome.
6. This test is also useful to determine fetal sex and fetal abnormalities in utero.

## NORMAL VALUES

Females: 44 autosomes and 2 X chromosomes.
Males: 44 autosomes and 1 X and 1 Y chromosome.

## COST

Medium.

## ADDITIONAL TESTS TO ORDER

Barr body analysis, serum FSH and LH, estrogen, progesterone and testosterone, and endocrinology consult.

# CISTERNOGRAPHY

## POSITIVE

This test is positive in congenital hydrocephalus, normal-pressure hydrocephalus, porencephalic and subarachnoid cysts, third ventricular tumors, and posterior fossa cysts. In clinical practice, it is most useful in diagnosing normal-pressure hydrocephalus and in differentiating it from Alzheimer's disease.

## NORMAL VALUES

Normal unobstructed flow of cerebrospinal fluid and normal reabsorption.

## COST

High.

## ADDITIONAL TESTS TO ORDER

CT scan and MRI.

# *CLOSTRIDIUM difficile* TOXIN ASSAY

## POSITIVE

Significant amounts of this toxin may be found in *pseudomembranous colitis,* and this is the best test to confirm the diagnosis.

## NORMAL VALUES

None present.

## COST

Low.

## ADDITIONAL TESTS TO ORDER

CBC, urinalysis, sedimentation rate, stool culture, tissue culture, colonoscopy, barium enema, ELISA and latex agglutination tests, and gastroenterology consult.

# CLOT RETRACTION

## DECREASED

Ask the following questions:

1. Is the platelet count decreased? If so, the patient has idiopathic or secondary thrombocytopenic purpura.
2. Is the RBC increased? If the patient has a decreased clot retraction and increased RBC in the face of a normal or increased platelet count, look for primary and secondary polycythemia. If both the platelet count and RBC are normal, the patient may have thrombasthenia.

## INCREASED

Clot retraction is increased in anemia and hypofibrinogenemia.

## NORMAL VALUES

Clot retraction is noticeable in 1 hour and almost complete in 4 hours.

## COST

Medium.

## ADDITIONAL TESTS TO ORDER

CBC, platelet count, chemistry panel, prothrombin consumption test, coagulation profile, bleeding time, fibrinogen, and hematology consult.

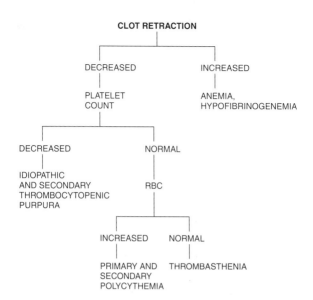

# COAGULANT FACTORS

## DECREASED

1. Factor VII: This factor is decreased in liver diseases and hypoproconvertinemia. To differentiate the two, order *liver function tests*. These are abnormal in liver disease.
2. Factor VIII: This factor is decreased in hemophilia A and von Willebrand's disease. To differentiate these two conditions, one should order a bleeding time. This is prolonged in von Willebrand's disease and is normal in hemophilia A. This factor is also decreased in consumptive coagulopathies.
3. Factor XI: This factor is decreased in liver disease, malabsorption syndrome, and hemophilia C. To differentiate these conditions, one should order liver function tests and a D-xylose absorption test.
4. Factor IX: This factor is decreased in liver disease, hemophilia B, and dicumarol drug administration. To differentiate these conditions, one should order liver function tests and take a careful history.
5. Other factor deficiencies: Factor XII is decreased in newborns, pregnancy, and nephrotic syndrome. Factor XIII is decreased in liver disease, multiple myeloma, pernicious anemia, lead poisoning, and macroglobulinemia. Factor VIII inhibitor is found in hemophilia A and immunologic conditions.

## NORMAL VALUES

Factor VII: 65–135%.
Factor VIII: 50–150%.
Factor IX: 60–140%.
Factor X: 45–155%.
Factor XI: 65–135%.
Factor XII: 50–150%.
Factor XIII: 45–140%.
Factor VIII: inhibitor-negative.

## COST

Medium to high.

## ADDITIONAL TESTS TO ORDER

CBC, chemistry panel, liver function tests, PTT, bleeding time, platelet count, prothrombin time, fibrin split products, thrombin time, and hematology consult.

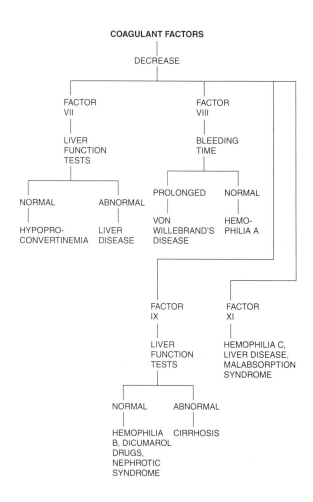

# COAGULATION TIME

## INCREASED

Ask the following questions:

1. Is the PTT increased? If it is, look for hemophilia and von Willebrand's disease. The PTT is also increased if the patient is receiving heparin therapy.
2. Is the prothrombin time increased? This occurs in vitamin K deficiency, warfarin sodium or dicumarol administration, and liver disease.
3. What is the thrombin time? The thrombin time is increased in afibrinogenemia, disseminated intravascular coagulation, liver disease, and heparin therapy.

## NORMAL VALUES

5–10 minutes.

## COST

Low.

## ADDITIONAL TESTS TO ORDER

Bleeding time, PTT, prothrombin time, thrombin time, fibrin split products, platelet count, capillary fragility test, and hematology consult.

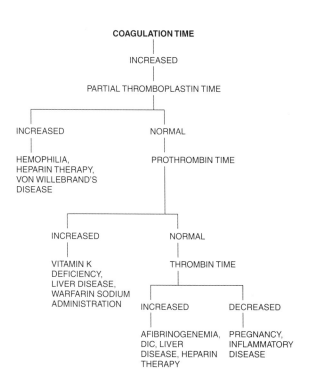

**COAGULATION TIME**
|
INCREASED
|
PARTIAL THROMBOPLASTIN TIME

INCREASED                    NORMAL
|                            |
HEMOPHILIA,                  PROTHROMBIN TIME
HEPARIN THERAPY,
VON WILLEBRAND'S
DISEASE

INCREASED              NORMAL
|                      |
VITAMIN K              THROMBIN TIME
DEFICIENCY,
LIVER DISEASE,
WARFARIN SODIUM        INCREASED          DECREASED
ADMINISTRATION         |                  |
                       AFIBRINOGENEMIA,   PREGNANCY,
                       DIC, LIVER         INFLAMMATORY
                       DISEASE, HEPARIN   DISEASE
                       THERAPY

# *COCCIDIOIDES* ANTIBODY TEST

## INCREASED

These antibodies are increased in the blood and CSF in coccidiomycosis. The tube precipitin test shows IgM antibodies and is positive during the first 2 to 3 months of illness. Later, the complement fixation test that demonstrates IgG antibodies becomes positive and may remain so indefinitely.

## NORMAL VALUES

Negative.

## COST

Low.

## ADDITIONAL TESTS TO ORDER

Sputum smear (cultures are dangerous), skin test, chest radiograph, sedimentation rate, animal inoculation, biopsy, and consultation with a pulmonologist.

# COCCIDIOIDOMYCOSIS SKIN TEST

## POSITIVE

A positive test indicates present or past infection with *Coccidioides immitis.* If a patient who was previously known to be negative becomes positive, active infection is likely.

## NORMAL VALUES

Negative. (The test may be negative in cavitary or disseminated disease.)

## COST

Low.

## ADDITIONAL TESTS TO ORDER

Smear and culture of sputum, urine, or exudates (handle carefully), serologic tests (especially complement fixation test), chest radiographs, sedimentation rate, CBC, chemistry panel, animal inoculation, biopsy, and consultation with a pulmonologist.

# COLD AGGLUTININS

## INCREASED

Ask the following questions:

1. Does the patient have a pneumonic infiltrate or upper respiratory symptoms? If these conditions are present, think of *Mycoplasma pneumoniae* or influenza.
2. Does the patient have hemoglobinuria? This finding suggests paroxysmal cold hemoglobinuria.
3. Are the serum haptoglobins decreased? If they are, look for hemolytic anemia and malaria. They may also be decreased in paroxysmal cold hemoglobinuria.
4. Is the VDRL positive? This finding points to congenital syphilis as a possible cause.
5. If the answers to the foregoing questions are not helpful, look for cirrhosis, lymphatic leukemia, listeriosis, subacute bacterial endocarditis, and lymphoma.

## NORMAL VALUES

A titer of less than 1:32.

## COST

Low.

## ADDITIONAL TESTS TO ORDER

CBC, chemistry panel, liver function tests, red cell fragility test, red cell survival test, enzyme immunoassay for *Mycoplasma* antibodies, bone marrow biopsy, blood smear for parasites, chest radiograph, ice water test, and hematology consult.

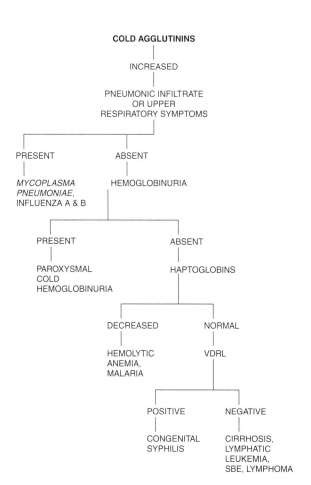

**COLD AGGLUTININS**
|
INCREASED
|
PNEUMONIC INFILTRATE
OR UPPER
RESPIRATORY SYMPTOMS

PRESENT

*MYCOPLASMA
PNEUMONIAE,*
INFLUENZA A & B

ABSENT

HEMOGLOBINURIA

PRESENT

PAROXYSMAL
COLD
HEMOGLOBINURIA

ABSENT

HAPTOGLOBINS

DECREASED

HEMOLYTIC
ANEMIA,
MALARIA

NORMAL

VDRL

POSITIVE

CONGENITAL
SYPHILIS

NEGATIVE

CIRRHOSIS,
LYMPHATIC
LEUKEMIA,
SBE, LYMPHOMA

# COLONOSCOPY

## POSITIVE

This test is used to diagnose polyps and carcinoma of the colon. It is also used to diagnose blood in the stool or causes of chronic diarrhea such as amebic colitis, ulcerative colitis, granulomatous colitis (Crohn's), diverticulitis, and pseudomembranous colitis. Biopsies are often taken.

## NORMAL VALUES

Normal mucosa without constriction or obstruction.

## COST

High.

## ADDITIONAL TESTS TO ORDER

CBC, chemistry panel, sedimentation rate, stool for occult blood, culture and ova and parasites times three, barium enema, CT scan of abdomen and pelvis, and gastroenterology consult.

# COLOR, URINE

1. *Colorless:* Nearly colorless urine may be found in diabetes insipidus, chronic nephritis, alcoholism, diabetes mellitus, and large fluid intake in a normal subject.
2. *Orange:* An orange color is found in dehydration and the ingestion of certain drugs (phenazopyridine and aminopyridine).
3. *Brown:* Brown urine is found in obstructive jaundice (bilirubin), porphyria, melanotic tumors, and the use of various drugs (e.g., sulfonamides).
4. *Red:* Red urine may indicate hematuria, hemoglobinuria, myoglobin, or porphyria. It may also be found in the use of phenazopyridine or ethoxazene.
5. *Black:* Black urine is found in alkaptonuria and melanotic tumors. Smoky urine may be due to red cells.
6. *Green:* Green urine is found in *Pseudomonas* infections and with the use of methylene blue, amitriptyline, and certain other drugs.

## NORMAL VALUES

Light to rich yellow.

## COST

Low.

## ADDITIONAL TESTS TO ORDER

CBC, sedimentation rate, urinalysis, urine culture, chemistry panel, urine porphyrins, urine melanin, urine bilirubin and urobilinogen, urine drug screen, Addis count, Fishberg concentration test, IVP, and nephrology consult.

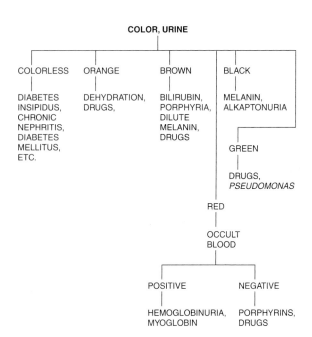

**COLOR, URINE**

**COLORLESS**

DIABETES
INSIPIDUS,
CHRONIC
NEPHRITIS,
DIABETES
MELLITUS,
ETC.

**ORANGE**

DEHYDRATION,
DRUGS,

**BROWN**

BILIRUBIN,
PORPHYRIA,
DILUTE
MELANIN,
DRUGS

**BLACK**

MELANIN,
ALKAPTONURIA

**GREEN**

DRUGS,
*PSEUDOMONAS*

**RED**

OCCULT
BLOOD

**POSITIVE**

HEMOGLOBINURIA,
MYOGLOBIN

**NEGATIVE**

PORPHYRINS,
DRUGS

# COLPOSCOPY

## POSITIVE

This test is positive in carcinoma of the cervix and vagina and leukoplakia. It is commonly used to evaluate abnormal Papanicolaou smears further. Biopsies and scrapings of the vagina and cervix are done during the procedure.

## NORMAL VALUES

Normal-appearing vaginal and cervical mucosa.

## COST

Medium.

## ADDITIONAL TESTS TO ORDER

Schiller test, D&C, endometrial biopsy, ultrasonography, CT scan of the pelvis, and gynecology consult.

# COMPLEMENT C3

## DECREASED

Ask the following questions:

1. Is the ASO titer increased? An increased ASO titer suggests that the decreased complement is due to acute glomerulonephritis.
2. Does the patient have a positive ANA? This suggests lupus erythematosus.

If neither of these tests are abnormal, the patient may have membranoproliferative glomerulonephritis, absence of C3b inactivator factor, recurrent bacterial or fungal infections, or subacute bacterial endocarditis.

## NORMAL VALUES

83–177 mg/dL.

## COST

Low.

## ADDITIONAL TESTS TO ORDER

CBC, urinalysis, complement C4, sedimentation rate, chemistry panel, blood cultures, RA test, serum protein electrophoresis, 24-hour urine protein, renal biopsy, nephrology consult, and rheumatology consult.

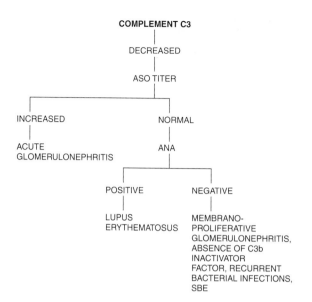

**COMPLEMENT C3**
|
DECREASED
|
ASO TITER

INCREASED — NORMAL

INCREASED:
ACUTE GLOMERULONEPHRITIS

NORMAL:
ANA

POSITIVE — NEGATIVE

POSITIVE:
LUPUS ERYTHEMATOSUS

NEGATIVE:
MEMBRANO-PROLIFERATIVE GLOMERULONEPHRITIS, ABSENCE OF C3b INACTIVATOR FACTOR, RECURRENT BACTERIAL INFECTIONS, SBE

# COMPUTED TOMOGRAPHY, ABDOMEN

## POSITIVE

This test is positive in tumors of the liver, pancreas, spleen, kidney, adrenal glands, and GI tract. It is useful in diagnosing malformations, abscesses, cysts, and chronic inflammatory disease of these organs, as well. Retroperitoneal lymphadenopathy, cancer of the pancreas, and metastatic liver disease are diagnosed by this method. It is *superior* to MRI because it can visualize the GI tract.

## NORMAL VALUES

Normal size, shape, and position of abdominal organs with homogeneous consistency of organs and tissue layers.

## COST

High.

## ADDITIONAL TESTS TO ORDER

CBC, urinalysis, chemistry panel, plain films of abdomen, upper GI series, small bowel series, barium enema, cholecystogram, IVP, ultrasonography, radionuclide scans, endoscopic procedures, exploratory laparotomy, and gastroenterology or surgical consult.

# COMPUTED TOMOGRAPHY, BRAIN

## POSITIVE

This test is positive in epidural, subdural, and intra-cerebral hematomas, neoplasms, cerebral infarct or hemorrhage, skull fractures, larger aneurysms, A-V malformations, degenerative diseases such as Alzheimer's and Pick's disease, and congenital malformations such as hydrocephalus. It may be positive in demyelinating diseases, but MRI is superior in this regard. Contrast enhancement is useful in diagnosing tumors, blood clots, aneurysms, and A-V malformations, but it carries the risk of allergic reaction.

## NORMAL VALUES

Homogeneous consistency of cerebral tissue, with no displacement of ventricles.

## COST

High.

## ADDITIONAL TESTS TO ORDER

MRI, EEG, MR angiography, spinal fluid analysis, myelin basic protein, CBC and chemistry panel, cerebral angiography, and neurology or neurosurgical consult.

# COMPUTED TOMOGRAPHY, CHEST

## POSITIVE

This test is positive in neoplasms of the lung and mediastinum, lung abscess, mediastinitis, interstitial lung disease, pulmonary embolism, and empyema. It is helpful in evaluating the solitary pulmonary nodule and in differentiating hilar adenopathy from pulmonary vasculature. It is also useful in diagnosing mediastinal masses.

## NORMAL VALUES

Normal size, shape, and consistency of lung and mediastinal structures, with no abnormal densities.

## COST

High.

## ADDITIONAL TESTS TO ORDER

CBC, urinalysis, chemistry panel, sedimentation rate, skin tests, sputum smear and culture, sputum for AFB and fungal smear and culture, chest radiograph, ECG, bronchoscopy, biopsy, RAI uptake and scan, and pulmonary consult.

# COMPUTED TOMOGRAPHY, EXTREMITIES AND JOINTS

## POSITIVE

The CT scan demonstrates acute fractures, hematomas, and hemorrhages into the joints. It is also helpful in diagnosing some tumors and assists in placing the needle for percutaneous needle biopsy.

## NORMAL VALUES

Normal size and shape of bones and joints. No fractures, mass, or hematoma.

## COST

High.

## ADDITIONAL TESTS TO ORDER

Plain films, CBC, chemistry panel, MRI, bone scan, arthroscopy, arthrography, arthrocentesis, and orthopedic consult.

# COMPUTED TOMOGRAPHY, HEAD

## POSITIVE

This test is often positive in acute craniofacial trauma demonstrating cranial, orbital, and sinus fractures, as well as intracranial hemorrhage. It is superior to MRI in detecting hemorrhage in the first 48 hours.

## NORMAL VALUES

Normal size, shape, and position of cranial and intra-cranial structures. No fracture, mass, or hematoma.

## COST

High.

## ADDITIONAL TESTS TO ORDER

CBC, chemistry panel, MRI, EEG, plain films, spinal fluid analysis, angiography, bone scan, and neurology or neurosurgical consult.

# COMPUTED TOMOGRAPHY, NECK

## POSITIVE

This test is positive in neoplasms of the thyroid, lymphomas, lymph node metastasis, aneurysms, and abscesses. It can help to evaluate disorders of the esophagus and larynx.

## NORMAL VALUES

Normal size, shape, and position of structures of the neck. No tumors present.

## COST

High.

## ADDITIONAL TESTS TO ORDER

Soft-tissue radiograph, esophagogram, MRI, esophagoscopy, laryngoscopy, RAI uptake and scan, ultrasonography of thyroid, biopsy of thyroid or lymph nodes, free $T_4$, thyroid antibodies, pulmonary consult, and endocrinology consult.

# COMPUTED TOMOGRAPHY, PELVIS

## POSITIVE

This test is positive in neoplasms of the uterus, tubes and ovaries, in prostatic, rectal, and bladder carcinoma, in abscess, and in hemorrhages in the cul-de-sac as in ruptured ectopic pregnancy and endometriosis. Because of the effects of radiation, it is not as useful as ultrasound or MRI in evaluating gynecologic disorders. It is useful in diagnosing diverticulitis and diverticular abscesses.

## NORMAL VALUES

Normal size, shape, and position of pelvic organs. No tumors or other masses noted.

## COST

High.

## ADDITIONAL TESTS TO ORDER

CBC, pregnancy test, urinalysis, chemistry panel, pelvic ultrasonography, sedimentation rate, urine culture, vaginal smears and cultures, Pap smear, PSA, cervical biopsy, endometrial biopsy, cystoscopy, colonoscopy, cystogram, barium enema, laparoscopy, gynecology consult, gastroenterology consult, and urology consult.

# COMPUTED TOMOGRAPHY, SPINE

## POSITIVE

This is positive in fractures, osteoarthritic spurs, herniated discs, tumors, abscesses, and hematomas. This method is useful in diagnosing subtle fractures. It is valuable in diagnosing *herniated discs* of the *lumbar spine,* but the accuracy in diagnosing herniated discs of the cervical and thoracic spine is poor compared with MRI. Combined CT scan and myelography markedly improve accuracy.

## NORMAL VALUES

Normal size, shape, and position of structures. No tumor found.

## COST

High.

## ADDITIONAL TESTS TO ORDER

Plain radiographs, MRI, combined CT scan and myelography, CBC, chemistry panel, EMG, NCV and evoked potential studies, PSA, discography, bone scan, and neurology or orthopedic consult.

# COOMBS' TEST, DIRECT AND INDIRECT

## POSITIVE

These tests are positive in transfusion reactions, autoimmune hemolytic anemia, and erythroblastosis fetalis. The direct Coombs' test is especially useful in differentiating acquired hemolytic anemia from hereditary hemolytic anemia (e.g., hereditary spherocytosis, sickle cell anemia). The direct Coombs' test is also positive in drug-induced hemolytic anemia (e.g., methyldopa, penicillin cephalosporins, sulfonamides).

## NORMAL VALUES

Negative.

## COST

Low.

## ADDITIONAL TESTS TO ORDER

CBC, sedimentation rate, urinalysis, chemistry panel, serum haptoglobins, ANA, serum protein electrophoresis, red cell survival time, hemoglobin electrophoresis, and hematology consult.

# COPPER AND CERULOPLASMIN

## DECREASED

In Wilson's disease, serum copper and ceruloplasmin are both decreased, whereas the urinary copper is increased.

## INCREASED

Copper and ceruloplasmin are increased in rheumatoid arthritis, thyrotoxicosis, biliary cirrhosis, patients using oral contraceptives, and pregnancy. To exclude biliary cirrhosis from this group, one should order a 24-hour urine copper. This value is increased in biliary cirrhosis.

## NORMAL VALUES

Copper: 65–150 $\mu$g/dL.
Ceruloplasmin: 25–45 mg/dL.

## COST

Low.

## ADDITIONAL TESTS TO ORDER

CBC, urinalysis, chemistry panel, sedimentation rate, RA test, mitochondrial antibodies, free $T_4$, serum protein electrophoresis, liver biopsy, and gastroenterology consult.

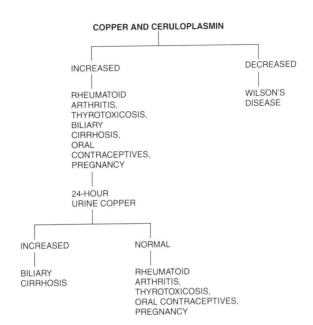

**COPPER AND CERULOPLASMIN**

INCREASED

RHEUMATOID ARTHRITIS, THYROTOXICOSIS, BILIARY CIRRHOSIS, ORAL CONTRACEPTIVES, PREGNANCY

DECREASED

WILSON'S DISEASE

24-HOUR URINE COPPER

INCREASED

BILIARY CIRRHOSIS

NORMAL

RHEUMATOID ARTHRITIS, THYROTOXICOSIS, ORAL CONTRACEPTIVES, PREGNANCY

# CORTISOL

## INCREASED

Cortisol is increased in Cushing's syndrome. To differentiate these conditions further, a high-dose dexamethasone suppression test is indicated. If the Cushing's syndrome is due to adrenal hyperplasia from a pituitary adenoma, the plasma cortisol will be suppressed. If it is due to an adrenal adenoma or carcinoma, it will not be suppressed. It is not suppressed in patients with ectopic ACTH-producing tumors, either.

## DECREASED

The plasma cortisol is decreased in Addison's disease, pituitary insufficiency, and adrenogenital syndrome. To distinguish these conditions, one should perform an ACTH-stimulation test. A positive response indicates pituitary insufficiency. A negative response indicates Addison's disease or congenital adrenal hyperplasia. To differentiate the latter from Addison's disease, one should determine the plasma 17-OH-progesterone level. This is elevated in congenital adrenal hyperplasia.

## NORMAL VALUES

8:00 AM: 5–20 $\mu$g/dL.

## COST

Low.

## ADDITIONAL TESTS TO ORDER

CBC, urinalysis, chemistry panel, electrolytes, dexamethasone suppression tests, ACTH stimulation test, plasma 17-OH-progesterone, androstenedione, dihydroepiandrosterone level, CT scan of brain, adrenal glands, and abdomen, and endocrinology consult.

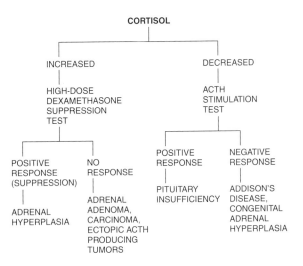

# C-PEPTIDE

## INCREASED

C-peptide is increased in insulinomas and in type II diabetes mellitus. These two can be distinguished by the blood sugar, which is elevated in type II diabetes and is decreased in insulinomas, especially after a 36- to 72-hour fast.

## DECREASED

C-peptide is decreased in type I diabetes mellitus and in factitious hypoglycemia. These two can be distinguished by the high blood sugar in type I diabetes and the low blood sugar in factitious hypoglycemia.

## NORMAL VALUES

0.9–4.2 mg/mL.

## COST

Low.

## ADDITIONAL TESTS TO ORDER

A 5-hour glucose tolerance test, plasma insulin, 36–72 hour fast, abdominal CT scan, arteriography, exploratory laparotomy, and endocrinology consult.

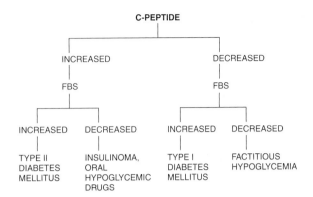

# C-REACTIVE PROTEIN (CRP)

## POSITIVE

Ask the following questions:

1. What is the ASO titer? An elevated ASO titer suggests rheumatic fever.
2. What is the rheumatoid factor? An increased RA titer suggests rheumatoid arthritis.
3. What is the MB–CPK? If this is elevated, look for a myocardial infarction.
4. Is the blood culture positive? Positive blood cultures are found in subacute bacterial endocarditis, septicemia, and other infectious diseases.

If none of these tests are positive, one should look for other causes of inflammation such as bacterial or viral infections, collagen diseases, malignant diseases, and tissue injury.

## NORMAL VALUES

Negative.

## COST

Low.

## ADDITIONAL TESTS TO ORDER

CBC, sedimentation rate, urinalysis and culture, chemistry panel, ANA, serum protein electrophoresis, culture of various body fluids, CEA, bone scan, CT scan of abdomen, chest radiograph, and consultation with an infectious disease expert or oncologist.

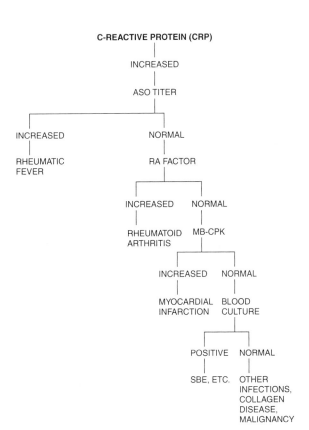

# CREATINE PHOSPHOKINASE

## INCREASED

This enzyme is increased in myocardial and muscle disease, regardless of the cause. Ask the following questions:

1. What is the MB–CPK? An elevated MB–CPK most likely indicates a myocardial infarction, especially if this value is significantly elevated or rising. A normal or slight elevation points to skeletal muscle disease and other disorders.
2. What is the EMG? A positive EMG enables one to distinguish among dermatomyositis, muscular dystrophy, and myxedema.
3. What is the ANA? The ANA is increased in three-fourths of patients with dermatomyositis.

## NORMAL VALUES

Men: 50–180 IU/L.
Women: 50–160 IU/L.

## COST

Low.

## ADDITIONAL TESTS TO ORDER

CBC, urinalysis, chemistry panel, MB–CPK, ECG, EMG, ANA, RA, muscle biopsy, radiograph of chest, MRI of skeletal muscle, sedimentation rate, ASO titer, cardiology consult, rheumatology consult, and neurology consult.

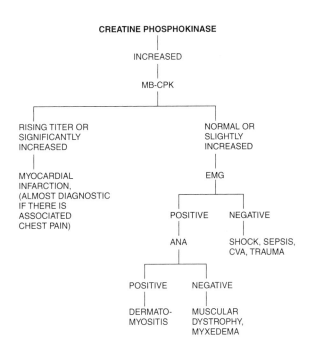

**CREATINE PHOSPHOKINASE**

INCREASED

MB-CPK

RISING TITER OR
SIGNIFICANTLY
INCREASED

MYOCARDIAL
INFARCTION,
(ALMOST DIAGNOSTIC
IF THERE IS
ASSOCIATED
CHEST PAIN)

NORMAL OR
SLIGHTLY
INCREASED

EMG

POSITIVE

NEGATIVE

ANA

SHOCK, SEPSIS,
CVA, TRAUMA

POSITIVE

NEGATIVE

DERMATO-
MYOSITIS

MUSCULAR
DYSTROPHY,
MYXEDEMA

# CREATININE

## INCREASED

Ask the following questions:

1. What is the BUN? An increase of both the creatinine and BUN usually means renal disease, but it may be due to dehydration or shock. A normal BUN with an increased creatinine may mean gigantism, hyperthyroidism, or the influence of drugs such as cephalosporins.
2. What is the BUN/creatinine ratio? An increased BUN/creatinine ratio in the presence of an increased BUN and creatinine points to prerenal azotemia, whereas a decreased BUN/creatinine ratio suggests renal and postrenal azotemia.

## DECREASED

Decreased creatinine is associated with muscle diseases such as muscular dystrophy and dermatomyositis.

## NORMAL VALUES

Females: 0.6–1.0 mg/dL.
Males: 0.8–1.7 mg/dL.

## COST

Low.

## ADDITIONAL TESTS TO ORDER

CBC, urinalysis, chemistry panel, sedimentation rate, serum and urine osmolality, blood volume, ANA, free T$_4$, plasma growth hormone, cystoscopy and retrograde pyelography, renal biopsy, muscle biopsy, and nephrology and urology consult.

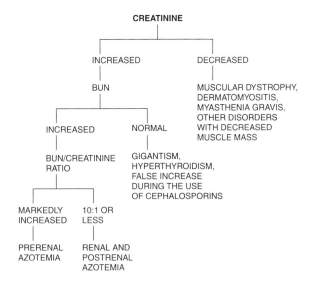

# CREATININE CLEARANCE

## DECREASED

The creatinine clearance is decreased in impaired renal function. It is most useful in determining the degree of malfunction in chronic glomerulonephritis and other forms of chronic renal disease before the BUN and creatinine become elevated. Therefore, it is useful in assessing the severity of these diseases and the prognosis. Determination of the creatinine clearance is also useful in estimating drug dosage in patients with renal disease.

## NORMAL VALUES

Males: 85–125 mL/minute.
Females: 75–115 mL/minute.

## COST

Low.

## ADDITIONAL TESTS TO ORDER

Urinalysis, CBC, chemistry panel, Addis count, Fishberg concentration test, serum complement, cystoscopy and retrograde pyelography, renal biopsy, ultrasonography, CT scan of abdomen, and nephrology consult.

# CRYOGLOBULINS

## TYPE I

These cryoglobulins are associated with multiple myeloma, macroglobulinemia, and other lymphoproliferative disorders.

## TYPES II AND III

These cryoglobulins are associated with infection, lupus erythematosus, rheumatoid arthritis and other collagen disorders, glomerulonephritis, chronic liver disease, and lymphoproliferative disorders.

## NORMAL VALUES

Negative.

## COST

Low.

## ADDITIONAL TESTS TO ORDER

CBC, urinalysis, sedimentation rate, chemistry panel, serum protein electrophoresis, ANA, RA test, ASO titer, antidouble-stranded DNA, liver function tests, Monospot test, VDRL, and hematology consult.

# CRYPTOCOCCUS ANTIGEN TITER

## POSITIVE

This test is positive in torulosis. A rising titer is more significant. False-positive and false-negative results occur.

## NORMAL VALUES

Negative.

## COST

Low.

## ADDITIONAL TESTS TO ORDER

India ink preparation, sputum and spinal fluid cultures, HIV antibody titer, biopsy, MRI of the brain, and neurology consult.

# CRYSTALS, URINE

1. Uric acid crystals: Although these may be a normal finding, one should consider gout and other conditions that cause increased blood uric acid levels.
2. Triple phosphate crystals: The presence of the crystals may be a sign of urinary tract infection.
3. Cystine crystals: These crystals are found in cystinuria.
4. Calcium phosphate and oxalate crystals: These are also found in normal urine but may indicate renal calculi.

## NORMAL VALUES

Uric acid crystals, calcium oxalate crystals, triple phosphate, calcium phosphate urate, and amorphous phosphate crystals.

## COST

Low.

## ADDITIONAL TESTS TO ORDER

CBC, chemistry panel, urinalysis, urine culture, 24-hour urine calcium, KUB, IVP, cystoscopy, synovianalysis, and urology consult.

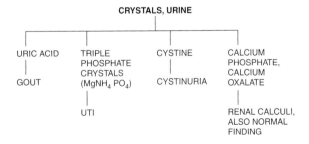

CRYSTALS, URINE

URIC ACID — GOUT

TRIPLE PHOSPHATE CRYSTALS ($MgNH_4 PO_4$) — UTI

CYSTINE — CYSTINURIA

CALCIUM PHOSPHATE, CALCIUM OXALATE — RENAL CALCULI, ALSO NORMAL FINDING

# CULTURES OF MISCELLANEOUS BODY FLUIDS

## NASAL CULTURES

These are done to screen hospital personnel, transplant recipients, dialysis patients, and other patients who are immunocompromised for *Staphylococcus aureus* and other infections.

## NASOPHARYNGEAL CULTURES

### Positive

Cultures are useful in detecting *Corynebacterium diphtheriae, Haemophilus influenzae,* β-hemolytic streptococci, *Bordetella pertussis, Streptococcus pneumoniae, Meningococcus,* and *Staphylococcus aureus.*

### Normal Flora

Normal flora include *Neisseria catarrhalis,* α-hemolytic streptococci, coagulase-negative staphylococci, diphtheroid bacilli, *Candida albicans,* and nonhemolytic streptococci.

## SKIN AND WOUND CULTURES

These are indicated when discharge is significant.

### Positive

Organisms recovered from the skin and wounds that may be pathologic are *Staphylococcus aureus, Strep-*

tococcus pyogenes, Pseudomonas, coliform bacilli, enterococci, Proteus, and Clostridium species.

## URETHRAL CULTURES

Any urethral discharge needs to be cultured. In males, prostatic massage should be performed to increase the chances for a positive culture.

### Positive

Organisms that may be considered pathologic are *Neisseria gonorrhoeae*, *Treponema pallidum*, *Haemophilus ducreyi*, *Chlamydia trachomatis*, and *Trichomonas vaginalis*.

### Normal Flora

Normal flora include coagulase-negative staphylococci, coliform bacilli, enterococci, and *Mycobacterium smegmatis*.

## VAGINAL CULTURES

A vaginal discharge needs to be cultured when a saline and KOH preparation fails to reveal the cause of the discharge or when there is good clinical evidence of gonorrhea. A specimen from the cervix and endocervical canal should be obtained if gonorrhea is suspected.

### Positive

Pathogenic organisms include *Neisseria gonorrhoeae*, *Haemophilus ducreyi*, *Trichomonas vaginalis*, *Candida albicans*, *Haemophilus vaginalis*, *Listeria monocytogenes*, and *Treponema pallidum*. *Chlamydia trachomatis* is also cultured using special media.

## Normal Flora

Normal flora are coliform bacilli, enterococci, anaerobic streptococci, *Bacteroides,* Döderlein bacillus, and coagulase-negative *Staphylococcus.*

## STOOL CULTURE

Stool cultures are useful in patients with acute and chronic diarrhea, especially when accompanied by fever and chills.

### Positive

Pathologic organisms that can be detected by stool cultures are *Salmonella* species, *Shigella, Vibrio cholerae, Escherichia coli,* staphylococci, *Clostridium botulinum* toxin, *Proteus* (in large numbers), *Pseudomonas* (in large numbers), *Candida albicans,* and *Clostridium difficile.*

### Normal Flora

These include enterococci, *Escherichia coli,* clostridia, staphylococci, *Proteus* species, *Pseudomonas,* and *Candida albicans. Salmonella* may be isolated in carriers.

## CEREBROSPINAL FLUID CULTURE

This is indicated in cases of fever or nuchal rigidity and any fever of unknown origin.

### Positive

Cultures are positive when any of the following organisms are found: *Streptococcus pneumoniae, Neisseria meningitidis, Haemophilus influenzae, Myco-*

*bacterium tuberculosis,* streptococci, coliform bacilli, *Listeria monocytogenes, Leptospira* species, *Bacteroides* species, and *Cryptococcus* and other fungi.

## Normal Flora

None, but may be contaminated by skin flora.

## PLEURAL FLUID

All specimens need to be cultured.

### Positive

Positive results may yield pneumococci, *Klebsiella, Haemophilus influenzae,* streptococci, *Mycobacterium tuberculosis, Yersinia pestis* and *Francisella tularensis, Staphylococcus aureus,* and fungi, including *Coccidioides immitis, Histoplasma capsulatum, Blastomyces dermatitidis,* and *Candida albicans.*

### Normal Flora

None, except the normal flora of the skin which may contaminate the specimen.

## PERITONEAL FLUID

Culture all specimens.

### Positive

The most common pathogenic organisms are pneumococci, *Neisseria gonorrhoeae,* and *Mycobacterium tuberculosis.* However, any organism from the stool may be cultured if the peritoneal fluid is due to a ruptured viscus (see Stool Culture).

## CONJUNCTIVAL CULTURE

This should be done in all cases of exudative conjunctivitis and hordeolum.

### Positive

Pathogenic organisms that may grow in culture include *Staphylococcus aureus, Neisseria gonorrhoeae, Streptococcus pneumoniae,* Koch—Weeks bacillus, *Chlamydia trachomatis, Pseudomonas* species, and $\beta$-hemolytic streptococci.

### Normal Flora

This is the same as the skin, discussed earlier in this section. One additional organism that may be found is *Corynebacterium xerosis.*

### EAR

Cultures are indicated whenever an exudate is present in the external canal. Occasionally, in acute otitis media without a rupture of the tympanic membrane, needle aspiration of the middle ear is indicated to obtain a specimen.

### Positive

Pathogenic organisms that may be obtained on culture include *Haemophilus influenzae, Streptococcus pneumoniae, Proteus* species, *Pseudomonas aeruginosa, Staphylococcus aureus,* $\alpha$- and $\beta$-hemolytic streptococci, coliform bacilli, and fungi.

## Normal Flora

These organisms include coagulase-negative diphtheroids, staphylococci, and *Peptostreptococcus tetradius.*

## COST

Low.

## ADDITIONAL TESTS TO ORDER

Repeat cultures, smears, dark-field examination, guinea pig inoculation, skin tests, serologic tests, tissue biopsy, cultures of other body fluids, repeated anaerobic cultures, and consultation with an infectious disease expert.

# CUTANEOUS IMMUNOFLUORESCENCE BIOPSY

## POSITIVE

This test is positive in lupus erythematosus, pemphigus, pemphigoid, dermatitis herpetiformis, and vasculitis. This test is therefore indicated when these conditions are suspected.

## NORMAL VALUES

No evidence of immunofluorescence of immunoglobulins or complement components. No evidence of intercellular epidermal antibody or basement membrane antibody. No evidence of IgA or fibrin in perilesional skin.

## COST

Medium.

## ADDITIONAL TESTS TO ORDER

ANA, anti-DNA tests, dermatology consult, and rheumatology consult.

# CYCLIC ADENOSINE MONOPHOSPHATE (cAMP), RENAL

## INCREASED

Renal cAMP is increased in primary hyperparathyroidism, vitamin D deficiency, malignant diseases associated with hypercalcemia, and hypercalciuria.

## DECREASED

Renal cAMP is decreased in hypoparathyroidism, pseudohypoparathyroidism, and hypocalcemic states.

## NORMAL VALUES

Check with the local laboratory. This is calculated from measurements of plasma and urine cyclic AMP.

## COST

Low to medium.

## ADDITIONAL TESTS TO ORDER

PTH assay, free T4, chemistry panel, 24-hour urine calcium, parathyroid ultrasonography, MRI of the thyroid, bone scan, radiograph of the teeth, skeletal survey, and endocrinology consult.

# CYSTINE

## INCREASED

Increased amounts of cystine appear in the urine in cystinuria and cystinosis.

## NORMAL VALUES

### Qualitative Test

Negative.

### Quantitative Test

Children under 8: 2–13 mg/24 hours.
Children over 8 and adults: 7–28 mg/24 hours.

## COST

Low.

## ADDITIONAL TESTS TO ORDER

Amino acids in urine.

# CYSTOMETRIC STUDIES

## POSITIVE

1. *Flaccid neurogenic bladder:* This result is found in lower motor neuron disorders such as tabes dorsalis, poliomyelitis, cauda equina syndrome, and diabetic neuropathy.
2. *Spastic neurogenic bladder:* This result is found in upper motor neuron disorders such as multiple sclerosis, syringomyelia, spinal cord tumors, transverse myelitis, spinal cord injury, and cervical spondylosis.
3. *Uninhibited bladder:* This result is found in cerebral disorders such as Alzheimer's disease, low-pressure hydrocephalus, and cerebral arteriosclerosis.

## NORMAL VALUES

Sensation of fullness at 100–450 mL; urge to void at 350–450 mL; filling pressure constant until urge to void occurs; good contraction on voiding, normal sensation.

## COST

Medium

## ADDITIONAL TESTS TO ORDER

Plain films of spine, MRI of the brain, cervical, thoracic or lumbar spine, NCV studies, EMG, glucose tolerance test, spinal fluid analysis, myelography, combined CT scan and myelography, cystoscopy, urology consult, and neurology consult.

# CYSTOSCOPY

## POSITIVE

This test can diagnose bladder polyps and carcinoma, stones, bladder diverticula, vesicle neck obstruction, prostatic hypertrophy, prostatitis, chronic cystitis, urethral strictures, and congenital anomalies of the genitourinary tract. Biopsies are usually taken of suspicious lesions. It is indicated to diagnose the cause of unexplained hematuria, recurrent urinary tract infection, urinary retention, and other urinary symptoms.

## NORMAL VALUES

Normal mucosa, no obstruction, no trabeculations or diverticula.

## COST

Medium.

## ADDITIONAL TESTS TO ORDER

Urinalysis, urine culture, prostatic massage and smear and culture of exudate, IVP, voiding cystogram, retrograde pyelography, ultrasonography, CT scan of pelvis, cystometric studies, and urology consult.

# CYTOLOGIC STUDIES

## NORMAL VALUES

Negative.

## BREAST

### Positive

Nipple discharge and the contents of breast cysts may show inflammatory cells in mastitis or abnormal cells in intraductal papillomas or cancer and intracystic infiltrating carcinoma.

### Cost

Low.

### Additional Tests to Order

Mammography, needle biopsy, ultrasonography, surgical consult.

## CEREBROSPINAL FLUID

### Positive

This test is positive in malignant gliomas, leukemia, ependymomas, and metastatic neoplasms.

### Cost

Low.

## Additional Tests to Order

Spinal fluid and analysis, MRI or CT scans, and neurology or neurosurgical consult.

## FEMALE GENITAL TRACT (PAPANICOLAOU SMEAR)

### Positive

This test is positive in carcinoma of the vagina, cervix, and endometrium. It is also useful in determining the level of circulating estrogen by its effect on the vaginal epithelium. This is done with the *maturation index*, which is the proportion of major cell types of each 100 cells counted. The more superficial cells present, the greater the estrogen effect, whereas the more parabasal cells present, the less the estrogen effect.

### Report Interpretation

Class I: Negative.
Class II: Atypical cytology, not neoplastic.
Class III: Suggestive of malignancy.
Class IV:Strongly suggestive of malignancy.
Class V: Malignancy.

### Cost

Low.

### Additional Tests to Order

Colposcopy, Schiller test, cervical and endometrial biopsy, ultrasonography, CT scan, laparoscopy, and gynecology consult.

### GASTROINTESTINAL TRACT

### Positive

This test is positive in esophageal and gastric carcinoma. Abnormal results may be found in chronic gastritis, pernicious anemia, and certain inflammatory disorders of the GI tract.

## Cost

Low.

## Additional Tests to Order

Upper GI series and esophagogram, esophagoscopy, gastroscopy and biopsy, gastric analysis, and gastroenterology consult.

# PERITONEAL EFFUSION

## Positive

Abnormal cells may be found in peritoneal metastasis or invasion from malignancies of the pancreas, GI tract, liver, kidney and ovary. Occasionally, abnormal cells are due to metastasis from a remote site such as the lung.

## Cost

Low.

## Additional Tests to Order

Liver function tests, CEA, C-125, CT scan of the abdomen and pelvis, laparoscopy, surgical consult, and oncology consult.

# PLEURAL EFFUSION

## Positive

Abnormal cells are found in carcinoma of the lung, mesothelioma, and metastasis from remote sites.

## Cost

Low.

## Additional Tests to Order

CBC, urinalysis, sputum for cytology, chest radiograph, CT scan of chest, bronchoscopy, and pulmonary consult.

## RESPIRATORY TRACT

### Positive

Abnormal cells are found in the sputum and bronchial washings obtained by bronchoscopy in patients with carcinoma of the lung and occasionally in patients with metastatic neoplasms.

## Cost

Low.

## Additional Tests to Order

CBC, urinalysis, chemistry panel, sputum culture and analysis, chest radiograph, CT scan of chest, bronchoscopy, needle biopsy, and pulmonary consult.

## URINARY TRACT

### Positive

Abnormal cells are found in the urine in patients with neoplasms of the bladder, renal pelvis, ureters, kidney, and prostate. Occasionally, abnormal cells are found in metastasis from remote sites.

## Cost

Low.

## Additional Tests to Order

CBC, urinalysis, chemistry panel, IVP, cystoscopy and biopsy, retrograde pyelogram, PSA, ultrasonography of prostate and bladder, CT scan, and urology consult.

# CYTOMEGALOVIRUS ANTIBODIES

## INCREASED

These antibodies are increased in cytomegalovirus infections. If the IgM is increased or if there is a fourfold or greater increase in IgG, an active infection with CMV should be suspected. Epstein—Barr virus infections may yield false-positive results.

## NORMAL VALUES

Negative.

## COST

Low.

## ADDITIONAL TESTS TO ORDER

CBC, chemistry panel, urinalysis, sedimentation rate, viral isolation, examination of stained urine sediment, CMV antigen testing, and consultation with an infectious disease expert.

# DEHYDRO-EPIANDROSTERONE SULFATE (DHEA-S)

## INCREASED

This substance is increased in the blood in adrenocortical neoplasms and hyperplasia, in polycystic ovaries, in ectopic ACTH-producing tumors, and in female patients with hirsutism and acne. The levels are especially high in adrenal carcinoma, and this helps to differentiate this form of Cushing's syndrome from adenoma and hyperplasia.

## DECREASED

DHEA-S is decreased in primary and secondary adrenal insufficiency.

## NORMAL VALUES

Less than 800 $\mu$g/dL, but values vary with age and sex. Check with your local laboratory.

## COST

Low.

## ADDITIONAL TESTS TO ORDER

Dexamethasone-suppression test, ACTH stimulation test, plasma cortisol, plasma ACTH, metyrapone test, CT scan of brain, CT scan of adrenal glands, abdomen, and pelvis, and endocrinology consult.

# DEXAMETHASONE-SUPPRESSION TEST

## LOW DOSE

### No Suppression

No suppression of plasma or urinary cortisol with low doses of dexamethasone (0.5 mg q6h for 2 days) is suggestive of Cushing's syndrome.

### Suppression

This is normal.

## HIGH DOSE

### No Suppression

No suppression of plasma or urinary cortisol with high doses of dexamethasone (2 mg q6h for 2 to 3 days) usually indicates either carcinoma or adenoma of the adrenal cortex.

### Suppression

If plasma or urinary cortisol is suppressed by high doses of dexamethasone, one should look for basophilic adenoma of the pituitary and adrenal cortical hyperplasia. Occasionally, an ectopic ACTH-producing tumor also causes suppression at the high dose.

## NORMAL VALUES

Suppression on low-dose dexamethasone.

## COST

Low.

## ADDITIONAL TESTS TO ORDER

ACTH stimulation test, androstenedione, DHEA-S, metyrapone test, CT scan of adrenal glands, and endocrinology consult.

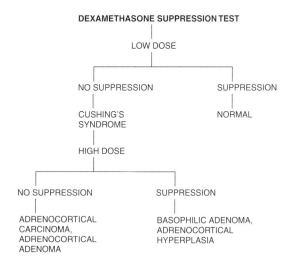

# DIGITAL SUBTRACTION ANGIOGRAPHY

## DEFINITION

This procedure uses a computer-based radiograph imaging method and venous catheterization. After placement of a catheter in the superior vena cava, a large bolus of contrast material is injected, and the aortic arch and its branches in the head, neck, and abdomen are visualized. Images are made and stored on video discs.

## POSITIVE

This study is positive in carotid stenosis, large cerebral aneurysms, carotid thrombosis, mesenteric thrombosis and insufficiency, renal artery stenosis, thoracic outlet syndrome, and pulmonary embolism. It may also be used to illuminate highly vascular tumors such as pheochromocytomas.

## NORMAL VALUES

No evidence of obstruction or malformations of the arteries visualized.

## COST

High.

## ADDITIONAL TESTS TO ORDER

Carotid duplex scan, MR angiography, four-vessel cerebral angiography, and conventional contrast angiography.

# DRUG SCREEN, SERUM OR URINE

## POSITIVE

This test is positive in patients who have overdosed or have become addicted to any of the many narcotics, tranquilizers, stimulants, antidepressants, and sedatives on the street or on the market. Most drug screens test for marijuana, ethanol, methanol, barbiturates, amphetamines, salicylates, PCP, acetaminophen, heroin and other narcotics, benzodiazepines, anticonvulsants, antihistamines, caffeine, theophylline, nicotine, phenothiazines, and the antidepressants.

## NORMAL VALUES

None detected.

## COST

Medium.

## ADDITIONAL TESTS TO ORDER

CBC, urinalysis, chemistry panel, serum osmolality, arterial blood gases, EEG, ECG, serial electrolytes, and consultation with a poison control center.

# DUODENAL ANALYSIS

## DEFINITION

In this procedure, a Miller–Abbott tube is passed into the duodenum, and samples of bile and pancreatic fluid are taken before and after the injection of cholecystokinin or secretin.

## POSITIVE

Patients suspected of having gallstones often show cholesterol and other crystals in the fluid. Patients with chronic pancreatitis have reduced or absent trypsin and other pancreatic enzymes in the fluid. The fluid may also show parasites such as *Giardia* or *Strongyloides.*

## NORMAL VALUES

Fluid contains normal amounts of pancreatic enzymes and no crystals or parasites.

## COST

Medium.

## ADDITIONAL TESTS TO ORDER

Stool for occult blood, fat, trypsin, and ova and parasites, cholecystography, gallbladder ultrasonography, transhepatic cholangiography, ERCP, pancreatic scan, pancreatic ultrasonography, CT scan of abdomen, and gastroenterology consult.

# *ECHINOCOCCUS* STAIN TEST

## POSITIVE

A positive test is suggestive of hydatid disease and is a clear indication for further testing. False-positive results do occur.

## NORMAL VALUES

Negative.

## COST

Low.

## ADDITIONAL TESTS TO ORDER

Sputum or urine smear, serologic tests, liver or bone biopsy, CT scan of abdomen, bone scan, and consultation with an infectious disease specialist.

# ECHOCARDIOGRAPHY

## POSITIVE

This test is positive in mitral stenosis and insufficiency, mitral valve prolapse, tricuspid stenosis and insufficiency, aortic stenosis, pericardial effusion, and congenital heart disease. It is also useful in diagnosing the myocardiopathies and *congestive heart failure* by determining the ejection fraction.

## NORMAL VALUES

Normal cardiac size and shape, normal movement of heart valves, normal movement and thickness of myocardium, and no effusion.

## COST

Medium.

## ADDITIONAL TESTS TO ORDER

ECG, chest radiograph (cardiac series), thallium scan, cardiac catheterization, angiocardiography, coronary angiography, exercise tolerance test, and cardiology consult.

# ECHOENCEPHALOGRAPHY

This study has largely been replaced by MRI (see Magnetic Resonance Imaging, Brain) and CT scans (see Computed Tomography, Brain) of the brain.

# ELECTROCARDIOGRAPHY

## ABNORMALITIES OF RATE AND RHYTHM (ALGORITHM A)

1. Rapid rate, regular rhythm, and normal QRS complexes suggest supraventricular tachycardia, sinus tachycardia, and atrial flutter with fixed AV conduction.
2. Rapid rate, regular rhythm, and wide QRS complexes suggest ventricular tachycardia or supraventricular tachycardia with bundle branch block.
3. Rapid rate, irregular rhythm and normal QRS complexes suggest auricular fibrillation or flutter with irregular AV conduction.
4. Rapid rate, irregular rhythm and wide QRS complexes suggest ventricular fibrillation.
5. Normal rate and irregular rhythm suggest VPCs, APCs, controlled auricular fibrillation, sinus arrhythmia, and AV dissociation with block.
6. Slow rate, regular rhythm, and normal QRS complexes suggest sinus bradycardia or AV nodal rhythm.
7. Slow rate, regular rhythm, and wide QRS complexes suggest complete AV block.
8. Slow rate and irregular rhythm may indicate second-degree heart block, AV dissociation with block, sick sinus syndrome, and APCs or VPCs.

## ABNORMALITIES OF THE P, QRS, ST, T, AND QT APPEARANCE AND INTERVALS (ALGORITHM B)

1. *P waves:* These may be notched in left atrial hypertrophy and peaked in right atrial hypertrophy and P-pulmonale. They are absent or inverted in conduction disturbances.
2. *PR interval:* This is prolonged in first-degree heart block and shortened in the WPW syndrome.
3. *QRS:* There are significant Q waves in myocardial infarction, deformed QRS in myocardial and bun-

dle branch block, low voltage in hypothyroidism, emphysema, beriberi heart disease, and myocardiopathy and high voltage in ventricular hypertrophy. The QRS interval is prolonged in bundle branch block and intraventricular conduction delay and appears to be prolonged in the WPW syndrome.

4. *ST interval:* This is elevated in myocardial infarction and acute pericarditis. It may be depressed by digitalis, other drugs, hypokalemia, myocardial ischemia or infarction, bundle branch block, or ventricular hypertrophy.

5. *T waves:* These waves are peaked in hyperkalemia and acute pericarditis. They are inverted in myocardial ischemia or infarct, ventricular hypertrophy, bundle branch block, drug use, hypokalemia, and chronic pericarditis.

6. *QT interval:* This is prolonged in hypokalemia, use of certain drugs, and hypocalcemia. It is shortened in hypercalcemia and digitalis toxicity.

## COST

Low.

## ADDITIONAL TESTS TO ORDER

CBC, sedimentation rate, chemistry panel, serial electrolytes, serial cardiac enzymes, echocardiography, Holter monitoring, thallium scan, Technetium-99m resting heart scan, chest radiograph, coronary angiography, His bundle electrocardiography, and cardiology consult.

# ECG (ALGORITHM A)

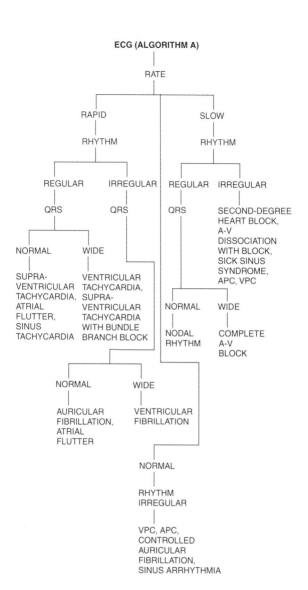

RATE

RAPID — RHYTHM
- REGULAR — QRS
  - NORMAL: SUPRA-VENTRICULAR TACHYCARDIA, ATRIAL FLUTTER, SINUS TACHYCARDIA
  - WIDE: VENTRICULAR TACHYCARDIA, SUPRA-VENTRICULAR TACHYCARDIA WITH BUNDLE BRANCH BLOCK
- IRREGULAR — QRS
  - NORMAL: AURICULAR FIBRILLATION, ATRIAL FLUTTER
  - WIDE: VENTRICULAR FIBRILLATION

SLOW — RHYTHM
- REGULAR — QRS
  - NORMAL: NODAL RHYTHM
  - WIDE: COMPLETE A-V BLOCK
- IRREGULAR: SECOND-DEGREE HEART BLOCK, A-V DISSOCIATION WITH BLOCK, SICK SINUS SYNDROME, APC, VPC

NORMAL — RHYTHM IRREGULAR: VPC, APC, CONTROLLED AURICULAR FIBRILLATION, SINUS ARRHYTHMIA

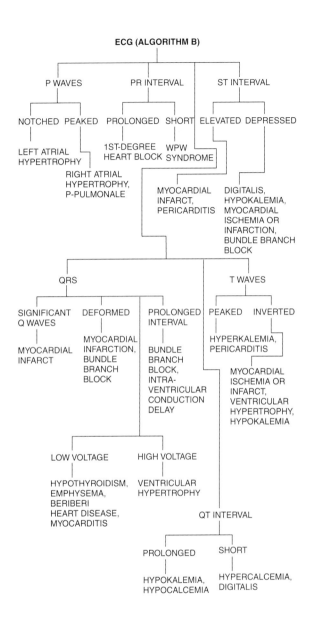

Algorithms A and B are merely a rapid refresher for the interpretation of electrocardiograms and require a basic knowledge of electrocardiography if they are to be applied to the patient.

# ELECTROENCEPHA-LOGRAPHY (EEG)

## ABNORMALITIES

1. Rapid rhythm (20–25 Hz), diffuse, suggests drug effects or toxicity such as barbiturates, phenothiazines, or benzodiazepines.
2. Rapid rhythm focal in location may be due to focal cortical epilepsy.
3. Slow rhythm ($\theta$, $\delta$), diffuse and constant suggests toxic or metabolic encephalopathy, encephalitis, severe concussion or degenerative disease such as Alzheimer's.
4. Slow rhythm, diffuse and paroxysmal, suggests centrancephalic epilepsy.
5. Slow rhythm, focal but constant, suggests neoplasm, abscess, hematoma, or infarction.
6. Slow rhythm, focal but paroxysmal, suggests focal cortical epilepsy.
7. Focal or diffuse spikes or spike waves are diagnostic of a seizure disorder.

The interpretation of an EEG is far more complicated than the foregoing list of abnormalities suggests, but it is hoped that this approach will provide the reader with a better understanding of this useful diagnostic test.

## NORMAL VALUES

### Awake

Adults: Background of symmetric $\alpha$ (8–13 Hz) or $\beta$ (14–17 Hz) activity, no focal or diffuse spike wave activity.
Children: As above, with increasing amounts of random diffuse slowing, depending on age.

## Sleep

Stage II sleep activity with 12–14 Hz spindles and parietal humps, symmetric. No focal or diffuse spike or wave activity.

## COST

Medium.

## ADDITIONAL TESTS TO ORDER

CBC, urinalysis, chemistry panel, sedimentation rate, CT scan, MRI, carotid duplex scans, cerebral angiography, and neurology or neurosurgical consult.

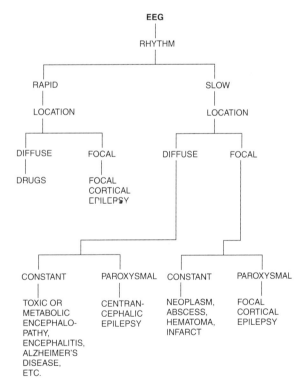

# ELECTROMYOGRAPHY

## POSITIVE

This test is positive in diseases of the anterior horn of the spinal cord (amyotrophic lateral sclerosis, poliomyelitis), nerve roots (herniated disc, radiculopathy), peripheral nerves (diabetic neuropathy), and muscle (muscular dystrophy, dermatomyositis). It is therefore indicated whenever disease is suspected in these portions of the nervous system. It also can be helpful in diagnosing myasthenia gravis.

## NORMAL VALUES

Muscles are electrically silent at rest, and on voluntary action, there is 15% or less polyphasic action potentials noted in each muscle tested.

## COST

Medium.

## ADDITIONAL TESTS TO ORDER

CBC, urinalysis, chemistry panel, sedimentation rate, heavy metal screen, glucose tolerance test, urine porphobilinogen, ANA, spinal fluid analysis, plain films of the spine and extremities, CT scan or MRI of the spine, myelography, nerve conduction velocity studies, muscle biopsy, and neurology consult.

# ENDOSCOPIC RETROGRADE CHOLANGIOPAN-CREATOGRAPHY (ERCP)

## POSITIVE

This test can diagnose the cause of obstructive jaundice by illuminating the biliary tree and direct examination of the ampulla of Vater. Consequently, common duct stones, carcinoma of the pancreas, carcinoma of the bile ducts, and ampulla of Vater can be ascertained. The test is also positive in chronic pancreatitis, pancreatic pseudocysts, biliary cirrhosis, and bile duct stricture.

## NORMAL VALUES

Normal appearance of the ampulla of Vater and biliary tree.

## COST

High.

## ADDITIONAL TESTS TO ORDER

Liver function tests, pancreatic function tests, intravenous cholangiography, transhepatic cholangiography, duodenal analysis, CT scan of the abdomen, exploratory laparotomy, GI consult, and surgical consult.

# EOSINOPHIL COUNT

## INCREASED

Eosinophils are increased in asthma, hay fever, parasitic disease, skin disorders, dermatomyositis and other collagen disease, hypersensitivity, pneumonitis, allergic bronchopulmonary aspergillosis, malignancies, myeloid metaplasia, fungal infections, and the use of certain drugs.

## NORMAL VALUES

Less than $450/mm^3$.

## COST

Low.

## ADDITIONAL TESTS TO ORDER

CBC, sedimentation rate, urinalysis, chemistry panel, stool for ova and parasites, blood smears for parasites, spirometry, nasal smears and sputum smears for eosinophils, skin biopsy, muscle biopsy, *Trichinella* skin test, and infectious disease consult.

# EPSTEIN–BARR ANTIBODY TEST

## POSITIVE VCA (VIRAL CAPSID)–IGM

The patient has an active infection (infectious mononucleosis or other Epstein–Barr infection).

## NEGATIVE VCA–IGM WITH POSITIVE VCA–IGG

The patient had infectious mononucleosis or another Epstein–Barr infection in the past, but has no active disease.

## NEGATIVE VCA–IGM AND NEGATIVE VCA–IGG

The patient has never been infected with Epstein–Barr virus and is susceptible.

## POSITIVE EA–D

The patient has possible nasopharyngeal carcinoma. Remember, a positive VCA or EBNA IgG titer does not diagnose chronic fatigue syndrome.

## NORMAL VALUES

VCA–IgM: negative.
VCA–IgG: negative.
EBNA–IgM: negative.
EBNA–IgG: negative.
EA–D: negative.

## COST

Low.

## ADDITIONAL TESTS TO ORDER

CBC, smear for atypical lymphocytes, sedimentation rate, heterophil antibody titer, chemistry panel, ASO titer, hematology consult, and infectious disease consult.

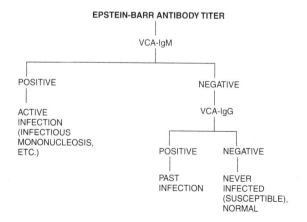

**EPSTEIN-BARR ANTIBODY TITER**

VCA-IgM

POSITIVE

NEGATIVE

ACTIVE INFECTION (INFECTIOUS MONONUCLEOSIS, ETC.)

VCA-IgG

POSITIVE

NEGATIVE

PAST INFECTION

NEVER INFECTED (SUSCEPTIBLE), NORMAL

# ERYTHROPOIETIN

## INCREASED

Ask the following questions:

1. Is the RBC increased? An *increase* of erythropoietin along with an *elevated RBC* suggests secondary polycythemia, hemangioblastoma, renal tumors, and pheochromocytomas. A *normal RBC* with an increased erythropoietin can be found in pheochromocytomas, hypernephromas, and polycystic disease, and elevated erythropoietin with a *decreased RBC* is found in aplastic anemia and iron-deficiency anemia.
2. Is the arterial oxygen decreased? This suggests secondary polycythemia caused by pulmonary disease.

## DECREASED

Ask the following questions:

1. Is the RBC increased or decreased? If it is increased, think of polycythemia vera. If it is decreased, think of chronic renal disease or simple chronic anemia from chronic inflammation.
2. What is the BUN? If the BUN is elevated, then chronic renal disease is most likely the cause.

## NORMAL VALUES

4–26 IU/L.

## COST

Low.

## ADDITIONAL TESTS TO ORDER

CBC, platelet count, chemistry panel, urinalysis, sedimentation rate, IVP, CT scan of brain and abdomen, spirometry, arterial oxygen saturation, and hematology consult.

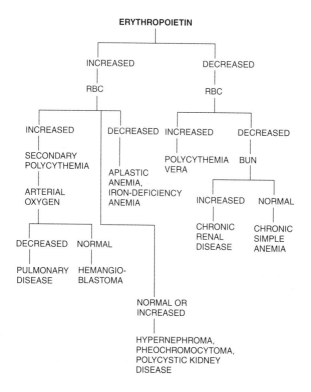

**ERYTHROPOIETIN**

INCREASED
RBC
- INCREASED — SECONDARY POLYCYTHEMIA — ARTERIAL OXYGEN
  - DECREASED — PULMONARY DISEASE
  - NORMAL — HEMANGIO-BLASTOMA
- DECREASED — APLASTIC ANEMIA, IRON-DEFICIENCY ANEMIA
- NORMAL OR INCREASED — HYPERNEPHROMA, PHEOCHROMOCYTOMA, POLYCYSTIC KIDNEY DISEASE

DECREASED
RBC
- INCREASED — POLYCYTHEMIA VERA
- DECREASED — BUN
  - INCREASED — CHRONIC RENAL DISEASE
  - NORMAL — CHRONIC SIMPLE ANEMIA

# ESOPHAGOGASTRO-DUODENOSCOPY (EGD)

## POSITIVE

This test is used to diagnose esophagitis, esophageal strictures and diverticula, esophageal carcinoma, Mallory–Weiss syndrome, hiatal hernia, gastritis, carcinoma of the stomach, lymphoma, benign tumors, gastric and duodenal ulcers, esophageal varices, stomal ulcers, and diverticula. It is indicated in the workup of hematemesis and melena. It is also diagnostic in Boerhaave's syndrome and hereditary telangiectasis. Biopsies are usually taken.

## NORMAL VALUES

Normal esophageal, gastric, and duodenal mucosa. No mass, strictures, or diverticula.

## COST

High.

## ADDITIONAL TESTS TO ORDER

CBC, chemistry panel, sedimentation rate, coagulation profile, stool for occult blood, gastric analysis, serum gastrin, upper GI series and esophagogram, esophageal manometry, CT scan, and gastroenterology consult.

# ESTRADIOL, BLOOD AND URINE

## INCREASED

When faced with an increased blood or urine estradiol, determine the FSH level. If the FSH level is increased, one should consider ectopic FSH, LH production, or precocious puberty. If the FSH is normal or decreased, one should consider ovarian tumors such as granulosa cell tumors or theca cell tumors and tumors of the adrenal cortex. The patient may also be taking estrogen-replacement therapy or contraceptives.

## DECREASED

When faced with a decreased estradiol level, one should determine the FSH level. If it is increased, one should consider menopause or Turner's syndrome. If it is decreased, one should consider the possibility of pituitary insufficiency or pituitary tumors.

## NORMAL VALUES

### Ovulating Female

Blood: 30–400 pg/mL.
Urine: 0–10 $\mu$g/24 hours.

### Menopause

Blood: 5–18 pg/mL.

## COST

Low.

## ADDITIONAL TESTS TO ORDER

Serum FSH and LH, plasma cortisol, free $T_4$, growth hormone, ACTH, CT scan of brain, CT scan of abdomen and pelvis, pelvic ultrasonography, endocrinology consult, and gynecology consult.

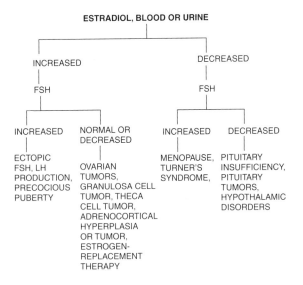

ESTRADIOL, BLOOD OR URINE

INCREASED
- FSH
  - INCREASED
    - ECTOPIC FSH, LH PRODUCTION, PRECOCIOUS PUBERTY
  - NORMAL OR DECREASED
    - OVARIAN TUMORS, GRANULOSA CELL TUMOR, THECA CELL TUMOR, ADRENOCORTICAL HYPERPLASIA OR TUMOR, ESTROGEN-REPLACEMENT THERAPY

DECREASED
- FSH
  - INCREASED
    - MENOPAUSE, TURNER'S SYNDROME,
  - DECREASED
    - PITUITARY INSUFFICIENCY, PITUITARY TUMORS, HYPOTHALAMIC DISORDERS

# ESTRIOL, BLOOD

## DECREASED

Decreasing levels of estriol during pregnancy signify fetal distress (rapid fall) and placental insufficiency (gradual fall).

## NORMAL VALUES

Consult with your laboratory.

## COST

Low.

## ADDITIONAL TESTS TO ORDER

Pelvic ultrasonography and obstetric consult.

# ESTROGEN AND PROGESTERONE RECEPTOR PROTEINS

## POSITIVE

Patients with breast cancer who test positive for both these receptor proteins have a good chance of responding to hormonal therapy, whereas those who test negative for both receptor proteins have only a minimal chance of response to hormonal therapy, and their prognosis is not as good. Patients who are estrogen receptor-positive but progesterone receptor-negative have a 40–50% chance of responding, whereas patients who are estrogen receptor-negative but progesterone receptor-positive have an even smaller chance of responding to hormonal therapy.

## NORMAL VALUES

Not applicable.

## COST

Low to medium.

## ADDITIONAL TESTS TO ORDER

Mammography, breast biopsy, lymph node biopsy, bone scans, CT scans, and oncology consult.

# EVOKED POTENTIAL STUDIES

1. *Brainstem-evoked potential:* This test is used to diagnose *multiple sclerosis,* acoustic neuromas, brainstem infarction, and other brainstem disorders.
2. *Visual-evoked potentials:* This test is used to diagnose *multiple sclerosis,* optic neuritis, and other prechiasmal and postchiasmal defects.
3. *Somatosensory-evoked potentials:* This test is also used primarily to diagnose *multiple sclerosis*, but it can help to diagnose brachial plexus neuropathy and nerve root and spinal cord lesions of many causes.
4. *Dermatomal somatosensory-evoked potentials (DSEP):* This test is primarily used to diagnose *radiculopathy* caused by herniated discs or other diseases of the spine.

## NORMAL VALUES

These vary with the laboratory performing the tests.

## COST

Medium.

## ADDITIONAL TESTS TO ORDER

CBC, urinalysis, chemistry panel, sedimentation rate, VDRL, ANA, spinal fluid analysis, plain films of the spine, MRI of the brain and spinal cord, myelography, nerve conduction velocity studies, EMG, audiogram, visual field examination, neurology consult, ophthalmology consult, and otology consult.

# EXERCISE TOLERANCE TESTING

## POSITIVE

This test is used primarily to diagnose coronary insufficiency or ischemic heart disease. The most common abnormality is ST depression of 80 milliseconds or longer. In addition, the test may induce a fall in blood pressure, cardiac arrhythmias, angina, or other symptoms and signs that may signify ischemic heart disease, myocardial disease, or congestive heart failure.

## NORMAL VALUES

No ST depression or deviation, no arrhythmia, and no abnormal symptoms or signs after achieving a predetermined heart rate based on age and sex.

## COST

Medium.

## ADDITIONAL TESTS TO ORDER

Resting ECG, chest radiograph, CBC, chemistry panel, echocardiography, thallium stress scan, Holter monitoring, coronary angiography, gated equilibrium heart scan, and cardiology consult.

# FEBRILE AGGLUTININS

## INCREASED

1. *Salmonella antibodies:* These are increased in typhoid fever, paratyphoid infections, and *Salmonella* A, B, C, D and E infections. O antigens are increased in 90–95% of patients by the end of the first 4 weeks and disappear within 6 to 12 months. H antigens are elevated later but persist for many years, so they are not specific for acute infections. A *rising titer* is much more significant than a single positive test. False-positive results occur in Enterobacteriaceae infections and any febrile illness.

2. *Proteus antibodies:* These are increased in rickettsial infection. High or rising titers of *Proteus* OX-K are present in scrub typhus, whereas high or rising titers of OX-19 are present in epidemic typhus and Rocky Mountain spotted fever. Numerous borderline false-positive results of these tests are seen. Moreover, two-thirds of patients with Rocky Mountain fever have false-negative results. That is why more specific serologic tests have gradually replaced these tests.

3. *Brucellosis antibodies:* These are elevated in *Brucella* infections. Once again, a rising titer is more significant. Many false-positive results are seen because many other disorders may stimulate antibodies that react with this antigen.

## NORMAL VALUES

Titers of 1:40 or less that do not rise.

## COST

Low.

## ADDITIONAL TESTS TO ORDER

CBC, urinalysis, chemistry panel, sedimentation rate, CRP, stool cultures, urine cultures, blood cultures, specific serologic tests for *Salmonella, Brucella,* and rickettsial diseases, and consultation with an infectious disease specialist.

# FERN TEST

## POSITIVE

A few drops of fluid placed on a slide and allowed
to dry produce a fern pattern that indicates *amniotic
fluid*. This is helpful in distinguishing amniotic fluid
from urine in pregnant women at term who have
ruptured their amniotic sac. Remember, blood in the
specimen inhibits the fern pattern.

## NORMAL VALUES

Amniotic fluid-positive; urine or other fluid-negative.

## COST

Low.

## ADDITIONAL TESTS TO ORDER

Pelvic ultrasonography, catheterization for residual
urine, and gynecology consult.

# FERRITIN

## DECREASED

Ferritin is decreased in iron-deficiency anemia and is the first biochemical change to occur in this disorder. No other condition is associated with a low serum ferritin.

## INCREASED

Ask the following questions:

1. What is the serum iron? If both the serum ferritin and iron are increased, hemochromatosis or hemosiderosis is the likely diagnosis.
2. What do the liver function tests show? If these are abnormal, consider acute hepatitis, chronic liver disease, and alcoholism.

If the ferritin is elevated but the foregoing tests are normal, one should consider malignant diseases, chronic inflammatory disease, hypothyroidism, and type II diabetes.

## NORMAL VALUES

Males: 20–300 ng/mL.
Females: 20–120 ng/mL.

## COST

Medium.

## ADDITIONAL TESTS TO ORDER

CBC, sedimentation rate, urinalysis, chemistry panel, CRP, RA titer, ANA, CT scan of abdomen and pelvis, chest radiograph, CEA, bone marrow examination, and hematology consult.

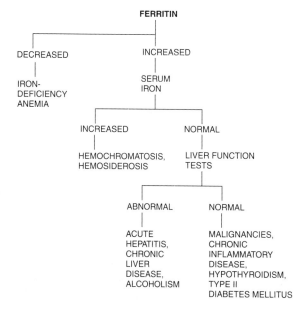

# FERROKINETIC STUDIES

## DEFINITION

Radioactive iron-59 is injected IV and blood samples are drawn at predetermined intervals for 3 hours, and additional samples are drawn three times a week for 3 weeks. This procedure allows one to determine the plasma clearance of radioactive iron. In addition, the uptake of radioactive iron is determined over various areas of the body during the procedure. This allows one to determine bone marrow activity.

## INCREASED UPTAKE

This is found in polycythemia vera, hemolytic anemia, iron-deficiency anemia, and anemia of blood loss.

## DECREASED UPTAKE

This is found in aplastic anemia, pernicious anemia, and myelofibrosis.

## DECREASED PLASMA CLEARANCE RATE

This is found in aplastic anemia, hemochromatosis, and myelofibrosis.

## INCREASED PLASMA CLEARANCE RATE

This is found in hemolytic anemia, iron-deficiency anemia, and polycythemia vera.

## NORMAL VALUES

### Uptake

85% of radioactive iron appears in the red cells within 10 days.

### Clearance

Radioactive iron disappears from the plasma within 1 to 2 hours.

## COST

Medium.

## ADDITIONAL TESTS TO ORDER

CBC, urinalysis, chemistry panel, sedimentation rate, serum iron and iron-binding capacity, serum $B_{12}$ and folic acid, serum haptoglobin, chromium tagged red cell survival time, bone marrow scan, bone marrow biopsy, and hematology consult.

# FETAL HEMOGLOBIN IN MATERNAL BLOOD

## INCREASED

An increase of hemoglobin F cells in maternal blood indicates anemia in the fetus and fetal–maternal hemorrhage. It also indicates that a Rh-negative or Du-negative mother has become immunized against fetal red cells of the Rho-positive type.

## NORMAL VALUES

Negative.

## COST

Low.

## ADDITIONAL TESTS TO ORDER

Direct and indirect Coombs' tests on mother and fetus, type and cross match of blood, fetal hemoglobin stain, amniocentesis, hemoglobin electrophoresis, chemistry panel of mother and fetus, pediatric consult, and hematology consult.

# FIBRIN SPLIT PRODUCTS

## INCREASED

Ask the following questions:

1. Is the WBC increased? This suggests leukemia or infection.
2. Has the patient had recent surgery or delivery? This suggests disseminated intravascular coagulation from a surgical or obstetric complication.
3. Does the patient have a history of drug use? Drugs may lead to prolonged coma and disseminated intravascular coagulation.
4. Does the patient have a known thrombotic event? Fibrin split products may be increased in venous thrombosis, pulmonary embolism, and snake bite.

If the answers to all these questions is no, one should look for burns, heat stroke, hypoxia and thrombotic thrombocytopenic purpura, and disseminated intravascular coagulation.

## NORMAL VALUES

0–4 $\mu$g/mL.

## COST

Low.

## ADDITIONAL TESTS TO ORDER

CBC, platelet count, blood smear, blood cultures, sedimentation rate, chemistry panel, PTT, prothrombin time, thrombin time, fibrinogen and D-dimer test, and hematology consult.

**FIBRIN SPLIT PRODUCTS**

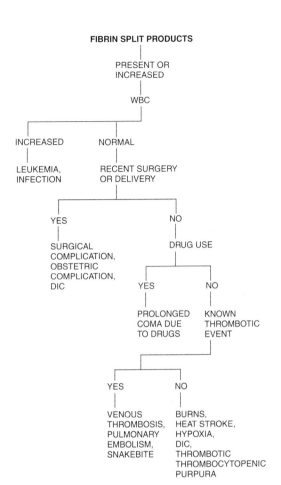

PRESENT OR
INCREASED

WBC

INCREASED — NORMAL

LEUKEMIA,
INFECTION

RECENT SURGERY
OR DELIVERY

YES — NO

SURGICAL
COMPLICATION,
OBSTETRIC
COMPLICATION,
DIC

DRUG USE

YES — NO

PROLONGED
COMA DUE
TO DRUGS

KNOWN
THROMBOTIC
EVENT

YES — NO

VENOUS
THROMBOSIS,
PULMONARY
EMBOLISM,
SNAKEBITE

BURNS,
HEAT STROKE,
HYPOXIA,
DIC,
THROMBOTIC
THROMBOCYTOPENIC
PURPURA

# FIBRINOGEN

## DECREASED

Fibrinogen is decreased in afibrinogenemia, dysfibrinogenemia, liver disease, disseminated intravascular coagulation, and hemorrhage.

## INCREASED

Increases in fibrinogen occur in pregnancy, oral contraceptive therapy, malignancy, and tissue damage and acute inflammation, but this test is rarely ordered to diagnose these conditions.

## NORMAL VALUES

200–400 mg/dL.

## COST

Low.

## ADDITIONAL TESTS TO ORDER

CBC, platelet count, coagulation profile, bleeding time, thrombin time, fibrin split products, liver function tests, sedimentation rate, chemistry panel, and hematology consult.

# FIBRINOLYSIS/ EUGLOBULIN LYSIS TIME

## INCREASED

Ask the following questions:

1. Is the pregnancy test positive? If so, look for an obstetric complication.
2. Has the patient had recent surgery? If so, look for a transfusion reaction or problems from extracorporeal circulation or from lung or pancreatic surgery.
3. Is the platelet count decreased? If so, look for thrombocytopenic purpura and leukemia.

## NORMAL VALUES

No lysis of clot in 3 hours.

## COST

Low.

## ADDITIONAL TESTS TO ORDER

CBC, platelet count, pregnancy test, coagulation profile, fibrin split products, fibrinogen, bone marrow examination, Coombs' test, ANA, liver–spleen scan, blood cultures, and hematology consult.

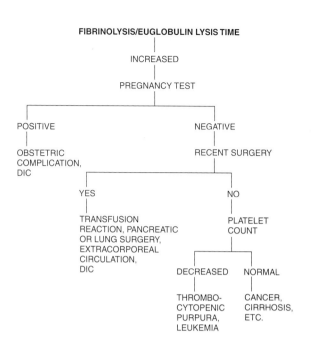

**FIBRINOLYSIS/EUGLOBULIN LYSIS TIME**

INCREASED

PREGNANCY TEST

POSITIVE

OBSTETRIC
COMPLICATION,
DIC

NEGATIVE

RECENT SURGERY

YES

TRANSFUSION
REACTION, PANCREATIC
OR LUNG SURGERY,
EXTRACORPOREAL
CIRCULATION,
DIC

NO

PLATELET
COUNT

DECREASED

THROMBO-
CYTOPENIC
PURPURA,
LEUKEMIA

NORMAL

CANCER,
CIRRHOSIS,
ETC.

# FISHBERG
# CONCENTRATION TEST

## ABNORMAL

The ability to concentrate the urine is diminished or absent in glomerulonephritis, chronic pyelonephritis, and other chronic renal diseases. This is the principal reason for ordering this test. Concentration powers are also diminished or lost in diabetes insipidus, renal diabetes insipidus, Fanconi's syndrome, hypercalcemia, and hypokalemia.

## NORMAL VALUES

Specific gravity of greater than 1.020 after fluid restriction.

## COST

Low.

## ADDITIONAL TESTS TO ORDER

CBC, urinalysis, Addis count, chemistry panel, serum osmolality, creatinine clearance, Hickey–Hare test, urine culture, ANA, ASO titer, CRP, serum complement, plasma ADH level, KUB, IVP, renal biopsy, ultrasonography, CT scan of abdomen and pelvis, and nephrology consult.

# FLUORESCEIN ANGIOGRAPHY

## POSITIVE

This test is positive in diabetic retinopathy, aneurysms, hemorrhagic macular degeneration, retinal artery occlusion, and carotid stenosis or thrombosis. A comparison of the time it takes for the fluorescein to appear in each eye helps to diagnose the last two disorders.

## NORMAL VALUES

No abnormalities of the retina, retinal vessels, and choroid are seen on color photographs taken of the fundus as the fluorescein passed through. No significant difference in the time of appearance of fluorescein in each eye.

## COST

Low to medium.

## ADDITIONAL TESTS TO ORDER

Carotid duplex scans, oculoplethysmography, carotid angiography, electroretinography, and ophthalmology consult.

# FLUORESCENT TREPONEMAL ANTIBODY ABSORPTION TEST (FTA–ABS)

## POSITIVE

A positive result is highly specific for syphilis. However, false-positive results occur in lupus erythematosus, macroglobulinemia, Lyme disease, leptospirosis, and relapsing fever. False-negative results occur, and HIV infections may delay the appearance of a positive test.

## NORMAL VALUES

Negative.

## COST

Low.

## ADDITIONAL TESTS TO ORDER

CBC, urinalysis, VDRL, sedimentation rate, chemistry panel, CSF analysis, MHA–TP test, TPI test, darkfield examination, and consultation with an infectious disease specialist.

# FOLIC ACID

## DECREASED

Ask the following questions:

1. Does the patient have a history of alcohol or drug use? Anticonvulsant drugs, chemotherapy, trimethoprim, and oral contraceptives interfere with folic acid metabolism.
2. What are the results of a D-xylose absorption test? Malabsorption syndrome is a frequent cause of folic acid deficiency.
3. What is the serum haptoglobin? A decreased serum haptoglobin suggests hemolytic anemia. If the foregoing tests are negative, the patient may have malnutrition, may be pregnant, may have a malignant diesease, or may have received long-term dialysis.

## NORMAL VALUES

5.5–25 $\mu$g/mL.

## COST

Medium.

## ADDITIONAL TESTS TO ORDER

CBC, urinalysis, chemistry panel, serum carotene, D-xylose absorption test, serum haptoglobins, mucosal biopsy, small bowel series, CT scan of abdomen, gastroenterology consult, and therapeutic trial.

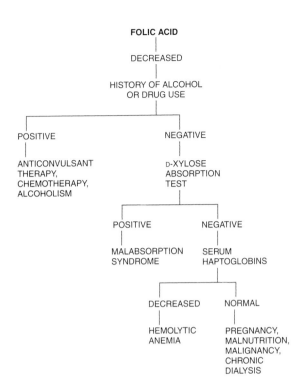

**FOLIC ACID**

DECREASED

HISTORY OF ALCOHOL
OR DRUG USE

POSITIVE

ANTICONVULSANT
THERAPY,
CHEMOTHERAPY,
ALCOHOLISM

NEGATIVE

D-XYLOSE
ABSORPTION
TEST

POSITIVE

MALABSORPTION
SYNDROME

NEGATIVE

SERUM
HAPTOGLOBINS

DECREASED

HEMOLYTIC
ANEMIA

NORMAL

PREGNANCY,
MALNUTRITION,
MALIGNANCY,
CHRONIC
DIALYSIS

# FOLLICLE-STIMULATING HORMONE (FSH), BLOOD AND URINE

## FEMALES

### Increased

FSH is increased in precocious puberty, Turner's syndrome, and menopause. To differentiate these conditions further, serum estradiol should be determined. Serum estradiol is increased in precocious puberty and decreased in Turner's syndrome and menopause.

### Decreased

FSH is decreased in hormone therapy, neoplasms of the ovary and adrenal gland, pituitary insufficiency, anorexia nervosa, and hypothalamic disorders. To differentiate these conditions further, a serum estradiol determination is indicated. Serum estradiol is increased in hormone therapy and neoplasms of the ovary and occasionally those of the adrenal glands. Serum estradiol is decreased in pituitary insufficiency, anorexia nervosa, and hypothalamic disorders.

## MALES

### Increased

FSH is increased in precocious puberty, in Klinefelter's syndrome, after orchiectomy (bilateral), and during the male climacteric. To separate these conditions, one should order a serum testosterone determination. Testosterone is increased in precocious puberty, whereas it is decreased in Klinefelter's syndrome, orchiectomy, and the male climacteric.

## Decreased

A decreased FSH is found in patients receiving hormone therapy, in pituitary insufficiency, and in hypothalamic disorders. To differentiate these conditions further, one should order a serum testosterone. Testosterone is increased in hormone therapy and is decreased in pituitary insufficiency and hypothalamic disorders.

## NORMAL VALUES

Serum, male: 1–10 mIU/mL.
Serum, female, ovulating: 2–22 mIU/mL (varies w/ cycle).
Serum, female, menopause: 20–138 mIU/mL.

## COST

Low.

## ADDITIONAL TESTS TO ORDER

Pregnancy test, serum and urine LH, plasma cortisol, serum estradiol and testosterone, vaginal smear, sperm count, pelvic ultrasound, gonadal ultrasound, laparoscopy, skull radiograph, CT scan of brain, CT scan of abdomen and pelvis, gynecology consult, and urology consult.

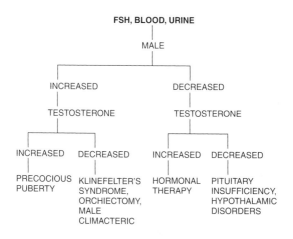

FSH, BLOOD, URINE
|
MALE

INCREASED
TESTOSTERONE

INCREASED — PRECOCIOUS PUBERTY

DECREASED — KLINEFELTER'S SYNDROME, ORCHIECTOMY, MALE CLIMACTERIC

DECREASED
TESTOSTERONE

INCREASED — HORMONAL THERAPY

DECREASED — PITUITARY INSUFFICIENCY, HYPOTHALAMIC DISORDERS

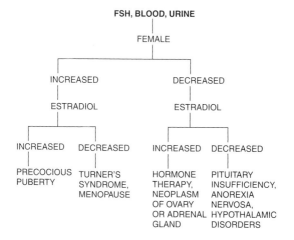

FSH, BLOOD, URINE
|
FEMALE

INCREASED
ESTRADIOL

INCREASED — PRECOCIOUS PUBERTY

DECREASED — TURNER'S SYNDROME, MENOPAUSE

DECREASED
ESTRADIOL

INCREASED — HORMONE THERAPY, NEOPLASM OF OVARY OR ADRENAL GLAND

DECREASED — PITUITARY INSUFFICIENCY, ANOREXIA NERVOSA, HYPOTHALAMIC DISORDERS

# FREE THYROXINE (T$_4$)

## INCREASED

The free T$_4$ is increased in subacute thyroiditis, Graves' disease, toxic nodular goiter, and iatrogenic hyperthyroidism. To differentiate these conditions further, a sedimentation rate is indicated. If this rate is *increased*, the patient probably has subacute thyroiditis. If this is normal, the patient has one of the other disorders in this group. An RAI uptake and scan should be performed. If the uptake is *increased*, the patient has Graves' disease or toxic nodular goiter. If it is *decreased,* the patient may have iatrogenic hyperthyroidism.

## DECREASED

A decreased free T$_4$ is usually due to myxedema, but it may also be caused by pituitary insufficiency, T$_3$ thyrotoxicosis, and tertiary hypothyroidism. To differentiate myxedema from the other members of the group, one should perform a TSH-sensitive assay. If this is increased, the patient has myxedema. Next, a TRF-stimulation test is indicated. If no response occurs, the patient has pituitary insufficiency. If a response is seen, the patient probably has tertiary hypothyroidism or T$_3$ thyrotoxicosis.

## NORMAL VALUES

1–2.3 ng/dL.

## COST

Low.

## ADDITIONAL TESTS TO ORDER

CBC, urinalysis, chemistry panel, sedimentation rate, free $T_3$, needle biopsy of thyroid, thyroid ultrasonography, CT scan of brain and thyroid, therapeutic trial, exploratory surgery, and endocrinology consult.

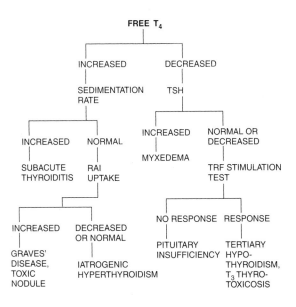

# FREE THYROXINE
# INDEX (FTI)

This test is being gradually replaced by the free $T_4$. However, for those clinicians who are in an area where the free $T_4$ is not available, it is probably the next best thing. The FTI excludes many false-positive results that occur because of a high or low TBG (see page 561). FTI can be calculated by the following formula:

$$FTI = T_4 \times T_3 \text{ uptake.}$$

## INCREASED

Hyperthyroidism, subacute thyroiditis.

## DECREASED

Primary hypothyroidism and pituitary insufficiency.

## COST

Low.

## ADDITIONAL TESTS TO ORDER

See page 269.

# FREE TRIIODOTHYRONINE (T$_3$)

## INCREASED

This is increased in Graves' disease and T$_3$ thyrotoxicosis. To differentiate these two conditions, one should obtain a free T$_4$ determination. If the free T$_4$ is *increased* also, the patient has *Graves' disease.* If it is normal or *decreased*, the patient may have T$_3$ *thyrotoxicosis.*

## DECREASED

The free T$_3$ is decreased in hypothyroidism.

## NORMAL VALUES

250–400 pg/dL.

## COST

Low.

## ADDITIONAL TESTS TO ORDER

Sedimentation rate, RAI uptake and scan, TSH-sensitive assay, ultrasonography of the thyroid, CT scan of thyroid, endocrinology consult, and exploratory surgery.

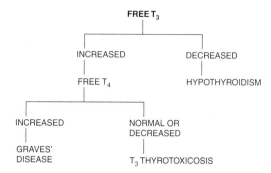

# FREI TEST

## POSITIVE

A positive test indicates present or past infection with lymphogranuloma venereum. False-positive reactions occur in people who are allergic to eggs or chicken.

## NORMAL VALUES

Negative.

## COST

Low.

## ADDITIONAL TESTS TO ORDER

Viral isolation from lymph nodes, rectum, urethra, or cervix, serologic tests, and consultation with a clinical pathologist or venereal disease specialist.

# FRUCTOSAMINE ASSAY

## INCREASED

Fructosamine is increased in diabetics with poor control of their blood sugar. As the diabetic's control of the blood sugar improves, the fructosamine returns to normal or near normal.

## NORMAL VALUES

205−285 $\mu$mol/L.

## COST

Low.

## ADDITIONAL TESTS TO ORDER

Chemistry panel, glucose tolerance tests, glycosylated hemoglobin, blood sugars twice daily, plasma acetone, arterial blood gases, insulin antibodies, and consultation with an endocrinologist.

# GALACTOSE-1-PHOSPHATE URIDYL TRANSFERASE

## DECREASED

A decrease of this enzyme occurs in galactosemia.

## NORMAL VALUES

19–30 U/g hemoglobin.

## COST

Medium.

## ADDITIONAL TESTS TO ORDER

Liver function tests, blood galactose levels, and pediatric consult.

# GALLBLADDER OR HEPATOIMINODIACETIC ACID (HIDA) SCAN

## POSITIVE

This scan is positive in acute and chronic cholecystitis, unusual biliary communications, and obstructive jaundice. If the patient has acute cholecystitis, the gallbladder will not fill.

## NORMAL VALUES

Good filling of the gallbladder and bile ducts and normal size and shape.

## COST

High.

## ADDITIONAL TESTS TO ORDER

Liver function tests, CBC, amylase and lipase, ERCP, ultrasonography of the gallbladder, transhepatic cholangiography, and gastroenterology or surgical consult.

# GALLBLADDER ULTRASONOGRAPHY

## POSITIVE

This test is positive in gallstones, gallbladder enlargement, cholecystitis, carcinoma, obstruction of the bile ducts, and common duct stones. It is especially useful in diagnosing gallstones in patients with obstructive jaundice. It can be used when oral cholecystography is contraindicated.

## NORMAL VALUES

Normal size, shape, and position of the gallbladder. No stones or other opacities.

## COST

Medium.

## ADDITIONAL TESTS TO ORDER

CBC, urinalysis, chemistry panel, oral cholecystography, intravenous cholangiography, HIDA scan, duodenal analysis, ERCP, percutaneous transhepatic cholangiography, exploratory laparotomy, surgical consult, and gastroenterology consult.

# GALLIUM SCAN

## POSITIVE

This scan is positive in abscesses, neoplasms, lymphomas, inflammation of body cavities (e.g., peritonitis), neoplasms and inflammation of the liver, bone, breast, or brain, and tuberculosis. It is especially useful in detecting abscesses anywhere in the body, particularly the abdomen. Remember, up to 40% of results may be false-negative.

## NORMAL VALUES

No focal increased uptake.

## COST

Medium to high.

## ADDITIONAL TESTS TO ORDER

CBC, sedimentation rate, CRP, urinalysis, chemistry panel, blood and urine cultures, CT scans, bone scan, Indium-III imaging, and consultation with an infectious disease expert or oncologist.

# GASTRIN

## INCREASED

Serum gastrin is increased in Zollinger–Ellison syndrome (marked increase), gastric and duodenal ulcers, pernicious anemia, atrophic gastritis, and gastric carcinoma. To separate these conditions into two groups, one should order a gastric analysis. Hydrochloric acid is normal or increased in Zollinger–Ellison syndrome, gastric ulcers, and duodenal ulcers, but it is decreased or absent in pernicious anemia, atrophic gastritis, and gastric carcinoma. The low serum vitamin $B_{12}$ usually separates pernicious anemia from the other two disorders. If not, a Schilling test can be ordered.

## NORMAL VALUES

90–280 pg/mL.

## COST

Low.

## ADDITIONAL TESTS TO ORDER

CBC, chemistry panel, serum $B_{12}$ and folic acid, stool for occult blood, upper GI series, gastroscopy, and gastroenterology consult.

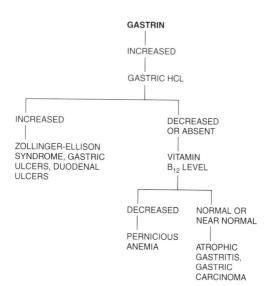

# GASTROINTESTINAL BLEEDING SCAN

## DEFINITION

Chromium-tagged red cells or labeled sulfur colloid are injected intravenously, and the GI tract is scanned for radioactivity.

## POSITIVE

Indicates bleeding in the upper or lower GI tract. Both the site and intensity can be determined so proper surgical intervention can be performed.

## NORMAL VALUES

No radioactive uptake in the GI tract.

## COST

High.

## ADDITIONAL TESTS TO ORDER

CBC, chemistry panel, gastric analysis, stool for occult blood, endoscopy, mesenteric angiography, string test, CT scan of abdomen, gastroenterology consult, and surgical consult.

# GLIADIN ANTIBODY

## INCREASED

These antibodies are increased in celiac disease, and therefore this test is a useful screening test for celiac disease in children. False-positive results occur in dermatitis herpetiformis.

## NORMAL VALUES

None detected.

## COST

Low.

## ADDITIONAL TESTS TO ORDER

CBC, urine, stool analysis, mucosal biopsy, D-xylose absorption, and gastroenterology consult.

# GLUCAGON

## INCREASED

Ask the following questions:

1. Is the blood sugar increased? This suggests acute pancreatitis, diabetic acidosis, pheochromocytoma, and glucagonoma.
2. Is the blood sugar normal or decreased? This suggests uremia, insulinoma, and infectious disease.
3. What is the serum amylase? An elevated serum amylase points to acute pancreatitis.
4. What are the catecholamines in blood or urine? If these are elevated, consider a pheochromocytoma.
5. What is the BUN? If the BUN is elevated, consider uremia as the possible cause.

## DECREASED

A decreased glucagon is found in chronic pancreatitis, in pancreatic carcinoma, and after pancreatectomy.

## NORMAL VALUES

50–200 pg/mL.

## COST

Low to medium.

## ADDITIONAL TESTS TO ORDER

CBC, urinalysis, chemistry panel, serum amylase and lipase, arterial blood gases, plasma or urine catecholamines, C-peptide, quantitative stool fat, and endocrinology consult.

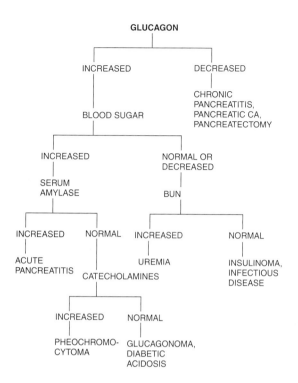

**GLUCAGON**

INCREASED

DECREASED
CHRONIC
PANCREATITIS,
PANCREATIC CA,
PANCREATECTOMY

BLOOD SUGAR

INCREASED
SERUM
AMYLASE

NORMAL OR
DECREASED
BUN

INCREASED
ACUTE
PANCREATITIS

NORMAL
CATECHOLAMINES

INCREASED
UREMIA

NORMAL
INSULINOMA,
INFECTIOUS
DISEASE

INCREASED
PHEOCHROMO-
CYTOMA

NORMAL
GLUCAGONOMA,
DIABETIC
ACIDOSIS

# GLUCOSE, BLOOD

## INCREASED

Ask the following questions:

1. Does the patient have acetone in the plasma or urine? This finding indicates diabetic acidosis.
2. What is the free $T_4$? If the free $T_4$ is increased, consider hyperthyroidism as the cause of the hyperglycemia.
3. What is the plasma cortisol? An increased plasma cortisol suggests Cushing's syndrome.
4. Are plasma or urine catecholamines increased? This finding suggests a pheochromocytoma. If none of the foregoing tests are abnormal, look for diabetes mellitus, glucagonoma, or acromegaly.

## DECREASED

Ask the following questions:

1. Is the patient taking oral hypoglycemic agents or insulin? If so, the dosage may be too high.
2. What is the D-xylose absorption? If this is abnormal, consider malabsorption syndrome.
3. What are the plasma cortisol levels? If this is decreased, consider Addison's disease or the various conditions associated with hypopituitarism.

If the foregoing questions fail to yield positive results, the patient may have an insulinoma, hypothyroidism, cirrhosis, or glycogen storage disease.

## NORMAL VALUES

70–100 mg/dL.

## COST

Low.

## ADDITIONAL TESTS TO ORDER

CBC, urinalysis, chemistry panel, glucose tolerance test, 72-hour fasting, C-peptide, plasma insulin, glycosylated hemoglobin, plasma cortisol, growth hormone, free $T_4$, TSH, plasma or urine catecholamines or VMA, liver biopsy, CT scan of abdomen, and endocrinology consult.

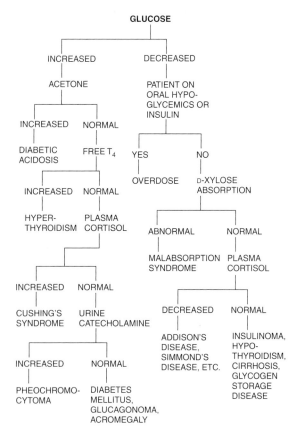

# GLUCOSE, CEREBROSPINAL FLUID

## INCREASED

Glucose is increased in the CSF in diabetes mellitus and after intravenous administration of glucose 5% and water.

## DECREASED

Glucose is decreased in the CSF in bacterial and fungal infections, leukemia, and lymphomas. It is also decreased in systemic disorders that cause hypoglycemia. To differentiate these conditions, one should obtain a smear and culture of CSF. These are positive in tuberculosis, bacterial meningitis and abscess, and fungal infections.

## NORMAL VALUES

45–85 mg/dL.

## COST

Low.

## ADDITIONAL TESTS TO ORDER

CBC, chemistry panel, sedimentation rate, lumbar puncture and CSF analysis, CT scan or MRI, spinal fluid smear and cultures, routine, AFB and fungal, neurology consult, blood cultures, and cultures of other body fluids and compartments.

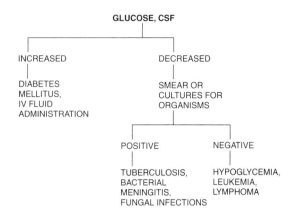

# GLUCOSE, URINE

## POSITIVE

Ask the following questions:

1. Is the blood sugar increased? If so, then the patient probably has diabetes mellitus or one of the other conditions associated with hyperglycemia (see page 285).
2. Does the patient have increased amino acids in the urine? If so, look for Fanconi's syndrome or associated disorders.
3. If one sees no hyperglycemia and no aminoaciduria, the patient may have a low renal threshold or other reducing substances or sugars (e.g., fructose) in the urine.

## NORMAL VALUES

Negative.

## COST

Low.

## ADDITIONAL TESTS TO ORDER

CBC, platelet, chemistry panel, thyroid profile, plasma cortisol, urine amino acids, urinalysis, plasma growth hormone, plasma acetone, and endocrinology consult.

**GLUCOSE, URINE**

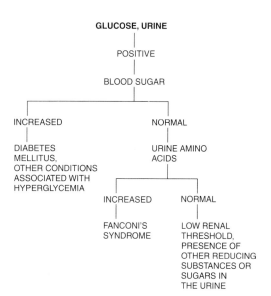

# GLUCOSE TOLERANCE TEST

## INCREASED GLUCOSE

Ask the following questions:

1. What is the plasma growth hormone? If growth hormone is increased, look for acromegaly or gigantism.
2. What is the plasma cortisol? If this is increased, consider Cushing's syndrome.
3. What is the free $T_4$? An increased free $T_4$ indicates hyperthyroidism.

If none of the foregoing are abnormal, one should consider starvation, pancreatic disease, pheochromocytoma, and glucagonoma.

## DECREASED GLUCOSE

Ask the following questions:

1. What is the C-peptide? An increased C-peptide suggests insulinoma.
2. What is the plasma cortisol? A decreased plasma cortisol suggests Addison's disease or pituitary insufficiency.
3. What is the growth hormone? A decreased growth hormone suggests pituitary insufficiency.

If the foregoing tests are normal, one should consider functional hypoglycemia, steatorrhea, and hypothyroidism.

## NORMAL VALUES

### Two-Hour Postprandial

$< 140$ mg/dL.

## Five-Hour Glucose Tolerance

$\frac{1}{2}$ hour, 1 hour: $< 200$ mg/dL.
2 hour: $< 140$ mg/dL.
3 hour: $< 125$ mg/dL.
4 hour: normal.
5 hour: normal.

## COST

Low.

## ADDITIONAL TESTS TO ORDER

CBC, urinalysis, chemistry panel, free $T_4$, plasma cortisol, growth hormone, C-peptide, liver function tests, D-xylose absorption, CT scan of brain, pituitary gland, and abdomen, and endocrinology consult.

**GLUCOSE TOLERANCE TEST**

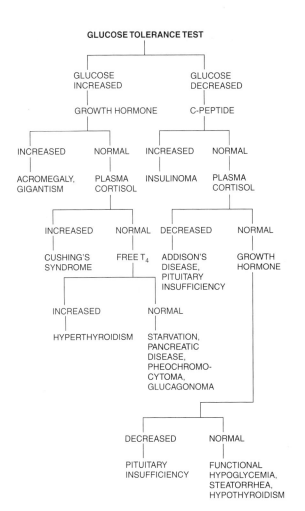

# GLUCOSE-6-PHOSPHATE DEHYDROGENASE (G6PD)

## INCREASED

G6PD is increased in pernicious anemia, Werlhof's disease, hepatic coma, hyperthyroidism, myocardial infarction, chronic blood loss, and other megaloblastic anemias.

## DECREASED

G6PD is decreased in hemolytic anemia resulting from G6PD deficiency. Several types of this condition are recognized.

## NORMAL VALUES

0.6–1.86 U/g hemoglobin.

## COST

Low.

## ADDITIONAL TESTS TO ORDER

CBC, red cell fragility, Coombs' test, red cell survival, serum haptoglobins, Heinz bodies, autohemolysis, and hematology consult.

## GLUCOSE-6-PHOSPHATE
DEHYDROGENASE

**DECREASED**

G6PD
DEFICIENCY,
HEMOLYTIC
ANEMIA

**INCREASED**

PERNICIOUS ANEMIA,
HEPATIC COMA,
HYPERTHYROIDISM,
MYOCARDIAL INFARCTION,
CHRONIC BLOOD LOSS,
OTHER MEGALOBLASTIC
ANEMIAS

# γ-GLUTAMYLTRANSFERASE

## INCREASED

Increase of this enzyme is most often caused by liver disease, particularly obstructive jaundice. Ask the following questions:

1. What are the amylase and lipase? If these are increased, look for pancreatitis and pancreatic CA.
2. What are the liver function tests? If these are positive, look for liver disease, cholecystitis, and obstructive jaundice.
3. What does the gallbladder ultrasound show? If this is positive, consider cholelithiasis and choledocholithiasis.

## NORMAL VALUES

10–40 U/L.

## COST

Low.

## ADDITIONAL TESTS TO ORDER

CBC, urinalysis, chemistry panel, liver function tests, sedimentation rate, amylase and lipase, gallbladder ultrasound, CT scan of abdomen, nuclear scan of liver, transhepatic cholangiography, ERCP, and gastroenterology consult.

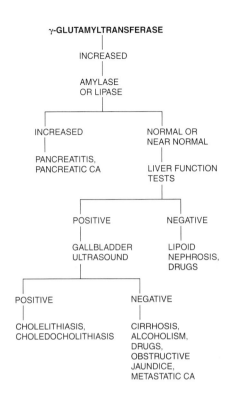

# GLYCOSYLATED HEMOGLOBIN

## INCREASED

An increase of glycosylated hemoglobin is good objective evidence that a diabetic has not maintained consistent control of the blood sugar. It is an excellent way to check on unreliable patients who may not be following their diet or taking insulin regularly.

## NORMAL VALUES

4–8%, but values vary with the laboratory.

## COST

Medium.

## ADDITIONAL TESTS TO ORDER

FBS, glucose tolerance test, plasma insulin, insulin antibodies, C-peptide, and endocrinology consult.

# GROWTH HORMONE

## INCREASED

Increased levels of plasma growth hormone (somatotropin) are found in gigantism and acromegaly. False-positive test results are found in patients on oral contraceptives and estrogen therapy. Some ectopic tumors produce growth hormone.

## DECREASED

Decreased levels of plasma growth hormone are found in dwarfism, obesity, and hypopituitarism. To differentiate these conditions, one should order an FSH and LH level. If these are also decreased, one should look for hypopituitarism and chromophobe adenoma of the pituitary.

## NORMAL VALUES

Men: 0–10 $\mu$g/mL.
Women: 0–15 $\mu$g/mL.
Children: 0–10 $\mu$g/mL.

## COST

Low.

## ADDITIONAL TESTS TO ORDER

Glucose tolerance test, glucose suppression of growth hormone, plasma ACTH, plasma cortisol, free $T_4$, TSH, CT scan or MRI of brain, and endocrine consult.

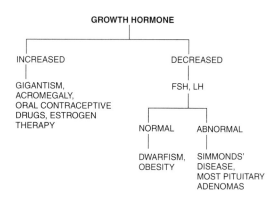

**GROWTH HORMONE**

INCREASED

GIGANTISM,
ACROMEGALY,
ORAL CONTRACEPTIVE
DRUGS, ESTROGEN
THERAPY

DECREASED

FSH, LH

NORMAL

DWARFISM,
OBESITY

ABNORMAL

SIMMONDS'
DISEASE,
MOST PITUITARY
ADENOMAS

# HAM TEST

## POSITIVE

A positive test indicates paroxysmal nocturnal hemoglobinuria. This condition is sometimes associated with iron-deficiency anemia, aplastic anemia, leukemia, and myelofibrosis.

## NORMAL VALUES

Negative.

## COST

Low.

## ADDITIONAL TESTS TO ORDER

CBC, sedimentation rate, serum iron and IBC, chemistry panel, bone marrow examination, and serum haptoglobins.

# HAPTOGLOBIN

## INCREASED

The serum haptoglobin is increased in any disease that causes tissue damage such as infection, neoplasm, or infarction. Among those disorders are nephritis, ulcerative colitis, rheumatic fever, myocardial infarction, and peptic ulcer disease.

## DECREASED

Serum haptoglobins are decreased in diseases associated with increased intravascular hemolysis. These include the hereditary and acquired hemolytic anemias, uremia, collagen disease, and red cell damage from prosthetic heart valves. To separate these disorders further, one should order a direct Coombs' test. This is positive in autoimmune hemolytic anemia, collagen disease, transfusion reactions, thrombotic thrombocytopenic purpura, and erythroblastosis fetalis.

## NORMAL VALUES

100–300 mg/100 mL.

## COST

Low.

## ADDITIONAL TESTS TO ORDER

CBC, chemistry panel, urinalysis, sedimentation rate, ANA, direct and indirect Coombs' test, red cell fragility test, chromium tagged red cell survival, sickle cell test, bone marrow examination, coagulation profile, ECG, chest radiograph, and hematology consult.

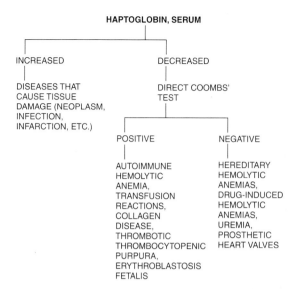

**HAPTOGLOBIN, SERUM**

INCREASED

DISEASES THAT
CAUSE TISSUE
DAMAGE (NEOPLASM,
INFECTION,
INFARCTION, ETC.)

DECREASED

DIRECT COOMBS'
TEST

POSITIVE

AUTOIMMUNE
HEMOLYTIC
ANEMIA,
TRANSFUSION
REACTIONS,
COLLAGEN
DISEASE,
THROMBOTIC
THROMBOCYTOPENIC
PURPURA,
ERYTHROBLASTOSIS
FETALIS

NEGATIVE

HEREDITARY
HEMOLYTIC
ANEMIAS,
DRUG-INDUCED
HEMOLYTIC
ANEMIAS,
UREMIA,
PROSTHETIC
HEART VALVES

# HEART SHUNT SCAN

## POSITIVE

This scan is positive in right-to-left and left-to-right cardiac shunts. It is useful in children with heart disease.

## NORMAL VALUES

Normal sequence of chamber filling.

## COST

Medium to high.

## ADDITIONAL TESTS TO ORDER

ECG, chest radiograph, arterial blood gases, echocardiography, cardiac catheterization, angiocardiography, and cardiology consult.

# HEAVY METALS

## HEAVY METAL SCREEN, URINE

This test is useful in diagnosing toxicity from numerous heavy metals, including antimony, arsenic, bismuth, cadmium, cobalt, copper, lead, mercury, selenium, thallium, and zinc.

### Normal Values

Negative.

## BLOOD LEAD LEVEL

This test is positive in lead poisoning. These patients may present with seizures, basophilic stippling of red cells, peripheral neuropathy such as Bell's palsy or wrist drop, and GI disturbances. They also may present with nephritis.

### Normal Values

Children: Less than 10 $\mu$g/dL.
Adults: Less than 40 $\mu$g/dL.

## ARSENIC, SERUM, URINE, HAIR, AND TOENAILS

These tests are *positive* in arsenic poisoning. The urine is the best test for acute poisoning, whereas the hair and toenails are useful in long-term exposure. Arsenic clears out of the serum in 4 days after acute exposure.

## Normal Values

Consult local laboratory.

## COPPER

See page 185.

## MERCURY, URINE

This test is positive in mercury poisoning, caused either by acute poisoning or by chronic occupational exposure.

## Normal Values

Up to 20 $\mu$g/L.

## ZINC, BLOOD

### Increased

Zinc is increased in the blood in accidental ingestion, overdosage, and occupational exposure.

### Decreased

Zinc is decreased in numerous disorders, including dwarfism, chronic liver disease, sickle cell anemia, neoplasms, stress, infection, pregnancy, malnutrition, pica, burns, and oral contraceptive use.

### Normal Values

60–130 $\mu$g/dL.

## COST

Low to medium.

## ADDITIONAL TESTS TO ORDER

CBC, urinalysis, sedimentation rate, chemistry panel, EEG, EMG, NCV study, ECG, liver function tests, and consultation with a poison control center.

# HEINZ BODIES

## INCREASED

These are increased in hemolytic anemias, especially G6PD deficiency. Drug poisoning may also significantly increase the number of cells with Heinz bodies inside. Heinz bodies are also increased in patients who have undergone splenectomy.

## NORMAL VALUES

None present.

## COST

Low.

## ADDITIONAL TESTS TO ORDER

See page 294.

# HEMATOCRIT

## INCREASED

An increased hematocrit suggests primary and secondary polycythemia. However, dehydration is an important cause. To help differentiate polycythemia from dehydration, one should order a serum protein or albumin and blood volume study.

## DECREASED

A decreased hematocrit is typical of anemia. To differentiate the type, look at the WBC. If the *WBC* is *increased,* one should look for leukemia, infectious disease, hemolytic anemia, hemorrhage, or myeloid metaplasia. What is the platelet count? If it is decreased in the face of a high WBC, one should look for leukemia and myeloid metaplasia. If the *WBC* is *decreased,* one should look for aplastic anemia, infiltrative disease of the bone marrow, and hypersplenism. A normal WBC suggests iron-deficiency anemia, anemia of chronic blood loss, and hemoconcentration.

## NORMAL VALUES

Adult males: 42–52%.
Adult females: 35–42%.
Children: 31–40%.
Infants: 35–54%.

## COST

Low.

## ADDITIONAL TESTS TO ORDER

CBL, blood smear, chemistry panel, sedimentation rate, serum haptoglobins, serum iron, serum $B_{12}$ and folic acid, hemoglobin electrophoresis, sickle cell preparation, bone marrow, and hematology consult.

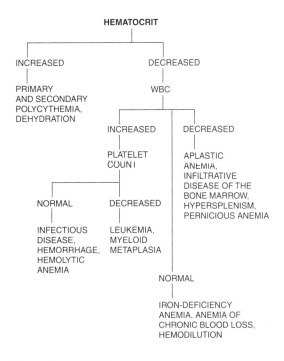

# HEMATURIA

## INCREASED RBCS

Ask the following questions:

1. Is the urine culture positive? If so, look for cystitis, pyelonephritis, and tuberculosis.
2. Are significant numbers of red cell casts present? This signifies glomerulonephritis, lower nephron nephrosis, renal embolism, and toxic nephritis.
3. If the cultures are negative and few or no red cell casts are present, look for polycystic kidneys, renal calculi, foreign body, or neoplasm. Is the patient taking warfarin sodium or heparin?

## HEMOGLOBIN OR MYOGLOBIN

Ask the following question: Are the serum haptoglobins decreased? This finding suggests that the hemoglobinuria results from hemolytic anemia, malaria, or a transfusion reaction. If the serum haptoglobins are normal, one should look for chemical intoxication, muscle injury, burns, or myocardial infarction as the cause.

## NORMAL VALUES

Negative.

## COST

Low.

## ADDITIONAL TESTS TO ORDER

CBC, platelet count, sedimentation rate, chemistry panel, coagulation profile, ANA, Ham test, blood smear for parasites, urine culture and colony count, IVP, CT scan of abdomen, serum complement, ASO titer, cystoscopy, renal biopsy, and nephrology or urology consult.

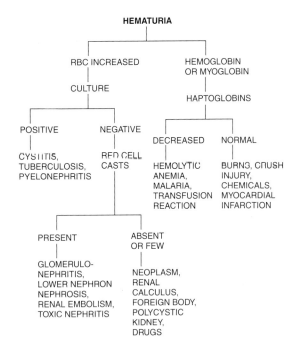

**HEMATURIA**

RBC INCREASED

CULTURE

POSITIVE
CYSTITIS, TUBERCULOSIS, PYELONEPHRITIS

NEGATIVE
RED CELL CASTS

PRESENT
GLOMERULO-NEPHRITIS, LOWER NEPHRON NEPHROSIS, RENAL EMBOLISM, TOXIC NEPHRITIS

ABSENT OR FEW
NEOPLASM, RENAL CALCULUS, FOREIGN BODY, POLYCYSTIC KIDNEY, DRUGS

HEMOGLOBIN OR MYOGLOBIN

HAPTOGLOBINS

DECREASED
HEMOLYTIC ANEMIA, MALARIA, TRANSFUSION REACTION

NORMAL
BURNS, CRUSH INJURY, CHEMICALS, MYOCARDIAL INFARCTION

# HEMOGLOBIN

## INCREASED

This is found in primary and secondary polycythemia and dehydration and other conditions associated with hemoconcentration.

## DECREASED

Is the WBC altered? If the WBC is *increased,* then the patient may have a hemolytic anemia, hemorrhage, infectious disease, leukemia, or myeloid metaplasia. Is the platelet count altered? If the platelet count is decreased, one should consider leukemia or myeloid metaplasia. If it is *normal,* one should consider hemolytic anemia, hemorrhage, or infectious disease. If the WBC is *decreased,* one should consider aplastic anemia, infiltrative disease of the bone marrow, hypersplenism, and megaloblastic anemia. If the WBC is *normal,* iron-deficiency anemia and anemia of chronic blood loss are possibilities.

## NORMAL VALUES

Men: 14–16.5 g/100 mL.
Women: 12–15 g/100 mL.
Newborn: 14–20 g/100 mL.
Children: Varies from 12–15 g/100 mL.

## COST

Low.

## ADDITIONAL TESTS TO ORDER

CBC, platelet count, blood smear, indices, reticulocyte count, serum haptoglobins, Coombs' test, serum iron and IBC, serum $B_{12}$ and folic acid, red cell survival test, bone marrow examination, stool for occult blood, liver–spleen scan, CT scan of abdomen, blood volume, and hematology consult.

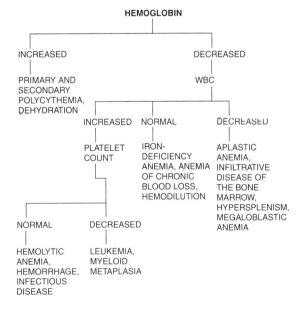

**HEMOGLOBIN**

INCREASED

PRIMARY AND SECONDARY POLYCYTHEMIA, DEHYDRATION

DECREASED

WBC

INCREASED

PLATELET COUNT

NORMAL

IRON-DEFICIENCY ANEMIA, ANEMIA OF CHRONIC BLOOD LOSS, HEMODILUTION

DECREASED

APLASTIC ANEMIA, INFILTRATIVE DISEASE OF THE BONE MARROW, HYPERSPLENISM, MEGALOBLASTIC ANEMIA

NORMAL

HEMOLYTIC ANEMIA, HEMORRHAGE, INFECTIOUS DISEASE

DECREASED

LEUKEMIA, MYELOID METAPLASIA

# HEMOGLOBIN, BART'S

## POSITIVE

Positive results are seen in homozygous $\alpha$-thalassemia (78%), heterozygous $\alpha$-thalassemia-2 trait (0.8–3%), heterozygous $\alpha$-thalassemia-1 trait (3–10%), homozygous $\alpha$-thalassemia-2 trait (3–10%), and hemoglobin H (20–30%).

## NORMAL VALUES

Less than 1%.

## COST

Low.

## ADDITIONAL TESTS TO ORDER

CBC, blood smear for morphology, red cell fragility test, chemistry panel, sickle cell preparation, hemoglobin electrophoresis, Coombs' test, and hematology consult.

# HEMOGLOBIN ELECTROPHORESIS

1. *Increased hemoglobin F:* This occurs in the newborn, HbH disease, leukemia, aplastic anemia, β-thalassemia major and minor, and sickle cell anemia. To differentiate these conditions further, a *red cell fragility test* is indicated. This value is decreased in sickle cell anemia and thalassemia.
2. *Increased hemoglobin S:* This is found in sickle cell anemia and sickle cell trait. In sickle cell anemia, 60–99% of the hemoglobin is HbS. In sickle cell trait, only 20–50% of the hemoglobin is HbS.
3. *Increased hemoglobin $A_2$:* This occurs in β-thalassemia major and minor.
4. *Increased hemoglobin C:* HbC is increased in hemoglobin C trait and disease. It is 30% in HbC trait and 95% or more in HbC disease.

## NORMAL VALUES

### Adults

$HbA_1$: 96–98.5%.
$HbA_2$: 1.5–4%.
HbF: 0–2.0%.

### Newborn

$HbA_1$: 20%.
$HbA_2$: 2%.
HbF: 80%.

## COST

Low.

## ADDITIONAL TESTS TO ORDER

HbF test, sickle cell preparation, red cell fragility, CBC and blood smear, serum iron and IBC, and hematology consult.

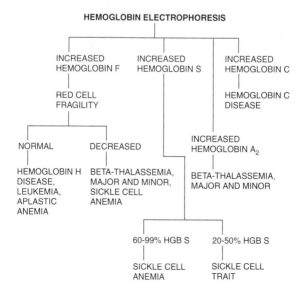

**HEMOGLOBIN ELECTROPHORESIS**

INCREASED HEMOGLOBIN F → RED CELL FRAGILITY

- NORMAL → HEMOGLOBIN H DISEASE, LEUKEMIA, APLASTIC ANEMIA
- DECREASED → BETA-THALASSEMIA, MAJOR AND MINOR, SICKLE CELL ANEMIA

INCREASED HEMOGLOBIN S

- 60-99% HGB S → SICKLE CELL ANEMIA
- 20-50% HGB S → SICKLE CELL TRAIT

INCREASED HEMOGLOBIN C → HEMOGLOBIN C DISEASE → INCREASED HEMOGLOBIN A$_2$ → BETA-THALASSEMIA, MAJOR AND MINOR

# HEMOGLOBIN F

## INCREASED

HbF is increased in the newborn (50–85%), thalassemia major (10–90%), thalassemia minor (2–12%), $\beta$-thalassemia-S disease (5–20%), and other less common hemoglobinopathies.

## NORMAL VALUES

Adult: Less than 2%.
Newborn: 50–85%.
1–6 Months: 8–75%.

## COST

Low.

## ADDITIONAL TESTS TO ORDER

Hb electrophoresis, red cell fragility, CBC and blood smear, sickle cell preparation, sedimentation rate, bone marrow examination, and hematology consult.

# HEPATITIS PANEL

1. *HBsAg:* HBsAg (hepatitis surface antigen) is present in hepatitis B infections.
2. *IgM anti-HBc:* If IgM anti-HBc (antibody to hepatitis B core antigen) is elevated, the patient has acute hepatitis. If IgM anti-HBc is not elevated but the HBsAg is elevated, the patient probably has chronic HBV hepatitis.
3. *IgM anti-HAV:* This is the antibody to hepatitis A. It is elevated in hepatitis A infections. If one sees simultaneous elevation of IgM anti-HAV and IgM anti-HBc, the patient has combined hepatitis A and B.
4. *Anti-HCV* is elevated in hepatitis C infections, however, it is only elevated 20–30% during the acute stage of the disease. In the chronic phase, more than 90% of the patients with HCV hepatitis have elevated anti-HCV antibodies.
5. *Anti-HDV:* This antibody is present in hepatitis D infections, but unfortunately, seroconversion may take 30–40 days. A negative result does not rule out HDV infection. Hepatitis D almost invariably occurs simultaneously with hepatitis B.
6. *Anti-HEV:* Currently, only research laboratories have the capability of testing for these antibodies.

## NORMAL VALUES

None detected.

## COST

Medium.

## ADDITIONAL TESTS TO ORDER

CBC, urinalysis, chemistry panel, sedimentation rate, serum protein electrophoresis, liver scan, CT scan of abdomen, and consultation with a gastroenterologist regarding liver biopsy (not usually recommended).

# HEPATITIS PANEL

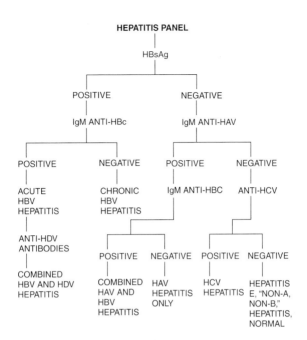

HBsAg

POSITIVE — IgM ANTI-HBc

- POSITIVE
  - ACUTE HBV HEPATITIS
  - ANTI-HDV ANTIBODIES
  - COMBINED HBV AND HDV HEPATITIS
- NEGATIVE
  - CHRONIC HBV HEPATITIS

NEGATIVE — IgM ANTI-HAV

- POSITIVE — IgM ANTI-HBC
  - POSITIVE
    - COMBINED HAV AND HBV HEPATITIS
  - NEGATIVE
    - HAV HEPATITIS ONLY
- NEGATIVE — ANTI-HCV
  - POSITIVE
    - HCV HEPATITIS
  - NEGATIVE
    - HEPATITIS E, "NON-A, NON-B," HEPATITIS, NORMAL

# HISTIOCYTE SMEAR, BLOOD

## POSITIVE

This test is positive in subacute bacterial endocarditis, typhoid fever, tuberculosis, leprosy, parasitic diseases, neoplasms such as Hodgkin's reticulocytosis and histiocytic leukemia, hemolytic anemia, and fat storage disease.

## NORMAL VALUES

None found.

## COST

Low.

## ADDITIONAL TESTS TO ORDER

Multiple blood cultures, culture of other tissue fluids, tuberculin test, stool for ova and parasites, blood smear for parasites, bone marrow examination, echocardiography, lymph node biopsy, serum haptoglobins, and consultation with an oncologist or infectious disease specialist.

# HISTOPLASMOSIS ANTIBODY TEST

## POSITIVE

This test is positive in histoplasmosis. It is the preferred method of establishing the diagnosis in most cases. False-negative results occur early in the disease and in severe or disseminated infection. False-positive results occur in patients with other fungal disease and tuberculosis.

## NORMAL VALUES

Negative.

## COST

Low.

## ADDITIONAL TESTS TO ORDER

Smear and culture of sputum, urine, blood and bone marrow, antigen tests of urine, serum and CSF, skin tests, chest radiograph, biopsy, and pulmonary consult.

# HISTOPLASMOSIS SKIN TEST

## POSITIVE

A positive test indicates present or past infection with *Histoplasma capsulatum.* False-negative results occur in patients who are seriously ill.

## NORMAL VALUES

Negative.

## COST

Low.

## ADDITIONAL TESTS TO ORDER

CBC, sedimentation rate, chemistry panel, sputum cultures, serologic tests, chest radiograph, CSF analysis and culture, and consultation with a pulmonologist.

# HIV ANTIBODY TESTS

## POSITIVE

A positive test for these antibodies means infection with HIV, which is the etiologic agent in AIDS. The EIA test is used first and is confirmed by Western blot analysis or the immunofluorescent antibody test. Reliability exceeds 99% when the confirmatory tests are used, as well.

## NORMAL VALUES

Negative.

## COST

Low.

## ADDITIONAL TESTS TO ORDER

CBC, T-lymphocyte CD4 and CD8 count, sedimentation rate, chest radiograph, sputum smear and cultures for *Pneumocystis carinii,* HIV-1 cultures, HIV antigen detection, and infectious disease consult.

# HLA TESTING

## HLA–B27

This antigen is found in patients with ankylosing spondylitis, Reiter's syndrome, juvenile rheumatoid arthritis, Graves' disease, and anterior uveitis. It is also associated with multiple sclerosis.

## HLA–B8

This antigen is associated with celiac disease, dermatitis herpetiformis, chronic active hepatitis, and myasthenia gravis.

## OTHERS

These antigens are associated with various other diseases, but the associations are not quite as specific.

## NORMAL VALUES

Not applicable.

## COST

Medium.

## ADDITIONAL TESTS TO ORDER

RA test, skeletal survey, bone scan, free $T_4$, sedimentation rate, acetylcholine receptor antibody titer, and consultation with a rheumatologist or other appropriate specialist.

# HOLTER MONITORING

## DEFINITION

This is essentially a 24–48 hour ECG. The patient is hooked up to a recording device in somewhat the same manner as a standard ECG machine, except the portable recording device is left attached for 24–48 hours. Then the material collected can be analyzed for abnormal data by a computer.

## POSITIVE

This test is positive in paroxysmal cardiac arrhythmias such as supraventricular tachycardia, various degrees of heart block, sick sinus syndrome, and APCs or VPCs. It is also helpful in diagnosing myocardial ischemia and providing a recording when the patient experiences chest pain.

## NORMAL VALUES

A limited number of premature contractions in 24 hours and no episodes of tachyarrhythmias, ST depression, or heart block during the recording period.

## COST

Medium.

## ADDITIONAL TESTS TO ORDER

ECG, exercise tolerance testing, thallium stress scan, echocardiography, chest radiograph, coronary angiography, cardiac catheterization and angiocardiography, and cardiology consult.

# HOMOGENTISIC ACID, URINE

## POSITIVE

A positive test for this substance is diagnostic of al-kaptonuria (ochronosis). The test is simple to perform: 10% sodium hydroxide solution is added to the urine. When homogentisic acid is present, the urine turns black.

## NORMAL VALUES

Negative.

## COST

Low.

## ADDITIONAL TESTS TO ORDER

Radiograph of the spine and long bones, bone scans, biopsy of cartilage, and orthopedic consult.

# HOMOVANILLIC ACID, URINE

## POSITIVE

A positive test for this substance is most likely the result of malignant pheochromocytoma, neuro-blastoma, or ganglioblastoma.

## NORMAL VALUES

Negative.

## COST

Low.

## ADDITIONAL TESTS TO ORDER

24-hour urine VMA or catecholamines, CT scan of the abdomen, and endocrinology consult.

# HYDROGEN BREATH ANALYSIS

## POSITIVE

A positive test is found in conditions associated with malabsorption of a carbohydrate such as lactase deficiency. This is because the sugar (i.e., lactose) is not broken down and absorbed in the small intestine and passes into the colon. There it is metabolized by bacteria, and this releases hydrogen that is picked up in the breath specimens during the test. Other conditions associated with a positive test include diabetic gastroparesis, blind loop syndrome, fistulae, jejunal diverticulosis, and irritable bowel syndrome.

## NORMAL VALUES

2–20 ppm.

## COST

Medium.

## ADDITIONAL TESTS TO ORDER

Lactose tolerance test, sucrose tolerance test, D-xylose absorption test, GI series and small bowel follow-through, small bowel biopsy, elimination diet, and gastroenterology consult.

# 5-HYDROXYINDOLEACETIC ACID (5-HIAA)

## INCREASED

This substance is increased in the urine in carcinoid tumors, particularly after they have metastasized. It is also increased in celiac disease and Whipple's disease. False-positive results may occur from numerous drugs, fruits (e.g., bananas, plums), nuts, and avocados. Some drugs may also cause false-negative results. Repeated testing is wise.

## NORMAL VALUES

Negative.

## COST

Low.

## ADDITIONAL TESTS TO ORDER

Repeated testing, chest radiograph, liver function tests, small bowel series, D-xylose absorption test, small bowel biopsy, exploratory laparotomy, and endocrinology consult.

# HYDROXYPROLINE, URINE

## INCREASED

Ask the following questions:

1. What is the alkaline phosphatase? If the alkaline phosphatase is increased and one sees increased hydroxyproline in the urine, the patient may have hyperparathyroidism, osteomalacia, metastatic cancer, Paget's disease, or a bone tumor.
2. What is the PTH assay? An increased PTH level suggests hyperparathyroidism and osteomalacia.
3. If the alkaline phosphatase is normal, what does the bone scan show? A normal alkaline phosphatase and abnormal bone scan suggest multiple myeloma. The bone scan is usually unremarkable in Marfan's syndrome, Klinefelter's syndrome, and osteoporosis. Acromegaly and rheumatoid arthritis may present some minor changes on bone scan.

## NORMAL VALUES

Total 22–77 mg/24 hours.

## COST

Low.

## ADDITIONAL TESTS TO ORDER

CBC, chemistry panel, urinalysis, sedimentation rate, RA test, plasma growth hormone after glucose suppression, bone scan, PTH, serum protein electrophoresis, serum testosterone and FSH, skeletal survey, bone densitometry, endocrine consult, and oncology consult.

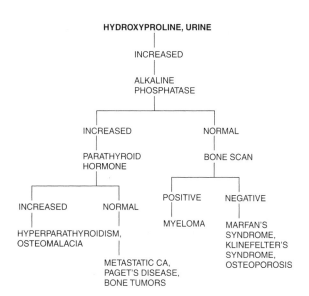

**HYDROXYPROLINE, URINE**

INCREASED

ALKALINE
PHOSPHATASE

INCREASED           NORMAL

PARATHYROID        BONE SCAN
HORMONE

INCREASED       NORMAL        POSITIVE    NEGATIVE

HYPERPARATHYROIDISM,        MYELOMA    MARFAN'S
OSTEOMALACIA                         SYNDROME,
                                     KLINEFELTER'S
           METASTATIC CA,        SYNDROME,
           PAGET'S DISEASE,     OSTEOPOROSIS
           BONE TUMORS

# HYSTEROSAL-PINGOGRAPHY

## POSITIVE

Abnormalities found on this test are obstruction of the fallopian tubes, endometrial polyps and carcinoma, uterine fibroids, and congenital anomalies of the female genital tract. The primary indication for this test is infertility. It may also help to diagnose the cause of abnormal uterine bleeding.

## NORMAL VALUES

Normal size, shape, and position of the uterus and fallopian tube. No obstruction or filling defects.

## COST

Medium.

## ADDITIONAL TESTS TO ORDER

CBC, urinalysis, chemistry panel, serum iron and IBC, free $T_4$, coagulation profile, ultrasonography, laparoscopy, CT scan of pelvis, and gynecology consult.

# IMMUNOELECTRO-PHORESIS

## IGA

This is *increased* in infections, cirrhosis, myeloma, hepatitis, IgA nephropathy, and Henoch–Schönlein purpura. IgA is *decreased* in selective hypo-IgA protein-losing enteropathies, hereditary telangiectasia, and nephrotic syndrome.

## IGE

This is *increased* in allergic disorders such as hay fever, asthma, atopic dermatitis, urticaria, and drug and food allergies. It is also *increased* in Wiskott–Aldrich syndrome, polyarteritis nodosa, and hypereosinophilic syndrome. *Decrease* occurs with the various hypogammaglobulinemias.

## IGG

This is *increased* in chronic infections, autoimmune diseases, and multiple myeloma. These globulins are *decreased* in hypogammaglobulinemia and agammaglobulinemia. They are also *decreased* in protein-losing enteropathy and nephrotic syndrome.

## IGM

An *increase* of this globulin occurs in viral infections, parasitic disease, nephrotic syndrome, hepatitis, and macroglobulinemia. A *decrease* occurs in selective hypo-IgM protein-losing enteropathies.

## NORMAL VALUES

IgA: 75–350 mg/dL.
IgD: Insignificant.
IgE: Insignificant.
IgG: 700–1350 mg/dL.
IgM: 35–200 mg/dL.

## COST

Low.

## ADDITIONAL TESTS TO ORDER

CBC, sedimentation rate, chemistry panel, eosinophil count, ANA, RA test, SIA water test, cryoglobulin test, blood smear for morphology, bone marrow examination, 24-hour urine protein, bone scan, stool for ova and parasites, and oncology and hematology consult.

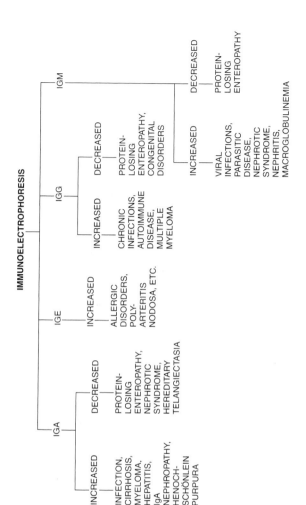

**IMMUNOELECTROPHORESIS**

- IGA
  - INCREASED
    - INFECTION, CIRRHOSIS, MYELOMA, HEPATITIS, IgA NEPHROPATHY, HENOCH-SCHÖNLEIN PURPURA
  - DECREASED
    - PROTEIN-LOSING ENTEROPATHY, NEPHROTIC SYNDROME, HEREDITARY TELANGIECTASIA
- IGE
  - INCREASED
    - ALLERGIC DISORDERS, POLY-ARTERITIS NODOSA, ETC.
- IGG
  - INCREASED
    - CHRONIC INFECTIONS, AUTOIMMUNE DISEASE, MULTIPLE MYELOMA
  - DECREASED
    - PROTEIN-LOSING ENTEROPATHY, CONGENITAL DISORDERS
- IGM
  - INCREASED
    - VIRAL INFECTIONS, PARASITIC DISEASE, NEPHROTIC SYNDROME, NEPHRITIS, MACROGLOBULINEMIA
  - DECREASED
    - PROTEIN-LOSING ENTEROPATHY

# IMPEDANCE PHLEBOGRAPHY

## DEFINITION

This test measures the drop in conductivity in an extremity (usually the leg) after release of a pneumatic cuff placed around the extremity to obstruct the venous flow. *Normally*, the conductivity drops rapidly after release of the cuff.

## POSITIVE

When venous flow is obstructed by a *deep vein thrombosis,* the conductivity does not drop significantly when the cuff is released or deflated.

## COST

Medium.

## ADDITIONAL TESTS TO ORDER

Venous Doppler study, iodine-125 fibrinogen venogram, phlebography, and cardiology consult.

# INSULIN

## INCREASED

Blood insulin is increased in diabetes mellitus type II, acromegaly, Cushing's syndrome, functional hypoglycemia, and insulinoma. Further differentiation is made with the blood sugar. It is increased in type II diabetes, acromegaly, and Cushing's syndrome, whereas it may be decreased in functional hypoglycemia and insulinoma.

## DECREASED

Endogenous insulin is decreased in type I diabetes mellitus.

## NORMAL VALUES

5–20 $\mu$U/mL.

## COST

Low.

## ADDITIONAL TESTS TO ORDER

CBC, urine, chemistry panel, C-peptide, plasma cortisol, growth hormone, glucose tolerance tests, tolbutamide tolerance tests, CT scan of brain and abdomen, and endocrinology consult.

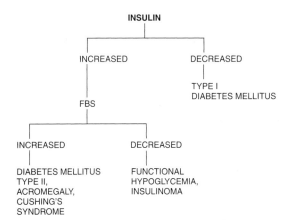

**INSULIN**

INCREASED — DECREASED

DECREASED:
TYPE I
DIABETES MELLITUS

INCREASED:
FBS

INCREASED:
DIABETES MELLITUS
TYPE II,
ACROMEGALY,
CUSHING'S
SYNDROME

DECREASED:
FUNCTIONAL
HYPOGLYCEMIA,
INSULINOMA

# INTRAVENOUS CHOLANGIOGRAPHY

## INDICATIONS

This test is indicated when visualization of the gall-bladder is unsuccessful with oral cholecystography or ultrasonography. It also may be possible to visualize the common duct and hepatic ducts with this procedure. ERCP and transhepatic cholangiography are more commonly used today.

## POSITIVE

This test shows gallstones, common duct stones, neoplasms, and congenital anomalies of the gallbladder and bile ducts.

## NORMAL VALUES

Normal size, shape, and position of the gallbladder and bile ducts without obstruction or filling defects.

## COST

Medium.

## ADDITIONAL TESTS TO ORDER

CBC, urinalysis, chemistry panel, gallbladder ultrasound, ERCP, transhepatic cholangiography, duodenal analysis, exploratory laparotomy, gastroenterology consult, and surgical consult.

# INTRAVENOUS PYELOGRAPHY

## POSITIVE

1. *Hydronephrosis:* This may be unilateral or bilateral. *Unilateral* hydronephrosis may result from renal calculus, papilloma of the renal pelvis, ureter, or bladder, malignant tumors of these structures, congenital bands, and extrinsic pressure from benign and malignant tumors elsewhere in the abdomen. Bilateral hydronephrosis is most often due to bladder neck obstruction, prostatic hypertrophy, and ureteroceles. It can also result from congenital bands, aberrant blood vessels, and extrinsic pressure from pelvic tumors.
2. *Bilateral kidney enlargement:* This is found most often from polycystic kidneys.
3. *Unilateral mass:* This suggests a tumor or simple cyst of the kidney. *Ultrasonography* differentiates these two conditions. If ultrasonography suggests a solid tumor, a *CT scan* should be done to confirm the diagnosis. A urologist should then be consulted.
4. *Calcifications:* Renal calcifications found on plain films of the abdomen must be confirmed by an IVP. These calcifications may result from stones, papillary necrosis, tuberculosis, or nephrocalcinosis.
5. *Delayed appearance of dye in one kidney:* This finding suggests renal artery stenosis. Renal angiography should be considered.
6. *Small kidneys:* These are found in chronic renal disease such as glomerulonephritis and pyelonephritis. An IVP is not usually successful in these conditions because of poor concentration of the dye. If only one kidney is small, one should consider unilateral renal artery stenosis.

## NORMAL VALUES

Normal size, shape, and position of the kidneys, ureters, and bladder without filling defects or obstruction.

## COST

Medium.

## ADDITIONAL TESTS TO ORDER

CBC, urinalysis, urine culture and colony count, chemistry panel, cytology, serum and urine osmolality, ultrasonography, CT scan of abdomen, urology consult, cystoscopy and retrograde pyelography, renal scan, renal angiography, and needle biopsy.

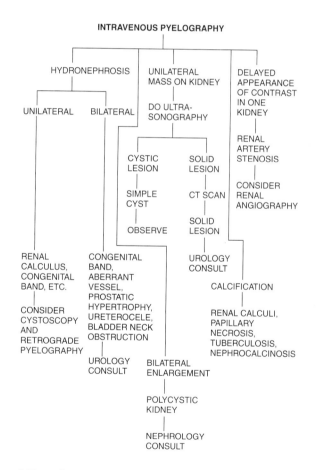

# IRON, SERUM

## INCREASED

Increased serum iron is associated with hemochromatosis, excessive iron therapy, vitamin $B_6$ therapy, aplastic anemia, and hemolytic anemia. To differentiate these conditions further, an RBC count is indicated. A significant decrease in the blood count is characteristic of aplastic anemia and hemolytic anemia.

## DECREASED

Decreased serum iron suggests iron-deficiency anemia. However, various chronic diseases (e.g., hepatitis, cirrhosis, neoplasm, and rheumatoid arthritis) can be associated with a decreased serum iron. To separate these conditions from iron-deficiency anemia, one should order a serum ferritin. This value is decreased in iron-deficiency anemia but increased in infectious and malignant conditions.

## NORMAL VALUES

20–150 ng/dL.

## COST

Low.

## ADDITIONAL TESTS TO ORDER

CBC, urinalysis, chemistry panel, liver function tests, serum protein electrophoresis, chest radiograph, bone marrow examination, iron-binding capacity, serum $B_{12}$ and folic acid, liver biopsy, and hematology consult.

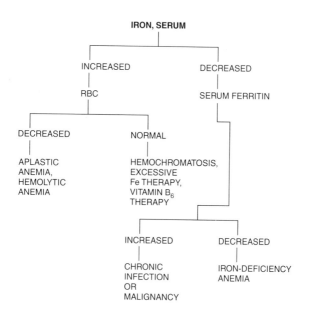

**IRON, SERUM**

INCREASED

RBC

DECREASED
APLASTIC
ANEMIA,
HEMOLYTIC
ANEMIA

NORMAL
HEMOCHROMATOSIS,
EXCESSIVE
Fe THERAPY,
VITAMIN $B_6$
THERAPY

DECREASED

SERUM FERRITIN

INCREASED
CHRONIC
INFECTION
OR
MALIGNANCY

DECREASED
IRON-DEFICIENCY
ANEMIA

# IRON-BINDING
# CAPACITY, TOTAL

## INCREASED

Ask the following questions:

1. What is the serum iron? If the serum iron is decreased, the patient most likely has iron-deficiency anemia, although the iron may also be decreased in pregnancy and chronic blood loss.
2. What do the liver function tests show? If results are abnormal, the patient may have acute hepatitis.

When the foregoing test results are normal, one should look for polycythemia and oral contraceptive use.

## DECREASED

Ask the following questions:

1. What is the serum iron? If this is increased, look for hemochromatosis or sideroblastic anemia.
2. What is the red cell fragility? If this is decreased, look for thalassemia and sickle cell anemia.

If the foregoing test results are normal, one should consider pernicious anemia, chronic infection, hepatic disease, malignant disease, uremia, and rheumatoid arthritis.

## NORMAL VALUES

250–450 mg/dL.

## COST

Low.

## ADDITIONAL TESTS TO ORDER

CBC, sedimentation rate, urinalysis, chemistry panel, RA titer, serum $B_{12}$ and folic acid, hemoglobin electrophoresis, sickle cell preparation, red cell survival time, liver biopsy, Schilling test, CT scan of abdomen and pelvis, and hematology consult.

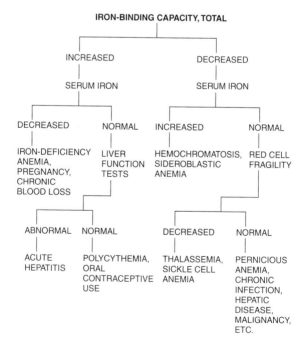

IRON-BINDING CAPACITY, TOTAL

INCREASED
SERUM IRON

DECREASED
IRON-DEFICIENCY ANEMIA, PREGNANCY, CHRONIC BLOOD LOSS

NORMAL
LIVER FUNCTION TESTS

ABNORMAL
ACUTE HEPATITIS

NORMAL
POLYCYTHEMIA, ORAL CONTRACEPTIVE USE

DECREASED
SERUM IRON

INCREASED
HEMOCHROMATOSIS, SIDEROBLASTIC ANEMIA

NORMAL
RED CELL FRAGILITY

DECREASED
THALASSEMIA, SICKLE CELL ANEMIA

NORMAL
PERNICIOUS ANEMIA, CHRONIC INFECTION, HEPATIC DISEASE, MALIGNANCY, ETC.

# 17-KETOSTEROIDS, 17-KETOGENIC STEROIDS, URINE

## INCREASED

These levels are increased in basophilic adenoma of the pituitary, ectopic ACTH syndrome, adrenocortical neoplasm or hyperplasia, and steroid therapy. To distinguish between basophilic adenoma and ectopic ACTH and the other conditions, a plasma ACTH is indicated. Plasma ACTH is elevated in both these conditions, but it is decreased in adrenocortical neoplasm or hyperplasia and steroid therapy.

## DECREASED

Urine 17-ketosteroids and 17-ketogenic steroids are decreased in Addison's disease, pituitary insufficiency, chromophobe adenomas, cretinism, and anorexia nervosa. To differentiate these conditions further, one should obtain a plasma ACTH level. The plasma ACTH level is increased in Addison's disease but decreased in the other conditions in this group. False increases and decreases occur during the use of many drugs.

## NORMAL VALUES

### 17-Ketosteroids

Men: 8–18 mg/24 hours.
Women: 5–15 mg/24 hours.

### 17-Ketogenic Steroids

Men: 5.5–23 mg/24 hours.
Women: 3–15 mg/24 hours.

## COST

Low.

## ADDITIONAL TESTS TO ORDER

CBC, urinalysis, chemistry panel, plasma cortisol, dexamethasone-suppression test, metyrapone test, plasma ACTH, CT scan of brain and adrenal and pituitary glands, and ACTH-stimulation test.

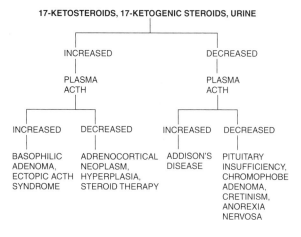

17-KETOSTEROIDS, 17-KETOGENIC STEROIDS, URINE

INCREASED — PLASMA ACTH

INCREASED: BASOPHILIC ADENOMA, ECTOPIC ACTH SYNDROME

DECREASED: ADRENOCORTICAL NEOPLASM, HYPERPLASIA, STEROID THERAPY

DECREASED — PLASMA ACTH

INCREASED: ADDISON'S DISEASE

DECREASED: PITUITARY INSUFFICIENCY, CHROMOPHOBE ADENOMA, CRETINISM, ANOREXIA NERVOSA

# LACTIC ACID, ARTERIAL BLOOD

## INCREASED

Lactic acid is increased in lactic acidosis because of shock, severe anemia, severe hypoxemia, diabetes mellitus, liver disease, sepsis, neoplasms, thiamine deficiency, carbon monoxide poisoning, hereditary enzyme abnormalities, drugs, and regional hypoperfusions.

## NORMAL VALUES

Less than 1.6 mmol/L.

## COST

Medium.

## ADDITIONAL TESTS TO ORDER

CBC, urinalysis, chemistry panel, sedimentation rate, chest radiograph, arterial blood gases, plasma acetone, serial electrolytes, pulmonary capillary wedge pressure, ECG, pulmonary function tests, and consultation with a pulmonologist and endocrinologist.

# LACTIC ACID DEHYDROGENASE (LDH)

## INCREASED

LDH is increased in liver, muscle, heart, lung, and blood diseases. To differentiate these disorders, ask the following questions:

1. What is the MB–CPK? This enzyme is increased in heart disease, particularly myocardial infarction. A rising titer associated with chest pain is almost diagnostic.
2. What is the transaminase (ALT)? An increase in the transaminase suggests liver disease and skeletal muscle disease.
3. What is the serum or urine creatine? If this is elevated, think of muscle disease.
4. What is the lung scan? A positive lung scan separates pulmonary infarction from the others in this group.

## NORMAL VALUES

63–160 units.

## COST

Low.

## ADDITIONAL TESTS TO ORDER

CBC, urinalysis, chemistry panel, sedimentation rate, ANA, urine or serum creatine, urine myoglobin, ECG, blood gases, liver function tests, LDH isozymes, chest radiograph, lung scan, EMG, cardiology consult, and neurology consult.

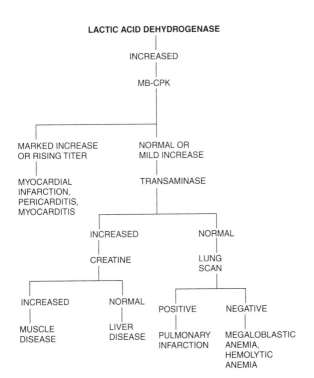

**LACTIC ACID DEHYDROGENASE**

INCREASED

MB-CPK

MARKED INCREASE
OR RISING TITER

MYOCARDIAL
INFARCTION,
PERICARDITIS,
MYOCARDITIS

NORMAL OR
MILD INCREASE

TRANSAMINASE

INCREASED

CREATINE

NORMAL

LUNG
SCAN

INCREASED

MUSCLE
DISEASE

NORMAL

LIVER
DISEASE

POSITIVE

PULMONARY
INFARCTION

NEGATIVE

MEGALOBLASTIC
ANEMIA,
HEMOLYTIC
ANEMIA

**Lactic Acid Dehydrogenase (LDH)**   351

# LACTIC ACID DEHYDROGENASE (LDH), CEREBROSPINAL FLUID (CSF)

## INCREASED

Increased levels of LDH are found in the CSF in bacterial meningitis, leukemia, lymphoma, metastatic carcinoma, subarachnoid hemorrhage, and occasionally viral meningitis. Positive cultures for bacteria separate bacterial meningitis from the other conditions in this group. Viral meningitis is associated with an increase of LDH-1,2 and LDH-3 isoenzymes, whereas bacterial meningitis is associated with an increase of LDH-4,5 isoenzymes.

## NORMAL VALUES

One-tenth of serum values.

## COST

Low.

## ADDITIONAL TESTS TO ORDER

CBC, chemistry panel, sedimentation rate, CSF analysis, CSF smear and cultures, acute and convalescent phase serum for viral studies, CT scan, and neurology consult.

**LACTIC ACID DEHYDROGENASE, CEREBROSPINAL FLUID**

```
LACTIC ACID DEHYDROGENASE, CEREBROSPINAL FLUID
                         |
        ┌────────────────┴────────────────┐
     INCREASED                          NORMAL
        |                                  |
     CULTURES                       VIRAL MENINGITIS
                                    (OCCASIONALLY
                                    MAY BE POSITIVE)
   ┌─────┴──────────────┐
POSITIVE              NEGATIVE
   |                     |
BACTERIAL          LEUKEMIA,
MENINGITIS         LYMPHOMA,
                   SUBARACHNOID
                   HEMORRHAGE,
                   METASTATIC
                   CARCINOMA
```

# LACTIC ACID DEHYDROGENASE (LDH) ISOZYMES

Separation of the lactic dehydrogenase isozymes is helpful in diagnosing myocardial infarction and pulmonary infarction.

## INCREASED LDH-1,2

This most likely results from a myocardial infarction, but hemolytic anemia, renal infarct, and pernicious anemia can also be the cause.

## INCREASED LDH-3

This is typical of pulmonary infarction but is also found in other pulmonary diseases.

## INCREASED LDH-4,5

This is typical of liver disease.

## NORMAL VALUES

Vary with the laboratory.

## COST

Low.

## ADDITIONAL TESTS TO ORDER

CBC, urinalysis, chemistry panel, liver function tests, MB–CPK, lung scan, chest radiograph, ECG, arterial blood gases, and cardiology or pulmonology consult.

## LACTIC ACID DEHYDROGENASE ISOZYMES

INCREASED
LDH-1, 2

INCREASED
LDH-3

INCREASED
LDH-4, 5

MYOCARDIAL
INFARCT,
HEMOLYTIC
ANEMIA,
RENAL INFARCT,
PERNICIOUS
ANEMIA

PULMONARY
INFARCT,
PNEUMONIA

LIVER DISEASE

# LACTOSE TOLERANCE

## POSITIVE

Glucose fails to rise after loading dose of oral lactose, indicating deficiency of the enzyme lactase in the intestine.

## NORMAL VALUES

A rise of at least 20 mg/dL in serum glucose between 30 minutes and an hour after a lactose load.

## COST

Low.

## ADDITIONAL TESTS TO ORDER

Analysis of respiratory hydrogen before and after lactose load (hydrogen breath analysis), D-xylose absorption, and other tests of malabsorption syndrome (see page 613). Consult a gastroenterologist.

# LAPAROSCOPY

## POSITIVE

Positive results are obtained with this test in endometriosis, salpingitis, tuberculous peritonitis, ovarian cysts and tumors, uterine fibroids, ectopic pregnancy, cirrhosis of the liver, metastatic carcinoma of the liver, and pancreatic conditions. The cause of ascites can often be found. This test may be useful in the infertility workup.

## NORMAL VALUES

Normal appearance of abdominal and pelvic organs.

## COST

High.

## ADDITIONAL TESTS TO ORDER

CBC, sedimentation rate, chemistry panel, liver function tests, plain films of abdomen, CT scan of abdomen and pelvis, ultrasonography, liver and pancreatic scan, peritoneal fluid analysis, gynecology consult, and gastroenterology consult.

# *LEGIONELLA* ANTIBODY

## INCREASED

This antibody is increased in *Legionella* infections. False-positive results occur in patients with *Yersinia, Bacteroides fragilis, Mycoplasma pneumoniae,* and other infections.

## NORMAL VALUES

Negative or no significant change in titer from one specimen to another.

## COST

Low.

## ADDITIONAL TESTS TO ORDER

CBC, sedimentation rate, sputum culture, cold agglutinins, chest radiograph, and pulmonary consult.

# LEPTOSPIROSIS ANTIBODY TITER

## INCREASED

These antibodies are increased in Weil's disease and aseptic meningitis from other forms of leptospirosis. This test is expensive, so one should have a high index of suspicion before ordering it.

## NORMAL VALUES

Negative.

## COST

Medium.

## ADDITIONAL TESTS TO ORDER

CBC, urinalysis, chemistry panel, sedimentation rate, blood smears, dark field examination, spinal fluid analysis, guinea pig inoculation, and consultation with an infectious disease expert.

# LEUCINE AMINOPEPTIDASE, (LAP), BLOOD, URINE

## INCREASED

Ask the following questions:

1. What is the transaminase (ALT, AST)? A significant elevation of the transaminase in the face of an increased leucine aminopeptidase (LAP) indicates hepatitis, cirrhosis, or infectious mononucleosis.
2. What is the direct bilirubin? A marked increase of the direct bilirubin suggests obstructive jaundice, pancreatic carcinoma, or other neoplasms of the biliary tree. A normal or modest increase of the direct bilirubin suggests choledocholithiasis or liver metastasis. A CT scan of the abdomen often differentiates these conditions. When attempting to differentiate the cause of an elevated alkaline phosphatase, one should order an LAP test. The LAP test is increased when the alkaline phosphatase elevation is caused by liver disease, but it is normal when it is caused by bone disease.

## NORMAL VALUES

Blood: Less than 50 U/L.
Urine: 2−18 U/24 hours.

## COST

Low.

## ADDITIONAL TESTS TO ORDER

CBC, chemistry panel, urinalysis, sedimentation rate, gallbladder ultrasound, hepatitis profile, HIDA test, CT scan of abdomen, ERCP, and gastroenterology consult.

**LEUCINE AMINOPEPTIDASE, BLOOD OR URINE**

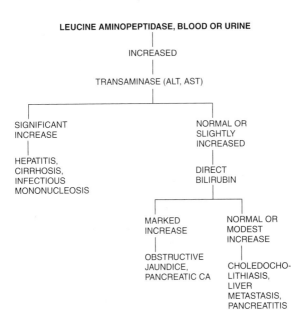

# LEUKOCYTE ALKALINE PHOSPHATASE

## INCREASED

Leukocyte alkaline phosphatase is increased in leukemoid reactions, polycythemia vera, and myeloid metaplasia. The *RBC* helps to differentiate these three conditions. This value is obviously increased in polycythemia vera, usually normal in leukemoid reactions, and decreased in myeloid metaplasia.

## DECREASED

Leukocyte alkaline phosphatase is decreased in acute and chronic myelogenous leukemia, a feature that makes it especially useful in differentiating this condition from myeloid metaplasia and leukemoid reactions. It is also decreased in infectious mononucleosis, hereditary hypophosphatasia, aplastic anemia, and paroxysmal nocturnal hemoglobinuria. To differentiate most of these conditions, one should look at the *WBC*. It is increased in myelogenous leukemia and infectious mononucleosis and is decreased in aplastic anemia. It is normal in the other two conditions.

## NORMAL VALUES

30–130 U/L (may vary from one laboratory to another).

## COST

Low.

## ADDITIONAL TESTS TO ORDER

CBC, platelet count, chemistry panel, Ham test, bone marrow examination, bone marrow biopsy, serum $B_{12}$

level, heterophil antibody titer, blood cultures, and
hematology consult.

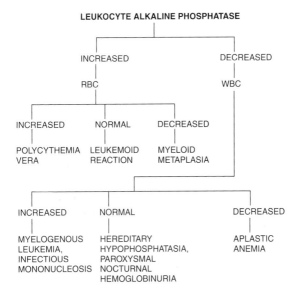

**LEUKOCYTE ALKALINE PHOSPHATASE**

# LIPASE

## INCREASED

Lipase is most often increased in acute pancreatitis. It is also increased in obstructive jaundice, cholecystitis, cirrhosis, chronic pancreatitis, pancreatic carcinoma, and the administration of certain drugs. To differentiate these conditions further, one should obtain a serum or urine amylase. If this value is markedly increased, the patient probably has acute pancreatitis.

A normal or slightly increased amylase associated with an increased lipase may mean liver disease, cholecystitis, or slowly developing pancreatic disease. To differentiate these further, liver function tests are indicated. If results are abnormal, one should consider liver disease or cholecystitis. If these are normal, one should consider occult pancreatic carcinoma or chronic pancreatitis.

## NORMAL VALUES

$< 125$ U/L.

## COST

Low.

## ADDITIONAL TESTS TO ORDER

CBC, urinalysis, chemistry panel, liver function tests, hepatitis panel, gallbladder ultrasonography, ERCP, flat plate and upright of the abdomen, duodenal analysis, liver biopsy, surgery consult, and gastroenterology consult.

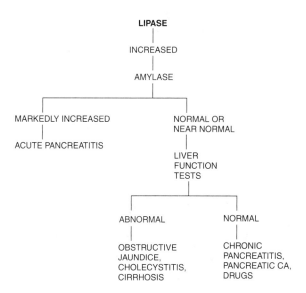

**LIPASE**

INCREASED

AMYLASE

MARKEDLY INCREASED

ACUTE PANCREATITIS

NORMAL OR
NEAR NORMAL

LIVER
FUNCTION
TESTS

ABNORMAL

OBSTRUCTIVE
JAUNDICE,
CHOLECYSTITIS,
CIRRHOSIS

NORMAL

CHRONIC
PANCREATITIS,
PANCREATIC CA,
DRUGS

# LIPOPROTEIN ELECTROPHORESIS

Lipoprotein electrophoresis can be used to separate the various types of cholesterol and in this way *diagnose* the *various types of lipoproteinemias.* Lipoprotein electrophoresis has replaced the more tedious and time-consuming method of separating these lipids, but the classification developed by ultracentrifugation remains. Consequently, cholesterol is separated into LDL, VLDL, and HDL. On electrophoresis, these separate into three bands: $\beta$, which is LDL, pre-$\beta$, which is VLDL, and $\alpha$, which is HDL. Chylomicrons also separate in this procedure.

## INCREASED CHYLOMICRONS

Chylomicrons are increased in type I and type II lipoproteinemia.

## INCREASED $\beta$ BAND (LDL)

LDL is increased in types IIa, IIb, and III lipoproteinemia. It is primarily triglycerides.

## INCREASED PRE-$\beta$ BAND (VLDL)

VLDL is increased in types IIb, IV, and V lipoproteinemia.

## INCREASED $\alpha$ BAND (HDL)

HDL is *increased* in liver disease and alcoholism and decreased in smokers and patients with increased risk of coronary disease.

## NORMAL VALUES

$\beta$ band (LDL): 25–50%.
Pre-$\beta$ band (VLDL): 60–185 mg/dL.
$\alpha$ band (HDL): 35–100 mg/dL.
Chylomicrons: Not present.

## COST

Low to medium.

## ADDITIONAL TESTS TO ORDER

Cholesterol, triglyceride, overnight refrigeration of plasma, chemistry panel, amylase and lipase, blood alcohol level, free $T_4$, 24-hour urine protein, liver biopsy, renal biopsy, coronary angiography, and consultation with a metabolic disease specialist or endocrinologist.

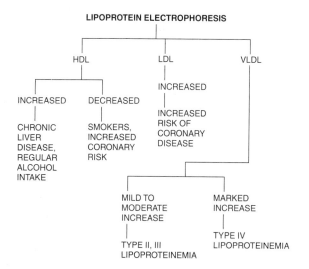

# LIVER SCAN

## POSITIVE

This scan is positive in liver tumors, abscesses, and cysts. It also can help to diagnose cirrhosis and the cause of jaundice. Metastases to the liver can frequently be detected. It is largely being replaced by the CT scan, but it is a cheaper test.

## NORMAL VALUES

Homogeneous uptake of radioactive material and no filling defects or deformities.

## COST

Medium.

## ADDITIONAL TESTS TO ORDER

Liver function tests, CT scan of abdomen, and gastro-enterology or surgical consult.

# LIVER ULTRASONOGRAPHY

## POSITIVE

This test is positive in cysts, abscess, and neoplasms of the liver. It is especially useful in differentiating a cyst or abscess from a tumor. It is also useful in diagnosing pleural effusion and ascites. A cirrhotic liver can be detected by multiple echoes. The gallbladder and biliary tree can be visualized in common duct obstruction.

## NORMAL VALUES

Normal size, shape, and position of liver and biliary tree, homogeneous parenchyma.

## COST

Medium.

## ADDITIONAL TESTS TO ORDER

Liver function tests, liver scan, CT scan of the liver, HIDA scan, gallbladder ultrasonography, oral cholecystography, ERCP, transhepatic cholangiography, liver biopsy, and gastroenterology consult.

# LONG-ACTING THYROID STIMULATOR (LATS)

## INCREASED

This substance is increased in Graves' disease and exophthalmos without hyperthyroidism.

## NORMAL VALUES

None is detected in 95% of healthy adults.

## COST

Low.

## ADDITIONAL TESTS TO ORDER

Free $T_4$, TSH, TRH stimulation test, RAI uptake and scan, endocrinology consult, and ophthalmology consult.

# LYME DISEASE ANTIBODY

## POSITIVE

This test is positive in Lyme disease. False-positives occur in syphilis, persons living in endemic areas, and tick-borne relapsing fever.

## NORMAL VALUES

Negative.

## COST

Low.

## ADDITIONAL TESTS TO ORDER

No other clinically useful tests are available at this time.

# LYMPHANGIOGRAPHY

## POSITIVE

This test demonstrates large lymph nodes in lymphoma, lymphosarcoma, and metastatic neoplasms. It also demonstrates abnormal lymphatics. Therefore, it can be used to diagnose unexplained edema of the lower extremities. It is also helpful in the staging of lymphomas.

## NORMAL VALUES

Normal-sized lymphatics and lymph nodes.

## COST

Medium.

## ADDITIONAL TESTS TO ORDER

CBC, chemistry panel, sedimentation rate, CT scan of abdomen, pelvis and chest, exploratory laparotomy, and oncology consult.

# LYSOZYME, BLOOD AND URINE

## INCREASED

This substance is increased in acute myelomonocytic leukemia, chronic myelogenous leukemia, sarcoidosis, Crohn's disease, tuberculosis, megaloblastic anemia, acute bacterial infections, and renal disease.

## NORMAL VALUES

Blood: 2.8–15.8 $\mu$g/mL.
Urine: 3 mg/24 hours.

## COST

Low.

## ADDITIONAL TESTS TO ORDER

CBC, chemistry panel, sedimentation rate, urinalysis, urine culture, bone marrow examination, lymph node biopsy, chest radiograph, Kveim test, tuberculin test, small bowel series, and hematology consult.

# MAGNESIUM

## INCREASED

Ask the following questions:

1. What is the BUN? Increased serum magnesium is common in acute and chronic renal failure.
2. What is the blood sugar? The magnesium is increased in diabetic acidosis and in elderly patients with controlled diabetes.

If the BUN and blood sugar are normal, one should consider Addison's disease, hypothyroidism, dehydration, diuretics, and lithium therapy as possible causes.

## DECREASED

Ask the following questions:

1. Are the liver function tests abnormal? A common cause of hypomagnesemia is alcoholism and cirrhosis.
2. Does the patient have significant diarrhea? The loss of magnesium in watery stools is remarkable in ulcerative colitis, chronic pancreatitis, hyperthyroidism, and malabsorption syndrome.

If the liver function tests are normal and the patient does not have significant diarrhea, one should consider toxemia of pregnancy, chronic nephritis, aldosteronism, diuretic use, and the use of other drugs.

## NORMAL VALUES

1.5–2.5 mEq/L.

## COST

Low.

## ADDITIONAL TESTS TO ORDER

CBC, urinalysis, chemistry panel, serial electrolytes, arterial blood gases, blood ammonia level, D-xylose absorption, plasma renin, 24-hour urine aldosterone, removal of all drugs, free $T_4$, endocrinology consult, and nephrology consult.

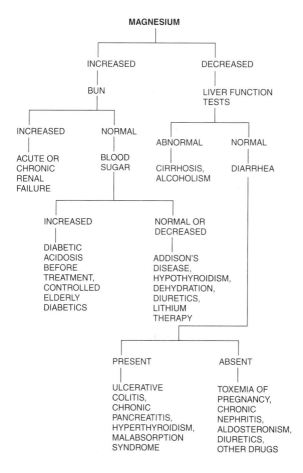

# MAGNETIC RESONANCE IMAGING (MRI), ABDOMEN

## POSITIVE

This test is positive in malignant diseases and abscess of the abdominal organs. In some circumstances, it is superior to the CT scan. It can help to differentiate *retroperitoneal lymph nodes* from other structures. It can be valuable in differentiating liver and adrenal tumors. It can distinguish benign cavernous hemangiomas from malignant tumors. It can show stenosis or obstruction of the aorta and its branches. The CT scan is superior in showing the GI tract.

## NORMAL VALUES

Normal size, shape, and position of abdominal organs, homogeneous parenchyma.

## COST

Very high.

## ADDITIONAL TESTS TO ORDER

Plain films of abdomen, upper GI series and esophagogram, small bowel series, barium enema, CT scan of abdomen, endoscopy, biopsy, cholecystography, ultrasonography, radionuclide scans, and gastroenterology consult.

# MAGNETIC RESONANCE IMAGING (MRI), BRAIN

## POSITIVE

This study can be used to diagnose almost all intracranial disorders, including hematomas, brain tumors, infarcts, large aneurysms and A-V malformations, degenerative disorders such as Alzheimer's disease, congenital disorders such as porencephalic cysts and hydrocephalus, multiple sclerosis and other demyelinating diseases, and infectious diseases. MRI is superior to CT scans in diagnosing multiple sclerosis.

MRI of the brain is indicated in determining the cause of headaches, vertigo, seizures, hemiparesis, paresthesias, memory disorders, speech disorders, and cranial nerve palsies. It is indicated to rule out intracranial bleeding after trauma to the head and neck, but it is not as valuable as the CT scan in the first 48 hours. MR angiography can be valuable in detecting smaller aneurysms and focal vascular lesions.

## NORMAL VALUES

Homogeneous cerebral, cerebellar, and brainstem tissue without displacement or mass lesions. Normal pituitary size and shape.

## COST

Very high.

## ADDITIONAL TESTS TO ORDER

CT scan, spinal fluid analysis and culture, cisternography, radioisotope brain scan, EEG, psychometric studies, and neurology or psychiatric consult.

# MAGNETIC RESONANCE IMAGING (MRI), CHEST

## POSITIVE

This test can enable one to diagnose mediastinal tumors, aortic aneurysms, congenital heart disease, rheumatic valvulitis, and other mediastinal masses. It is useful in staging of tumors.

## NORMAL VALUES

Normal size, shape, and position of structures of the chest. No tumor or other mass lesions.

## COST

Very high.

## ADDITIONAL TESTS TO ORDER

Chest radiograph, mediastinoscopy, CT scan of chest, echocardiography, cardiology consult, and consultation with a thoracic surgeon.

# MAGNETIC RESONANCE IMAGING (MRI), JOINTS

## POSITIVE

MRI is superior to CT in diagnosis of pathologic processes in the joints. Positive findings may be torn meniscus, torn anterior or posterior cruciate ligament, torn rotator cuff, synovial inflammation, malignant tumors of the joint, aseptic necrosis, and septic arthritis.

## NORMAL VALUES

Normal tissue layers, normal architecture of joint, no mass or inflammation.

## COST

Very high.

## ADDITIONAL TESTS TO ORDER

CBC, chemistry panel, RA test, ANA, sedimentation rate, ASO titer, CRP, synovial analysis, plain films of the joint, CT scan of joint, arthrography, arthroscopy, bone scan, and orthopedic consult.

## COST CONSIDERATIONS

The MRI is usually double the price of a CT scan and other imaging studies. The clinician must be certain that this extra cost is worthwhile. For example, in screening patients presenting with neurologic symptoms but no objective neurologic findings for possible brain tumor, a CT scan usually provides adequate information. Unfortunately, too often the patient is not satisfied unless the more sophisticated study is done.

# MAGNETIC RESONANCE IMAGING (MRI), NECK

## POSITIVE

This test is positive in malignant tumors of the neck, lymphadenopathy, thyroid tumors, parathyroid adenomas, brachial plexopathy, aneurysms, retropharyngeal abscess, and esophageal diverticula. MR angiography can show carotid stenosis.

## NORMAL VALUES

Normal size, shape, and position of cervical structures. No mass lesions noted.

## COST

Very high.

## ADDITIONAL TESTS TO ORDER

RAI uptake and scan, ultrasonography, carotid duplex scan, biopsy, endocrinology consult, surgical consult, and oncology consult.

# MAGNETIC RESONANCE IMAGING (MRI), PELVIS

## POSITIVE

This is especially valuable in diagnosing gynecologic malignant diseases (cervical, endometrial and vaginal). It is also of assistance in diagnosing prostate, bladder, and rectal carcinoma and their spread. It is useful in detecting retroperitoneal lymphadenopathy.

## NORMAL VALUES

Normal size, shape, and position of pelvic organs. No mass lesions.

## COST

Very high.

## ADDITIONAL TESTS TO ORDER

Urinalysis, CT scan of abdomen, Pap smear, colposcopy, cystoscopy, sigmoidoscopy, ultrasonography, laproscopy, hysterosalpingography, gynecology consult, and urology consult.

# MAGNETIC RESONANCE IMAGING (MRI), SPINE

## POSITIVE

This test is positive in spinal cord tumors, herniated discs, cervical spondylosis, transverse myelitis, multiple sclerosis, congenital anomalies, vascular disorders, and degenerative disease of the spinal cord. It is not superior to the CT scan in detecting fractures, osteophytic spurs, and calcification. It is superior to the CT scan in the diagnosis of herniated discs and radiculopathy.

## NORMAL VALUES

Normal size, shape, and position of spinal cord, nerve roots, and structures of the spine. No mass lesions noted.

## COST

Very high.

## ADDITIONAL TESTS TO ORDER

CBC, urinalysis, chemistry panel, sedimentation rate, EMG, nerve conduction studies, dermatomal somatosensory-evoked potential (DSEP) study, bone scan, plain films of spine, CT scan, and neurology or neurosurgical consult.

# MAMMOGRAPHY

## POSITIVE

This test is positive in benign and malignant tumors of the breast. It is useful in diagnosing the cause of breast masses, nipple discharges, and breast pain. Patients with a definite lump in the breast should have a diagnostic mammogram, not just a screening mammogram.

## NORMAL VALUES

Homogeneous breast tissue with no mass identified.

## COST

Medium.

## ADDITIONAL TESTS TO ORDER

Ultrasonography, fine-needle aspiration, MRI, ductography, breast biopsy, surgical consult, and oncology consult.

# MEAN CORPUSCULAR HEMOGLOBIN (MCH)

## INCREASED

An increased MCH suggests sprue, malabsorption syndrome, folic acid deficiency, and pernicious anemia. To differentiate pernicious anemia from the other disorders, a Schilling test is performed. This is abnormal in pernicious anemia.

## DECREASED

A decreased MCH is typical of thalassemia, sickle cell anemia, iron-deficiency anemia, and anemia of chronic blood loss. To further differentiate this group, a serum iron determination should be obtained. Serum iron is decreased in iron-deficiency anemia and anemia of chronic blood loss, whereas it is increased in thalassemia and sickle cell anemia.

## NORMAL VALUES

27–32 pg.

## COST

Low.

## ADDITIONAL TESTS TO ORDER

CBC, platelet count, sedimentation rate, red cell fragility, serum haptoglobins, red-cell survival, serum iron and IBC, stool for occult blood, serum B$_{12}$ and folic acid, Schilling test, bone marrow, and hematology consult.

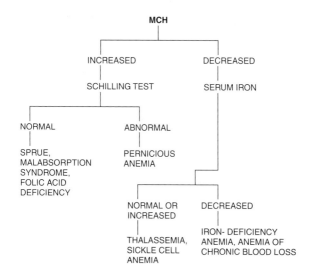

# MEAN CORPUSCULAR HEMOGLOBIN CONCENTRATION (MCHC)

## INCREASED

An MCHC suggests hereditary spherocytosis.

## DECREASED

A decreased MCHC suggests iron-deficiency anemia, anemia of chronic blood loss, sideroblastic anemia, and thalassemia. To differentiate these, a serum iron determination should be obtained. If the serum iron is decreased, one should consider iron-deficiency anemia or anemia of chronic blood loss. If the serum iron is normal or increased, one should consider sideroblastic anemia or thalassemia.

## NORMAL VALUES

32–36%.

## COST

Low.

## ADDITIONAL TESTS TO ORDER

CBC, platelet count, blood smear, indices, serum iron and IBC, sedimentation rate, serum haptoglobins, hemoglobin electrophoresis, stool for occult blood, red cell fragility, bone marrow examination, and hematology consult.

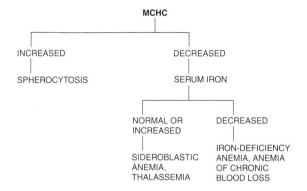

# MEAN CORPUSCULAR VOLUME (MCV)

## INCREASED

If the MCV is increased, one should look for a large liver. If present, alcoholism, cirrhosis, folic acid deficiency, and sideroblastic anemia should be considered. If absent, one should consider pernicious anemia, sprue, folic acid deficiency, hemolytic anemia, and hypothyroidism.

## DECREASED

A decreased MCV is associated with iron-deficiency anemia, anemia of chronic blood loss, thalassemia, and sickle cell disease. To differentiate these, one should order a serum iron and IBC. If these values are decreased, then the patient probably has iron-deficiency anemia or anemia of chronic blood loss. If not, the patient may have thalassemia or sickle cell anemia. Red cell fragility testing further confirms the latter two diagnoses.

## NORMAL VALUES

07–103 cu $\mu$m/rod coll.

## COST

Low.

## ADDITIONAL TESTS TO ORDER

CBC, chemistry panel, platelet count, blood smear, MCH, MCHC, serum $B_{12}$ and folic acid, stool for occult blood, sickle cell preparation, reticulocyte count, serum iron and IBC, bone marrow examination, free $T_4$, Schilling test, and hematology consult.

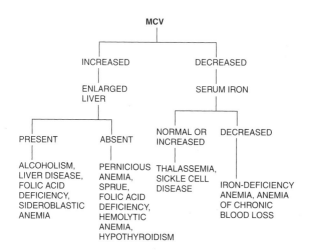

# MELANIN, URINE

## POSITIVE

The presence of melanin in the urine should make one suspect metastatic melanoma.

## NORMAL VALUES

Negative.

## COST

Low.

## ADDITIONAL TESTS TO ORDER

Skin biopsy, lymph node biopsy, nuclear scans, CT scans, dermatology consult, and oncology consult.

# MEDIASTINOSCOPY

## POSITIVE

This test helps to diagnose mediastinitis, sarcoidosis, tuberculosis, fungal diseases of the lung, Hodgkin's disease, thymoma, and carcinoma of the lungs. It can also be used to assess the extent of carcinoma of the lung. Biopsies are often taken.

## NORMAL VALUES

No evidence of infection, neoplasm, or lymphadenopathy.

## COST

High.

## ADDITIONAL TESTS TO ORDER

CBC, urinalysis, chemistry panel, sedimentation rate, tuberculin test, Kveim test, fungal skin tests, sputum analysis and culture, sputum cytology, chest radiograph, bronchoscopy, CT scan of chest, needle biopsy, scalene node biopsy, pulmonary consult, and surgical consult.

# METHEMOGLOBIN

## INCREASED

1. Does the patient have a history of drug or chemical ingestion? This suggests toxic methemoglobinemia caused by nitrites, nitrates, chlorates, chloroquine, quinones, benzenes, toluene, sulfonamides, aniline dye, and phenacetin, for example.
2. Does the patient have a family history? This suggests enzymatic or metabolic disorders such as NADH-methemoglobin reductase deficiency, as well as HgM disease.
3. If none of the foregoing questions is positive, blackwater fever and paroxysmal hemoglobinuria should be suspected.

## NORMAL VALUES

0.5–1.5%.

## COST

Low.

## ADDITIONAL TESTS TO ORDER

CBC, blood smear, urine drug screen, hemoglobin electrophoresis, urinalysis, chemistry panel, VDRL, serum haptoglobins, and toxicology consult.

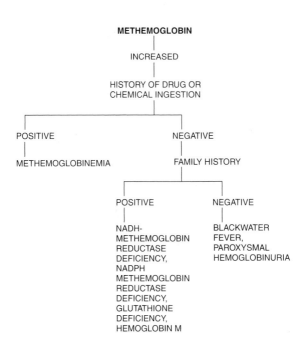

**METHEMOGLOBIN**
|
INCREASED
|
HISTORY OF DRUG OR
CHEMICAL INGESTION

POSITIVE
|
METHEMOGLOBINEMIA

NEGATIVE
|
FAMILY HISTORY

POSITIVE
|
NADH-
METHEMOGLOBIN
REDUCTASE
DEFICIENCY,
NADPH
METHEMOGLOBIN
REDUCTASE
DEFICIENCY,
GLUTATHIONE
DEFICIENCY,
HEMOGLOBIN M

NEGATIVE
|
BLACKWATER
FEVER,
PAROXYSMAL
HEMOGLOBINURIA

# METYRAPONE TEST

1. *No response:* No response to the administration of 3g metyrapone means that the plasma cortisol, ACTH and 11-deoxycortisol do not change significantly, and an adrenal tumor should be suspected.
2. *Decreased plasma cortisol and increased ACTH and 11-deoxycortisol:* This signifies either Cushing's disease (marked increase of ACTH and 11-deoxycortisol) or a normal response (mild increase in ACTH and 11-deoxycortisol).
3. *Decreased plasma cortisol, no increase of ACTH or 11-deoxycortisol:* This signifies pituitary insufficiency.

## NORMAL VALUES

See item No. 2 above.

## COST

Low to medium.

## ADDITIONAL TESTS TO ORDER

CBC, eosinophil count, plasma cortisol, plasma ACTH, dexamethasone suppression test, ACTH-stimulation test, CT scan of brain and abdomen, and endocrinology consult.

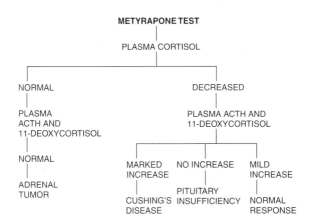

**METYRAPONE TEST**

PLASMA CORTISOL

NORMAL

PLASMA
ACTH AND
11-DEOXYCORTISOL

NORMAL

ADRENAL
TUMOR

DECREASED

PLASMA ACTH AND
11-DEOXYCORTISOL

MARKED
INCREASE

CUSHING'S
DISEASE

NO INCREASE

PITUITARY
INSUFFICIENCY

MILD
INCREASE

NORMAL
RESPONSE

# MINIMUM INHIBITORY CONCENTRATION (MIC)

## INTERPRETATION

Once a positive blood culture is obtained, the organism can be grown in a solution containing various antibiotics in various dilutions. The MIC is the lowest concentration that inhibits the growth of the organism in the solution. By this means, the clinician can determine the antibiotic of choice and the dosage.

## INDICATIONS

This test is indicated whenever blood culture is positive for a pathogenic organism.

## NORMAL VALUES

The lowest concentration that prevents the growth of the organism in question.

## COST

Low to medium.

# MONOSPOT TEST

## POSITIVE

A positive test indicates acute infectious mononucleosis.

## NEGATIVE

A negative test does not rule out infectious mononucleosis. The clinician should order a heterophil antibody test with guinea pig absorption.

## POSITIVE HETEROPHIL ANTIBODY TEST

This indicates acute infectious mononucleosis.

## NEGATIVE HETEROPHIL ANTIBODY TEST

The patient may still have infectious mononucleosis. One should obtain an Epstein–Barr antibody titer for both IgM and IgG antibodies. IgM antibodies indicate active disease. IgG antibodies are not an indication of infectious mononucleosis. If no IgM antibodies are present, serologic tests should be done for cytomegalovirus and toxoplasmosis.

## NORMAL VALUES

Negative.

## COST

Low.

## ADDITIONAL TESTS TO ORDER

CBC, look for atypical lymphocytes, chemistry panel, hepatitis profile, liver biopsy, and consultation with an infectious disease specialist.

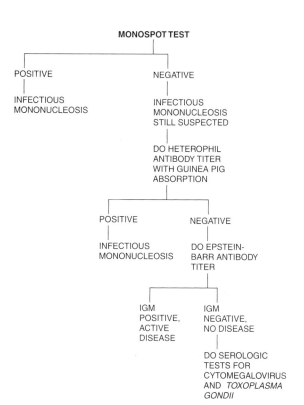

**MONOSPOT TEST**

POSITIVE

INFECTIOUS
MONONUCLEOSIS

NEGATIVE

INFECTIOUS
MONONUCLEOSIS
STILL SUSPECTED

DO HETEROPHIL
ANTIBODY TITER
WITH GUINEA PIG
ABSORPTION

POSITIVE

INFECTIOUS
MONONUCLEOSIS

NEGATIVE

DO EPSTEIN-
BARR ANTIBODY
TITER

IGM
POSITIVE,
ACTIVE
DISEASE

IGM
NEGATIVE,
NO DISEASE

DO SEROLOGIC
TESTS FOR
CYTOMEGALOVIRUS
AND *TOXOPLASMA
GONDII*

# MUCOPOLYSACCHARIDE SCREEN, URINE

## POSITIVE

This test is positive in Hurler's syndrome and other rare mucopolysaccharidoses.

## NORMAL VALUES

Negative.

## COST

Low.

## ADDITIONAL TESTS TO ORDER

Tissue culture of skin biopsy fibroblasts with an assay for the specific enzyme that causes the disorder, skull radiograph and skeletal survey, and consultation with an expert in metabolic or genetic disorders.

# MUCOPROTEINS

## INCREASED

Ask the following questions:

1. What is the RA test? An increased RA factor distinguishes rheumatoid arthritis from the rest of the group.
2. What is the HLA−B27? A positive HLA−B27 distinguishes ankylosing spondylitis from the rest of the group. Neoplasms and infections can also cause increased serum mucoproteins.

## DECREASED

Mucoproteins are decreased in liver disease.

## NORMAL VALUES

85−205 mg/L.

## COST

Low.

## ADDITIONAL TESTS TO ORDER

CBC, urinalysis, chemistry panel, RA test, HLA−B27 antigen, sedimentation rate, CT scan of abdomen, liver biopsy, radiograph of joints, and oncology consult.

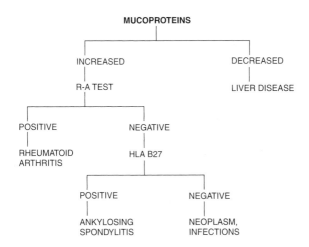

**MUCOPROTEINS**

INCREASED

R-A TEST

POSITIVE

RHEUMATOID
ARTHRITIS

NEGATIVE

HLA B27

POSITIVE

ANKYLOSING
SPONDYLITIS

NEGATIVE

NEOPLASM,
INFECTIONS

DECREASED

LIVER DISEASE

# MYELIN BASIC PROTEIN, CEREBROSPINAL FLUID

## INCREASED

This substance is increased in the CSF in *multiple sclerosis* and numerous other demyelinating diseases.

## NORMAL VALUES

Less than 4 ng/mL.

## COST

Low to medium.

## ADDITIONAL TESTS TO ORDER

Spinal fluid γ-globulin, visual evoked potentials, somatosensory evoked potentials, MRI of brain and spinal cord, and neurology consult.

# MYELOGRAPHY

## POSITIVE

This test is used to diagnose ruptured or herniated discs, spinal cord and cauda equina neoplasms, subarachnoid block, syringomyelia, cervical spondylosis, vertebral fractures, epidural abscess, spinal cord hematomas, and many congenital anomalies of the spine. Three types of examinations are requested: lumbar, thoracic, and cervical myelography. When this procedure is combined with a CT scan, the accuracy and yield of positive results increase.

## NORMAL VALUES

Normal size, shape, and position of spinal cord, nerve roots and spinal structures. No obstruction or filling defects.

## COST

High.

## ADDITIONAL TESTS TO ORDER

CSF analysis, CT scan of spine, MRI of spine (specify which level), bone scans, plain radiograph films of spine, chemistry panel, PSA, EMG, nerve conduction studies, dermatomal somatosensory-evoked potential (DSEP) study, and neurology or neurosurgical consult.

# MYOGLOBIN, BLOOD AND URINE

## INCREASED

The blood and urine myoglobin is increased in myocardial infarction and skeletal muscle disorders such as trauma, myopathies, polymyositis, burns, alcoholic myopathy, surgical trauma, acute alcoholism, epileptic seizures, and viral and bacterial infections. To separate these disorders from myocardial infarction, one should order an MB–CPK. This value is elevated in myocardial infarction and is normal or near normal in skeletal muscle disorders.

## NORMAL VALUES

Blood: 30–90 ng/mL.
Urine: 0–2 $\mu$g/mL.

## COST

Low.

## ADDITIONAL TESTS TO ORDER

CBC, urinalysis, chemistry panel, MB–CPK, ECG, sedimentation rate, ANA, CRP, blood cultures, and cardiology consult.

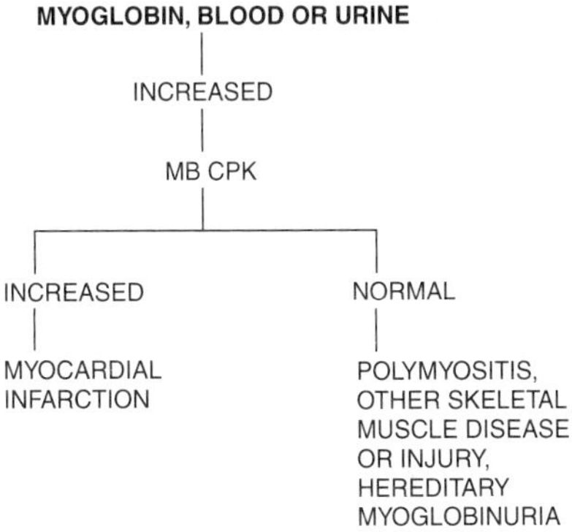

**MYOGLOBIN, BLOOD OR URINE**

INCREASED

MB CPK

INCREASED

MYOCARDIAL
INFARCTION

NORMAL

POLYMYOSITIS,
OTHER SKELETAL
MUSCLE DISEASE
OR INJURY,
HEREDITARY
MYOGLOBINURIA

# NERVE CONDUCTION STUDIES

## POSITIVE

These studies are positive in peripheral neuropathy (e.g., diabetic neuropathy, alcoholic neuropathy) and entrapment syndromes such as carpal tunnel syndrome, tarsal tunnel syndrome, and tardy ulnar palsy. They are indicated whenever disease of the peripheral nerves are suspected. The algorithm separates the abnormalities found in nerve conduction studies into two groups. Increased distal latencies are found in entrapment neuropathy such as carpal tunnel syndrome. Decreased velocity is found in neuropathy. If the neuropathy is focal, one should consider trauma, mononeuritis multiplex, diabetes, and lead intoxication. If the neuropathy is diffuse, one should consider diabetes mellitus, hypothyroidism, alcohol, nutrition, and hereditary disorders.

## NORMAL VALUES

Velocity: 40–60 m/second, depending on nerve studied.
Distal Latency: 3.0–4.5 milliseconds, depending on nerve tested (check with the laboratory).

## COST

Medium.

## ADDITIONAL TESTS TO ORDER

See page 233.

**NERVE CONDUCTION STUDIES**

```
                    NERVE CONDUCTION STUDIES
          |                         |
    DISTAL                      VELOCITY
    LATENCY                         |
          |                     DECREASED
    INCREASED                       |
          |              _____|_____
    ENTRAPMENT          |                       |
    NEUROPATHY       FOCAL                   DIFFUSE
          |             |                       |
    CARPAL TUNNEL   MONONEUROPATHY         POLYNEUROPATHY
    SYNDROME,
    TARSAL TUNNEL
    SYNDROME, ETC.
```

DISTAL
LATENCY

INCREASED

ENTRAPMENT
NEUROPATHY

CARPAL TUNNEL
SYNDROME,
TARSAL TUNNEL
SYNDROME, ETC.

VELOCITY

DECREASED

FOCAL

MONONEUROPATHY

CONSIDER
TRAUMA,
MONONEURITIS
MULTIPLEX,
DIABETES
MELLITUS,
LEAD
INTOXICATION,
TARDY ULNAR
PALSY, PERONEAL
NEUROPATHY, ETC.

DIFFUSE

POLYNEUROPATHY

CONSIDER
DIABETES MELLITUS,
HYPOTHYROIDISM,
ALCOHOLISM,
MALNUTRITION,
PORPHYRIA,
HEREDITARY
NEUROPATHY,
GUILLAIN-BARRÉ
SYNDROME, ETC.

# NITRITE TEST

## POSITIVE

This test is positive in urinary tract infections. It is reliable when it is positive. However, false-negative results may occur, especially when a random specimen is used. Random specimens may not have had enough time for conversion of nitrate to nitrite. An overnight specimen is preferred. In addition, on rare occasions, a strain of bacteria does not produce enzymes necessary to convert nitrate to nitrite.

## NORMAL VALUES

Negative.

## COST

Low.

## ADDITIONAL TESTS TO ORDER

Urinalysis, examination of urinary sediment, urine culture and colony count, anaerobic urine culture, IVP, cystoscopy, and urology consult.

# OBSTETRIC ULTRASONOGRAPHY

## POSITIVE

Positive findings include multiple pregnancies, abnormal fetal position, hydrocephalus and other cranial abnormalities of the fetus, placenta previa, abruptio placentae, fetal growth retardation and death, and polyhydramnios. This test can also be used as a pregnancy test (it is positive as early as 4 weeks) and to determine fetal age.

## NORMAL VALUES

Normal size, shape, and position of fetus and placenta.

## COST

Medium.

## ADDITIONAL TESTS TO ORDER

Pregnancy test of blood or urine, urine pregnanediol, serum estriol, amniocentesis, and obstetric consult.

# ORBITAL AND OCULAR ULTRASONOGRAPHY

## POSITIVE

This test is positive in orbital mass lesions, vitreous opacities, hemangiomas, retinal detachment, orbital abscess, foreign bodies, orbital cysts, and alkali burns of the cornea. It is useful in diagnosing the cause of exophthalmos, especially the unilateral type.

## NORMAL VALUES

Normal retinal and other layers of the eyeball, normal retro-orbital tissue.

## COST

Medium.

## ADDITIONAL TESTS TO ORDER

Free $T_4$, radiographs of the orbits, CT scan of the sinuses, brain and orbits, cerebral angiography, and ophthalmology consult.

# OSMOLALITY, SERUM

## INCREASED

Serum osmolality is increased in dehydration, starvation, high-protein diet, cirrhosis, diabetes mellitus, diabetic acidosis, aldosteronism, diabetes insipidus, and hypercalcemia. To differentiate these conditions, urine osmolality should be determined. If the urine osmolality is also increased, then dehydration, starvation, high-protein diet, cirrhosis, and diabetes mellitus are the more likely causes of the increased serum osmolality.

## DECREASED

Decreased serum osmolality occurs in inappropriate ADH secretion, congestive heart failure, Addison's disease, acute renal failure, chronic renal failure, hypokalemia, and compulsive water drinking. A urine osmolality determination shows an increase in inappropriate ADH secretion, congestive heart failure, Addison's disease, and acute renal failure. Urine osmolality is decreased, along with decreased serum osmolality, in chronic renal failure, hypokalemia, and compulsive water drinking.

## NORMAL VALUES

Serum: 285–295 mOsm/L.
Urine: 600–800 mOsm/L.

## COST

Low.

## ADDITIONAL TESTS TO ORDER

CBC, chemistry panel, urinalysis, serum electrolytes, arterial blood gases, blood volume, intake and output,

Fishberg concentration test, Addis count, serum ADH, plasma cortisol, plasma renin, 24-hour urine aldosterone, endocrinology consult, and nephrology consult.

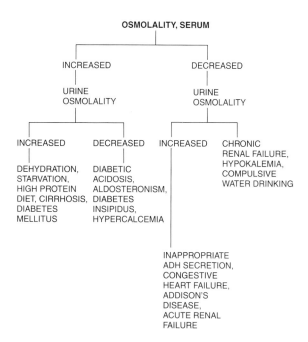

# OVAL FAT BODIES AND FATTY CASTS

## PRESENT

The finding of these bodies and casts is typical of nephrotic syndrome. Nephrotic syndrome may be associated with glomerulonephritis, Kimmelstiel-Wilson disease, lupus erythematosus, and primary lipoid nephrosis.

## NORMAL VALUES

Negative.

## COST

Low.

## ADDITIONAL TESTS TO ORDER

CBC, urinalysis, chemistry panel, ASO titer, CRP, serum complement, ANA, glucose tolerance test, Addis count, Fishberg concentration test, 24-hour urine protein, serum protein electrophoresis, renal biopsy, and nephrology consult.

# OXYGEN, ARTERIAL

## DECREASED

Ask the following questions:

1. What is the carbon dioxide? If the carbon dioxide is *increased*, look for emphysema, asthma, pickwickian syndrome, respiratory paralysis, CNS disease, kyphoscoliosis, and disorders of the chest wall and thoracic spine and drug effects.
2. What does spirometry show? If spirometry shows a *decreased* 1-second timed vital capacity with an increased carbon dioxide, consider emphysema and asthma. If the timed vital capacity is *normal,* look for pickwickian syndrome, respiratory paralysis, CNS disease, chest wall and thoracic spine disorders, and drug effects.
3. If the carbon dioxide is normal or decreased, what does the chest radiograph show? A *focal infiltrate* suggests pulmonary infarction, congestive heart failure, or pneumonia. A *diffuse infiltrate* and *negative* findings suggest congestive heart failure, pulmonary fibrosis, shock, pulmonary or intracardiac shunt, sarcoidosis, or alveolar proteinosis.
4. What does the perfusion lung scan show? If this is positive, consider pulmonary infarction.
5. What does the pulmonary capillary wedge pressure show? If this is increased, consider congestive heart failure. If it is decreased, the patient may have hypovolemic shock. If it is normal, consider a right-to-left shunt or pulmonary fibrosis, pneumoconiosis, or sarcoidosis.

## NORMAL VALUES

83–100 mm.

## COST

Low.

## ADDITIONAL TESTS TO ORDER

Repeated arterial blood gases, CBC, urinalysis, chemistry panel, methemoglobin, sulfhemoglobin, carboxyhemoglobin, venous pressure and circulation time, blood volume, ECG, CT scan of chest, lung biopsy, additional pulmonary function studies, pulmonary consult, and cardiology consult.

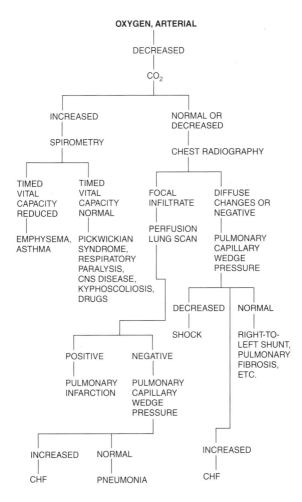

# PANCREATIC SCAN

## POSITIVE

This test is positive in chronic pancreatitis, carcinoma of the pancreas, and pancreatic pseudocysts. It has been largely replaced by the CT scan of the abdomen. Many false-positive results are seen, but few false-negatives.

## NORMAL VALUES

Homogeneous uptake.

## COST

High.

## ADDITIONAL TESTS TO ORDER

CBC, chemistry panel, amylase and lipase, CT scan of abdomen, duodenal analysis, ERCP, ultrasonography, and gastroenterology and surgical consult.

# PANCREATIC ULTRASONOGRAPHY

## POSITIVE

This test is positive in chronic pancreatitis, pancreatic pseudocysts, and pancreatic carcinoma. This may be the best method available to visualize the pancreas.

## NORMAL VALUES

Homogeneous pancreatic tissue with normal size and shape.

## COST

Medium to high.

## ADDITIONAL TESTS TO ORDER

Liver function tests, amylase and lipase, stool for fat and trypsin, duodenal analysis, pancreatic scan, CT scan of abdomen, ERCP, exploratory laparotomy, and gastroenterology consult.

# PARANASAL SINUS RADIOGRAPHY

## ABNORMALITIES

These include fluid levels typical of acute sinusitis, thickening of the wall, which is more typical of chronic sinusitis, polyps, mucoceles, tumors, fractures, and foreign bodies.

## NORMAL VALUES

Sinuses are well aerated and contain no mass or fluid.

## COST

Medium.

## ADDITIONAL TESTS TO ORDER

CBC, sedimentation rate, aspiration and culture, CT scan, nasopharyngoscopy, and ENT consult.

# PARATHYROID HORMONE (PTH)

## INCREASED

PTH is increased in hyperparathyroidism, ectopic parathyroid-producing tumor, renal disease, pseudohypoparathyroidism, vitamin D deficiency with or without rickets or osteomalacia, and malabsorption syndrome. To differentiate among these conditions, one should order a serum calcium. This value is elevated in hyperparathyroidism and ectopic PTH production, but it is decreased in renal disease, pseudohypoparathyroidism, vitamin D deficiency, and malabsorption syndrome.

## DECREASED

PTH is decreased in hypoparathyroidism, sarcoidosis, milk-alkali syndrome, hypervitaminosis D, and Graves' disease. Once again, a serum calcium determination helps to differentiate some of these conditions. This value is low in hypoparathyroidism but normal or increased in the other conditions in this group.

## NORMAL VALUES

10–65 pg/mL.

## COST

Medium.

## ADDITIONAL TESTS TO ORDER

CBC, urinalysis, urine calcium, chemistry panel, C-terminal PTH, skeletal survey, radiograph of teeth, bone scan, ultrasonography of parathyroid glands, free $T_4$, and endocrinology consult.

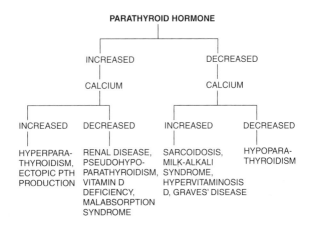

PARATHYROID HORMONE

INCREASED

CALCIUM

INCREASED

HYPERPARA-
THYROIDISM,
ECTOPIC PTH
PRODUCTION

DECREASED

RENAL DISEASE,
PSEUDOHYPO-
PARATHYROIDISM,
VITAMIN D
DEFICIENCY,
MALABSORPTION
SYNDROME

DECREASED

CALCIUM

INCREASED

SARCOIDOSIS,
MILK-ALKALI
SYNDROME,
HYPERVITAMINOSIS
D, GRAVES' DISEASE

DECREASED

HYPOPARA-
THYROIDISM

# PARATHYROID ULTRASONOGRAPHY

## POSITIVE

This test is positive in adenomas of the parathyroid gland and helps to differentiate them from hyperplasia and carcinoma.

## NORMAL VALUES

Homogeneous parathyroid glands of equal size and normal position.

## COST

Medium.

## ADDITIONAL TESTS TO ORDER

Chemistry panel, serial calcium, phosphorus and alkaline phosphatase determinations, serum PTH assay, renal cyclic AMP, skeletal survey, radiographs of teeth, urine calcium, and endocrinology consult.

# PARTIAL THROMBOPLASTIN TIME (PTT) AND ACTIVATED PARTIAL THROMBOPLASTIN TIME (APTT)

## INCREASED

Ask the following questions:

1. Is the bleeding time prolonged? An increased PTT combined with a prolonged bleeding time is found in von Willebrand's disease and disseminated intravascular coagulation.
2. Is the prothrombin time increased? An increased PTT and prothrombin time suggest liver disease, heparin therapy, vitamin K deficiency, and disseminated intravascular coagulation.
3. If both the bleeding time and prothrombin time are normal, look for hemophilia and disorders with circulatory anticoagulants such as tuberculosis, glomerulonephritis, lupus erythematosus, and drug reactions.

## NORMAL VALUES

PTT: 30–45 seconds.
APTT: 16–25 seconds.

## COST

Low.

## ADDITIONAL TESTS TO ORDER

Prothrombin time, bleeding time, platelet count, thrombin time, fibrin split products, ANA, sedimentation rate, and hematology consult.

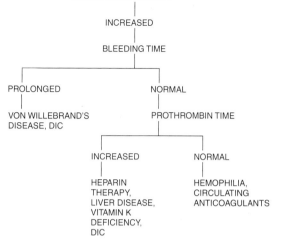

**PARTIAL THROMBOPLASTIN TIME
AND ACTIVATED PARTIAL
THROMBOPLASTIN TIME**

INCREASED

BLEEDING TIME

PROLONGED

VON WILLEBRAND'S
DISEASE, DIC

NORMAL

PROTHROMBIN TIME

INCREASED

HEPARIN
THERAPY,
LIVER DISEASE,
VITAMIN K
DEFICIENCY,
DIC

NORMAL

HEMOPHILIA,
CIRCULATING
ANTICOAGULANTS

# PELVIC ULTRASONOGRAPHY

## POSITIVE

This test is positive in ectopic pregnancy, salpingitis, ovarian cysts and tumors, uterine fibroids, and endometriosis. It is also useful in diagnosing intrauterine pregnancy (see page 409) and in determining the position of intrauterine contraceptive devices.

## NORMAL VALUES

Normal size, shape, and position of uterus, tubes, and ovaries. No mass.

## COST

Medium.

## ADDITIONAL TESTS TO ORDER

CBC, sedimentation rate, urinalysis, chemistry panel, pregnancy test of blood or urine, CT scan of pelvis, hysterosalpingography, laparoscopy, serum estradiol and FSH, prolactin, and gynecology consult.

# PELVIMETRY

## POSITIVE

This test is positive in cephalopelvic disproportion. It is indicated to determine whether a cesarean section is necessary because the fetal head cannot pass through the mother's pelvis.

## NORMAL VALUES

Normal size, shape, and position of the fetal head and mother's pelvis.

## COST

Medium.

## ADDITIONAL TESTS TO ORDER

Pelvic ultrasonography, obstetric consult.

# PERITONEAL FLUID ANALYSIS

Ask the following questions:

1. Is it a transudate? If the specific gravity is less than 1.015, it is a transudate. This suggests cirrhosis of the liver, congestive heart failure, nephrotic syndrome, constrictive pericarditis, or Meigs' syndrome.
2. If it is a transudate, are the liver function tests abnormal? If the answer is yes, the patient probably has cirrhosis.
3. Is it an exudate? If the specific gravity is over 1.018, the fluid is an exudate. This signifies peritonitis, malignant peritoneal disease, or pancreatitis.
4. If it is an exudate, is the WBC markedly increased? This differentiates bacterial and tuberculous peritonitis from the other conditions.
5. If it is an exudate, what do the cytologic studies show? If these are positive, consider metastatic carcinoma, lymphoma, mesothelioma, and hepatoma as the cause of the ascites.
6. If the foregoing conditions are eliminated, one is left with chronic peritonitis, bile peritonitis, and trauma as possible causes.

## NORMAL VALUES

Little or no fluid, specific gravity less than 1.015, WBC less than 500 cells/mm$^3$, and protein less than 3 g/dL.

## COST

Low.

## ADDITIONAL TESTS TO ORDER

CBC, urinalysis, chemistry panel, cultures of ascitic fluid, radiograph of chest and abdomen, ECG, CT scan of abdomen, laparoscopy, gastroenterology consult, and surgical consult.

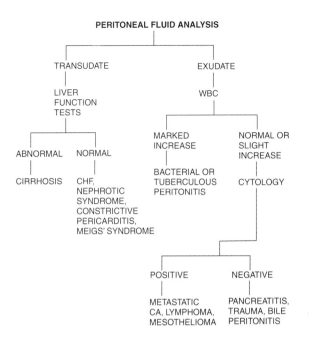

PERITONEAL FLUID ANALYSIS

TRANSUDATE

LIVER
FUNCTION
TESTS

ABNORMAL

CIRRHOSIS

NORMAL

CHF,
NEPHROTIC
SYNDROME,
CONSTRICTIVE
PERICARDITIS,
MEIGS' SYNDROME

EXUDATE

WBC

MARKED
INCREASE

BACTERIAL OR
TUBERCULOUS
PERITONITIS

NORMAL OR
SLIGHT
INCREASE

CYTOLOGY

POSITIVE

METASTATIC
CA, LYMPHOMA,
MESOTHELIOMA

NEGATIVE

PANCREATITIS,
TRAUMA, BILE
PERITONITIS

**Peritoneal Fluid Analysis    427**

# pH

## INCREASED

Ask the following question: What is the bicarbonate level? If the bicarbonate is increased, then the patient has metabolic alkalosis. If the bicarbonate is decreased, the patient has respiratory alkalosis. If the bicarbonate is normal, the patient has early (uncompensated) respiratory alkalosis.

## DECREASED

Ask the following question: What is the bicarbonate level? If the bicarbonate level is increased, the patient has respiratory acidosis. If the bicarbonate level is decreased, the patient has metabolic acidosis. If the bicarbonate level is normal, the patient has early (uncompensated) respiratory alkalosis.

## NORMAL

A normal pH in the face of a significant increase in the bicarbonate level suggests a compensated respiratory acidosis, whereas a normal pH in the face of decreased bicarbonate indicates a compensated respiratory alkalosis.

## NORMAL VALUES

7.35- 7.45.

## COST

Low.

## ADDITIONAL TESTS TO ORDER

CBC, chemistry panel, electrolytes, arterial blood gas analysis, serum and urine ketones, lactic acid, pulmonary function tests, ECG, and consultation with a pulmonologist or endocrinologist.

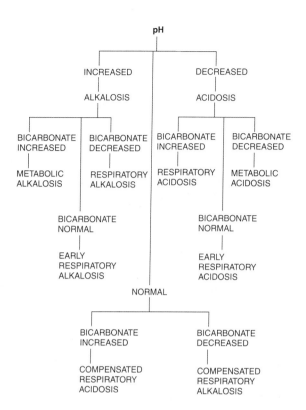

# pH, URINE

## INCREASED

Urine pH is increased in pyelonephritis, salicylate intoxication, metabolic alkalosis, renal tubular acidosis, Cushing's disease, chronic renal failure, and respiratory alkalosis. Certain drugs (e.g., acetazolamide) can increase urine pH.

## DECREASED

Urine pH is decreased in metabolic acidosis, respiratory acidosis, alkaptonuria, diarrhea, diabetes mellitus, and dehydration. Certain drugs (e.g., methenamine mandelate) may decrease urine pH.

## NORMAL VALUES

4.6–8.0.

## COST

Low.

## ADDITIONAL TESTS TO ORDER

CBC, urinalysis, chemistry panel, sedimentation rate, urine culture and colony count, IVP, cystogram, cystoscopy, arterial blood gases, renal biopsy, and urology consult.

**pH, URINE**

INCREASED

INFECTION,
SALICYLATE
INTOXICATION,
METABOLIC
ALKALOSIS,
RENAL TUBULAR
ACIDOSIS,
CHRONIC RENAL
FAILURE,
RESPIRATORY
ALKALOSIS,
DRUGS

DECREASED

METABOLIC
ACIDOSIS,
RESPIRATORY
ACIDOSIS,
DIARRHEA,
DIABETES
MELLITUS,
DEHYDRATION,
DRUGS

# PHARYNGEAL SMEAR

This test can be used to detect streptococci and to give a rapid diagnosis of streptococcal pharyngitis. A pharyngeal smear may also detect gonococci. A clinical pathologist or microbiologist should be consulted for assistance.

## COST

Low.

## ADDITIONAL TESTS TO ORDER

CBC, culture, streptozyme test, ASO titer, CRP, sedimentation rate, rapid slide test for streptococcal cell wall antigens, therapeutic trial, and ENT consult.

# PHENYLALANINE, BLOOD

## INCREASED

This substance is increased in the blood of patients with PKU. This test is used to screen newborn infants for PKU.

## NORMAL VALUES

Less than 2 mg/dL in first 48 hours of life.

## COST

Low.

## ADDITIONAL TESTS TO ORDER

The test may be repeated after feeding of protein. Heterozygotes may be detected by loading tests with phenylalanine orally or intravenously.

# PHONOCARDIOGRAPHY

## DEFINITION

In this test, heart sounds are recorded simultaneously with ECG and jugular pulse to determine the character and timing of murmurs in the cardiac cycle accurately. Recordings are made over the apex, pulmonic area, aortic area, and left sternal border at the fourth intercostal space.

## POSITIVE

This test is helpful in diagnosing valvular heart disease and various congenital cardiac anomalies such as ASD and VSD and tetralogy of Fallot. It cannot, however, exceed the diagnostic accuracy of a stethoscope in the hands of a skilled clinician.

## NORMAL VALUES

Normal heart sounds, no murmurs.

## COST

Medium.

## ADDITIONAL TESTS TO ORDER

ECG, echocardiography, cardiac catheterization and cardioangiography, and cardiology consult.

# PHOSPHORUS

## INCREASED

Ask the following questions:

1. What is the serum calcium? An increased phosphorus with decreased calcium means that the patient probably has either renal disease or hypoparathyroidism.
2. What is the alkaline phosphatase? An increased alkaline phosphatase with increased phosphorus and decreased calcium means that the patient most likely has renal disease, whereas a normal alkaline phosphatase is most compatible with hypoparathyroidism. Increased phosphorus and normal or increased calcium suggest milk-alkali syndrome, hypervitaminosis D, bone tumors, and Addison's disease.

## DECREASED

Ask the following questions:

1. What is the serum calcium? Decreased phosphorus and increased calcium suggest hyperparathyroidism and sarcoidosis. A decreased phosphorus with decreased calcium suggests malabsorption syndrome, vitamin D deficiency, renal tubular acidosis, and hypoproteinemia.
2. What is the alkaline phosphatase? An increased alkaline phosphatase with low phosphorus and high calcium is most likely caused by hyperparathyroidism. If the alkaline phosphatase is normal in the face of low phosphorus and high calcium, the patient probably has sarcoidosis, but a serum PTH level should be determined anyway. If both phosphorus and calcium are decreased but alkaline phosphatase is increased, the patient most likely has malabsorption syndrome, vitamin D deficiency, or renal tubular acidosis. On the other

hand, if these two electrolytes are low but the alkaline phosphatase is normal, one should suspect hypoproteinemia.

## NORMAL VALUES

Adults: 2.5–4.8 mg/dL.
Children: 3.5–5.8 mg/dL.

## COST

Low.

## ADDITIONAL TESTS TO ORDER

CBC, urinalysis, sedimentation rate, chemistry panel, serum PTH, ultrasonogram of the parathyroid glands, bone scan, 1,25-dihydroxyvitamin D D-xylose absorption test, endocrinology consult, and nephrology consult.

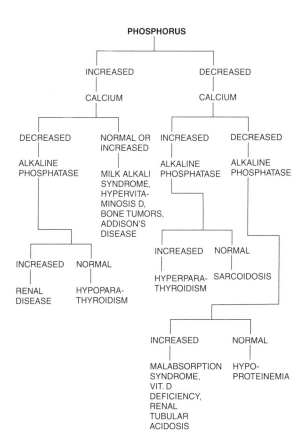

**PHOSPHORUS**

- INCREASED
  - CALCIUM
    - DECREASED
      - ALKALINE PHOSPHATASE
        - INCREASED
          - RENAL DISEASE
        - NORMAL
          - HYPOPARA-THYROIDISM
    - NORMAL OR INCREASED
      - MILK ALKALI SYNDROME, HYPERVITA-MINOSIS D, BONE TUMORS, ADDISON'S DISEASE
- DECREASED
  - CALCIUM
    - INCREASED
      - ALKALINE PHOSPHATASE
        - INCREASED
          - HYPERPARA-THYROIDISM
        - NORMAL
          - SARCOIDOSIS
    - DECREASED
      - ALKALINE PHOSPHATASE
        - INCREASED
          - MALABSORPTION SYNDROME, VIT. D DEFICIENCY, RENAL TUBULAR ACIDOSIS
        - NORMAL
          - HYPO-PROTEINEMIA

# PLATELET AGGREGATION

## DECREASED

Platelet aggregation is decreased in idiopathic thrombocytopenic purpura, von Willebrand's disease, aspirin use, acute leukemia, infectious mononucleosis, and Glanzmann's thrombasthenia.

## NORMAL VALUES

Aggregation of platelets in 5 minutes or less.

## COST

Medium.

## ADDITIONAL TESTS TO ORDER

CBC, platelet count, bleeding time, capillary fragility, blood smear, platelet antibody titer, Monospot test, and hematology consult.

# PLATELET ANTIBODIES

## PRESENT

Platelet antibodies are found in 90% of children with *idiopathic thrombocytopenic purpura,* so it is a useful test to differentiate this disorder. These antibodies are also found in posttransfusion purpura and drug-induced thrombocytopenia.

## NORMAL VALUES

Negative.

## COST

Medium.

## ADDITIONAL TESTS TO ORDER

CBC, platelet count, platelet aggregation, bleeding time, capillary fragility test, coagulation profile, and hematology consult.

# PLATELET COUNT

## INCREASED

The platelet count is increased in various disorders, most notably polycythemia vera and chronic myelogenous leukemia. To differentiate these disorders further, one should order an RBC and WBC. An increase in both the RBC and WBC distinguishes polycythemia vera, whereas an increase in the WBC suggests chronic myelogenous leukemia. If both the RBC and WBC are normal or near normal, one should look for cancer, cirrhosis, heart disease, iron-deficiency anemia, tuberculosis, and other disorders.

## DECREASED

A decrease in the platelet count is also associated with numerous disorders, but most notably idiopathic thrombocytopenic purpura. To distinguish these disorders, a WBC should be ordered. It is increased in leukemia, acute infections, and hemolytic anemia, but it is decreased in bone marrow suppression, aplastic anemia, myelophthisic anemia, and pernicious anemia. A normal WBC is more typical of idiopathic thrombocytopenic purpura.

## NORMAL VALUES

150,000–350,000 mm$^3$.

## COST

Low.

## ADDITIONAL TESTS TO ORDER

CBC, blood smear, red cell indices, serum haptoglobins, serum iron and IBC, serum $B_{12}$ and folic acid, bone marrow examination, liver–spleen scan, CT scan of abdomen, liver function tests, and hematology consult.

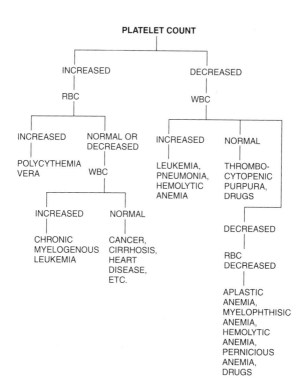

PLATELET COUNT

INCREASED
- RBC
  - INCREASED
    - POLYCYTHEMIA VERA
  - NORMAL OR DECREASED
    - WBC
      - INCREASED
        - CHRONIC MYELOGENOUS LEUKEMIA
      - NORMAL
        - CANCER, CIRRHOSIS, HEART DISEASE, ETC.

DECREASED
- WBC
  - INCREASED
    - LEUKEMIA, PNEUMONIA, HEMOLYTIC ANEMIA
  - NORMAL
    - THROMBO-CYTOPENIC PURPURA, DRUGS
  - DECREASED
    - RBC DECREASED
      - APLASTIC ANEMIA, MYELOPHTHISIC ANEMIA, HEMOLYTIC ANEMIA, PERNICIOUS ANEMIA, DRUGS

# PLEURAL FLUID ANALYSIS

Ask the following questions:

1. Is it a transudate? If the specific gravity is less than 1.015 (i.e., transudate) the patient may have congestive heart failure, cirrhosis, nephrosis, or Meigs' syndrome.
2. If it is a transudate, what is the venous pressure and circulation time? If these values are increased, the patient probably has congestive heart failure.
3. If it is a transudate, what do the liver function tests show? If these are abnormal, look for cirrhosis. If these are normal, consider nephrosis or Meigs' syndrome.
4. If it is an exudate, what is the WBC? A marked increase in the WBC suggests empyema or tuberculosis.
5. If it is an exudate, what is the RBC? If this is increased, consider pulmonary infarct, mesothelioma, and trauma as likely possibilities.
6. If it is an exudate, what do cytologic studies show? If these are positive, consider bronchogenic carcinoma, metastases, mesothelioma, and lymphoma as likely possibilities. If cytologic results are normal, consider the possibility of collagen disease, chylous effusion, and chronic pancreatitis.

## NORMAL VALUES

Little or no fluid; transudate.

## COST

Low.

## ADDITIONAL TESTS TO ORDER

CBC, urinalysis, chemistry panel, sedimentation rate, sputum smear and culture routine and AFB, tuberculin and fungal skin tests, sputum cytology, chest radiograph, ECG, ultrasonography, CT scan of chest, bronchoscopy, needle biopsy, pulmonary consult, and cardiology consult.

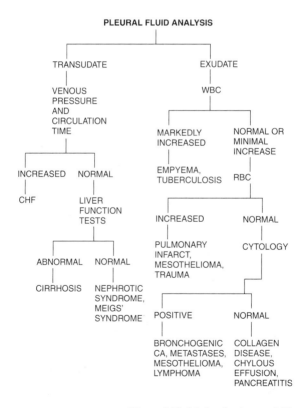

**PLEURAL FLUID ANALYSIS**

- TRANSUDATE
  - VENOUS PRESSURE AND CIRCULATION TIME
    - INCREASED
      - CHF
    - NORMAL
      - LIVER FUNCTION TESTS
        - ABNORMAL
          - CIRRHOSIS
        - NORMAL
          - NEPHROTIC SYNDROME, MEIGS' SYNDROME
- EXUDATE
  - WBC
    - MARKEDLY INCREASED
      - EMPYEMA, TUBERCULOSIS
    - NORMAL OR MINIMAL INCREASE
      - RBC
        - INCREASED
          - PULMONARY INFARCT, MESOTHELIOMA, TRAUMA
        - NORMAL
          - CYTOLOGY
            - POSITIVE
              - BRONCHOGENIC CA, METASTASES, MESOTHELIOMA, LYMPHOMA
            - NORMAL
              - COLLAGEN DISEASE, CHYLOUS EFFUSION, PANCREATITIS

# PORPHYRINS, URINE

## INCREASED

*Porphyrins* are *increased* in the urine in porphyria hepatica, porphyria cutanea tarda, porphyria erythropoietica, lead poisoning, cirrhosis, neoplasms, CNS disorders, and exposure to other toxic substances. Porphyria hepatica (intermittent abdominal form) is distinguished from the other diseases by an *increased* porphobilinogen in the urine. Certain drugs (e.g., barbiturates, sulfonamides), menstruation, and pregnancy may cause false-positive test results.

## NORMAL VALUES

Porphyrins: 50–300 mg/24 hours.
Porphobilinogen: Negative.

## COST

Low.

## ADDITIONAL TESTS TO ORDER

CBC, urinalysis, chemistry panel, stool porphobilinogen, urine $\delta$-aminolevulinic acid, HMB synthase in erythrocytes, URO decarboxylase activity in erythrocytes, blood lead level, liver function tests, and referral to a center experienced in the diagnosis and treatment of these disorders.

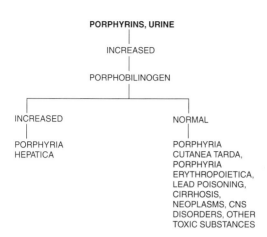

**PORPHYRINS, URINE**

INCREASED

PORPHOBILINOGEN

INCREASED

PORPHYRIA
HEPATICA

NORMAL

PORPHYRIA
CUTANEA TARDA,
PORPHYRIA
ERYTHROPOIETICA,
LEAD POISONING,
CIRRHOSIS,
NEOPLASMS, CNS
DISORDERS, OTHER
TOXIC SUBSTANCES

# POTASSIUM

## INCREASED

Ask the following questions:

1. What is the BUN? An increased potassium level is often caused by acute renal failure.
2. What is the plasma cortisol? Addison's disease is associated with increased potassium.
3. What is the bicarbonate? Metabolic acidosis, especially diabetic acidosis, is a cause of hyperkalemia.
4. Is there hemolysis in the test tube?

## DECREASED

Ask the following questions:

1. What is the sodium? If the sodium level is normal or increased, think of aldosteronism, Cushing's syndrome, periodic paralysis, and IV fluid administration without supplemental potassium.
2. What is the bicarbonate? An increased bicarbonate suggests that the low potassium is due to a metabolic alkalosis such as occurs in pyloric obstruction, severe vomiting, and mercurial diuretics. Decreased sodium and bicarbonate, along with a decreased potassium, are found in diabetic acidosis, diarrhea, renal tubular acidosis, starvation, malabsorption syndrome, and the use of many diuretics.

## NORMAL VALUES

3.5–5 mEq/L.

## COST

Low.

**446**

## ADDITIONAL TESTS TO ORDER

CBC, urinalysis, chemistry panel, serial electrolytes, plasma cortisol, plasma renin, 24-hour urine aldosterone, D-xylose absorption, endocrinology consult, nephrology consult.

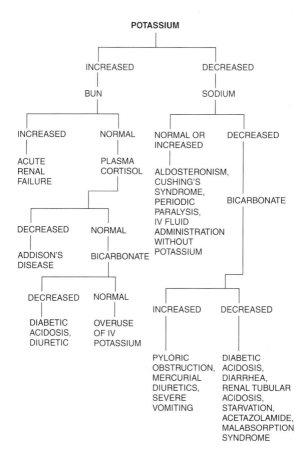

# POTASSIUM, URINE 24-HOUR

## INCREASED

Ask the following question: What is the urine volume? An increased urine volume, along with an increased potassium suggests chronic renal failure, diabetic acidosis, aldosteronism, Cushing's disease, diuretic use, and renal tubular acidosis. A decreased urine volume with an increased urine potassium suggests dehydration, starvation, vomiting, salicylate toxicity, and inappropriate ADH secretion (SIADH).

## DECREASED

Ask the following question: What is the urine volume? An increased urine volume with a decreased potassium may be associated with malabsorption syndrome and diabetes insipidus. A decreased urine volume with a decreased potassium suggests prolonged diarrhea, acute renal failure, and adrenal insufficiency.

## NORMAL VALUES

40–80 mEq/24 hours.

## COST

Low.

## ADDITIONAL TESTS TO ORDER

CBC, chemistry panel, urinalysis, serum and urine osmolality, repeated serum electrolytes, urine culture, Fishberg concentration test, serum ADH, plasma aldosterone, plasma cortisol, blood volume, plasma renin, nephrology consult, and endocrine consult.

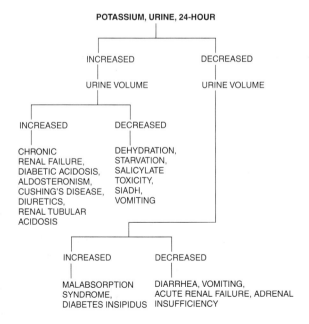

**POTASSIUM, URINE, 24-HOUR**

INCREASED

URINE VOLUME

INCREASED

CHRONIC RENAL FAILURE, DIABETIC ACIDOSIS, ALDOSTERONISM, CUSHING'S DISEASE, DIURETICS, RENAL TUBULAR ACIDOSIS

DECREASED

DEHYDRATION, STARVATION, SALICYLATE TOXICITY, SIADH, VOMITING

DECREASED

URINE VOLUME

INCREASED

MALABSORPTION SYNDROME, DIABETES INSIPIDUS

DECREASED

DIARRHEA, VOMITING, ACUTE RENAL FAILURE, ADRENAL INSUFFICIENCY

# PREGNANCY TEST, BLOOD AND URINE

## POSITIVE

### Male

This suggests a testicular tumor such as a seminoma.

### Female

A positive test in a female suggests pregnancy. To determine whether the pregnancy is intrauterine or ectopic and to differentiate pregnancy from other conditions, *pelvic ultrasonography* is performed. If ultrasonography is negative, one should consider cancer of other organs, menopause, and ovarian dysgenesis. If ultrasonography is positive, is the mass intrauterine or extrauterine? An intrauterine mass may indicate pregnancy, choriocarcinoma, or hydatiform mole. An extrauterine mass may indicate an ectopic pregnancy, salpingitis, or ovarian tumor.

## NORMAL VALUES

Negative blood and urine.

## COST

Low.

## ADDITIONAL TESTS TO ORDER

CBC, urinalysis, chemistry panel, sedimentation rate, serum estradiol, culdocentesis, CT scan of abdomen and pelvis, laparoscopy, and gynecology consult.

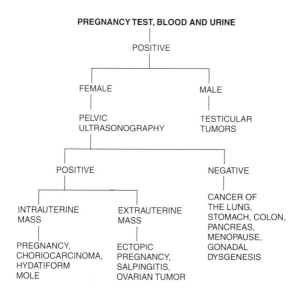

**PREGNANCY TEST, BLOOD AND URINE**

POSITIVE

FEMALE — MALE

FEMALE:
PELVIC ULTRASONOGRAPHY

MALE:
TESTICULAR TUMORS

PELVIC ULTRASONOGRAPHY → POSITIVE / NEGATIVE

POSITIVE:
- INTRAUTERINE MASS → PREGNANCY, CHORIOCARCINOMA, HYDATIFORM MOLE
- EXTRAUTERINE MASS → ECTOPIC PREGNANCY, SALPINGITIS, OVARIAN TUMOR

NEGATIVE:
CANCER OF THE LUNG, STOMACH, COLON, PANCREAS, MENOPAUSE, GONADAL DYSGENESIS

# PREGNANEDIOL, URINE

## INCREASED

*Pregnanediol* is *increased* in corpus luteum cysts, arrhenoblastoma of the ovary, and adrenal neoplasms. *Plasma cortisol* is *elevated* in most adrenal neoplasms, thus differentiating them from ovarian tumors.

## DECREASED

*Pregnanediol* is *decreased* in fetal death, threatened abortion, ovarian failure, toxemia of pregnancy, and pituitary insufficiency. The serum *FSH* and *LH* help to distinguish pituitary insufficiency from the other conditions. It is *decreased* in pituitary insufficiency and is *normal* or *increased* in the other conditions.

## NORMAL VALUES

Follicular phase: 0.5–1.5 mg/24 hours.
Luteal phase: 2–7 mg/24 hours.
Menopause: 0.2–1.0 mg/24 hours.
Pregnancy: 5–63 mg/24 hours.

## COST

Low.

## ADDITIONAL TESTS TO ORDER

Serum FSH and LH, serum estradiol and progesterone, plasma cortisol, pregnancy test, pelvic ultrasound, laparoscopy, CT scan of brain, abdomen, and pelvis, exploratory laparotomy, and gynecology consult.

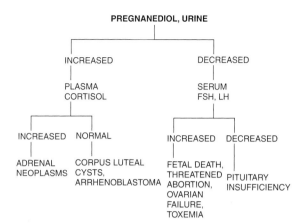

**PREGNANEDIOL, URINE**

INCREASED — PLASMA CORTISOL
- INCREASED → ADRENAL NEOPLASMS
- NORMAL → CORPUS LUTEAL CYSTS, ARRHENOBLASTOMA

DECREASED — SERUM FSH, LH
- INCREASED → FETAL DEATH, THREATENED ABORTION, OVARIAN FAILURE, TOXEMIA
- DECREASED → PITUITARY INSUFFICIENCY

# PREGNANETRIOL, URINE

## INCREASED

This substance is increased in the urine in congenital adrenocortical hyperplasia and Stein–Leventhal syndrome.

## NORMAL VALUES

Children: less than 1.0 mg/24 hours.
Adults: less than 2.0 mg/24 hours.

## COST

Low.

## ADDITIONAL TESTS TO ORDER

Serum FSH and LH, plasma cortisol, plasma ACTH, CT scan of abdomen and pelvis, laparoscopy, exploratory laparotomy, gynecology consult, and endocrinology consult.

# PROLACTIN

## INCREASED

Ask the following questions:

1. Does the patient have a history of drug ingestion? Many drugs, including phenothiazines, antidepressants, antihypertensives, and marijuana cause elevated prolactin levels.
2. What does the CT scan of the pituitary show? If this is positive, consider a prolactin-secreting pituitary tumor.
3. If the foregoing information and testing are negative, look for hypothalamic disorders, ectopic prolactin-producing tumors, and hypothyroidism and renal failure.

## NORMAL VALUES

Females: 0–23 ng/mL.
Males: 0–20 ng/mL.

## COST

Low.

## ADDITIONAL TESTS TO ORDER

Repeat test after withdrawal of drugs, pregnancy test, tests of other pituitary hormones (ACTH, LH, FSH), MRI of the brain, and endocrinology consult.

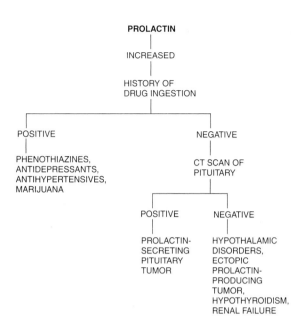

**PROLACTIN**

INCREASED

HISTORY OF
DRUG INGESTION

POSITIVE

PHENOTHIAZINES,
ANTIDEPRESSANTS,
ANTIHYPERTENSIVES,
MARIJUANA

NEGATIVE

CT SCAN OF
PITUITARY

POSITIVE

PROLACTIN-
SECRETING
PITUITARY
TUMOR

NEGATIVE

HYPOTHALAMIC
DISORDERS,
ECTOPIC
PROLACTIN-
PRODUCING
TUMOR,
HYPOTHYROIDISM,
RENAL FAILURE

# PROSTATE-SPECIFIC ANTIGEN (PSA)

## POSITIVE

This test is positive in prostatic carcinoma. False-positive results occur after digital examination of the prostate, prostatitis, and benign prostatic hypertrophy. The PSA can also be used to follow-up patients with prostatic carcinoma.

## NORMAL VALUES

Less than 4 $\mu$g/L.

## COST

Low.

## ADDITIONAL TESTS TO ORDER

CBC, urinalysis, chemistry panel, acid phosphatase, bone scan, prostatic biopsy, transrectal ultrasonography, CT scan of pelvis, and urology consult.

# PROTEIN, CEREBROSPINAL FLUID

## INCREASED

Increased CSF protein is found in cerebral hemorrhage, subarachnoid hemorrhage, meningitis, encephalitis, leukemia, brain or spinal cord tumors, Guillain–Barré syndrome, hypothyroidism, diabetes mellitus, and syphilis. To differentiate these conditions, one should look for RBCs and WBCs. If numbers of RBCs are significant, one should consider cerebral hemorrhage, subarachnoid hemorrhage, or a traumatic tap. If *RBCs are absent* (or few) *and WBCs are increased,* one should consider meningitis, encephalitis, or leukemia. If both RBCs and WBCs are absent or are present in normal numbers, one should consider brain or spinal cord tumor, Guillain–Barré syndrome, hypothyroidism, diabetes mellitus, and syphilis.

## NORMAL VALUES

15–45 mg/dL.

## COST

Low.

## ADDITIONAL TESTS TO ORDER

CBC, urinalysis, free $T_4$, chemistry panel, lumbar puncture and CSF analysis, blood culture, CSF smear and culture, India ink preparation, CT scan, MRI, and neurology consult.

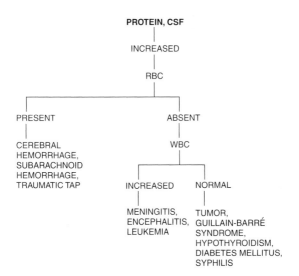

**PROTEIN, CSF**

INCREASED

RBC

PRESENT

CEREBRAL
HEMORRHAGE,
SUBARACHNOID
HEMORRHAGE,
TRAUMATIC TAP

ABSENT

WBC

INCREASED

MENINGITIS,
ENCEPHALITIS,
LEUKEMIA

NORMAL

TUMOR,
GUILLAIN-BARRÉ
SYNDROME,
HYPOTHYROIDISM,
DIABETES MELLITUS,
SYPHILIS

# PROTEIN, URINE

## INCREASED

Ask the following questions:

1. Are the WBCs increased? Proteinuria and an increase of WBCs without a significant increase in RBCs make cystitis or pyelonephritis likely.
2. Are the RBCs increased? Proteinuria and increased RBCs with a normal or only slight increase in WBCs suggest glomerulonephritis, polycystic kidney disease, tuberculosis, renal calculus, trauma, neoplasm, and collagen disease.
3. Is glucose present in the urine? This finding associated with proteinuria suggests diabetic nephritis or nephrosis.
4. Rarely, proteinuria without increased WBCs, RBCs, or glycosuria suggests hypertension, toxemia of pregnancy, fever, cardiac disease, poisoning, orthostatic proteinuria, or multiple myeloma.

## NORMAL VALUES

Negative.

## COST

Low.

## ADDITIONAL TESTS TO ORDER

CBC, urinalysis, chemistry panel, sedimentation rate, ANA, serum protein electrophoresis, urine for Bence Jones protein, 24-hour urine protein, urine culture, Addis count, ASO titer, IVP, CT scan of abdomen, renal biopsy, cystoscopy and retrograde pyelography, and nephrology or urology consult.

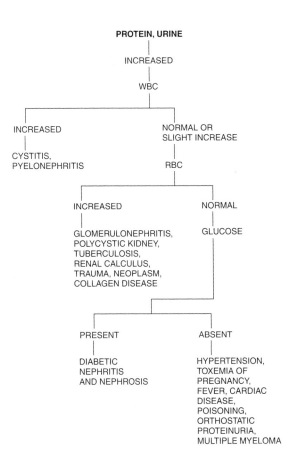

**PROTEIN, URINE**
|
INCREASED
|
WBC

INCREASED → CYSTITIS, PYELONEPHRITIS

NORMAL OR SLIGHT INCREASE
|
RBC

INCREASED → GLOMERULONEPHRITIS, POLYCYSTIC KIDNEY, TUBERCULOSIS, RENAL CALCULUS, TRAUMA, NEOPLASM, COLLAGEN DISEASE

NORMAL
|
GLUCOSE

PRESENT → DIABETIC NEPHRITIS AND NEPHROSIS

ABSENT → HYPERTENSION, TOXEMIA OF PREGNANCY, FEVER, CARDIAC DISEASE, POISONING, ORTHOSTATIC PROTEINURIA, MULTIPLE MYELOMA

# PROTEIN ELECTROPHORESIS

## ALBUMIN

Changes in albumin are covered elsewhere (see page 15).

## $\alpha_1$-GLOBULIN

This is *decreased* in alpha$_1$-antitrypsin deficiency and nephrosis.

## $\alpha_2$-GLOBULIN

This is *increased* in nephrotic syndrome, burns, trauma, biliary cirrhosis, ulcerative colitis, and rarely multiple myeloma. It is *decreased* in acute hemolytic anemia.

## $\beta$-GLOBULINS

*Increased* in liver disease, multiple myeloma, and obstructive jaundice, *decreased* in nephrosis.

## $\gamma$-GLOBULINS

These are *increased* in multiple myeloma, macroglobulinemia, lymphoma, collagen disease, chronic infection, and monoclonal and polyclonal gammopathies. They are *decreased* in agammaglobulinemia, nephrotic syndrome, leukemia, lymphoma, and protein-losing enteropathy.

## NORMAL VALUES

Total protein: 6.5–8.5 g/dL.
Albumin: 3.5–5.2 g/dL.
$\alpha_1$-Globulin: 0.15–0.45 g/dL.
$\alpha_2$-Globulin: 0.5–1.00 g/dL.
$\beta$-Globulin: 0.5–1.20 g/dL.
$\gamma$-Globulin: 0.6–1.60 g/dL.

## COST

Low.

## ADDITIONAL TESTS TO ORDER

CBC, urinalysis, sedimentation rate, immunoelectrophoresis, ANA, RA, chemistry panel, liver function tests, skeletal survey, chest radiograph, bone scan, bone marrow examination, liver biopsy, 24-hour urine protein, and oncology and hematology consult.

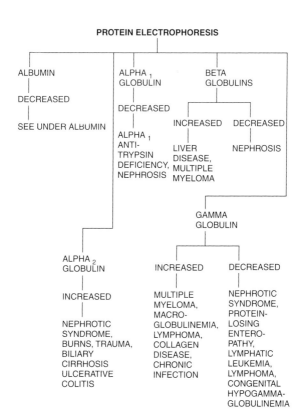

PROTEIN ELECTROPHORESIS

ALBUMIN

DECREASED

SEE UNDER ALBUMIN

ALPHA₁ GLOBULIN

DECREASED

ALPHA₁ ANTI-TRYPSIN DEFICIENCY, NEPHROSIS

BETA GLOBULINS

INCREASED

LIVER DISEASE, MULTIPLE MYELOMA

DECREASED

NEPHROSIS

ALPHA₂ GLOBULIN

INCREASED

NEPHROTIC SYNDROME, BURNS, TRAUMA, BILIARY CIRRHOSIS ULCERATIVE COLITIS

GAMMA GLOBULIN

INCREASED

MULTIPLE MYELOMA, MACRO-GLOBULINEMIA, LYMPHOMA, COLLAGEN DISEASE, CHRONIC INFECTION

DECREASED

NEPHROTIC SYNDROME, PROTEIN-LOSING ENTERO-PATHY, LYMPHATIC LEUKEMIA, LYMPHOMA, CONGENITAL HYPOGAMMA-GLOBULINEMIA

# PROTEIN ELECTROPHORESIS, CEREBROSPINAL FLUID

## INCREASED IGG

An increased IgG as determined by spinal fluid protein electrophoresis is helpful in the diagnosis of *multiple sclerosis.* It is also found in neurosyphilis and other CNS infections.

## INCREASED IGM

This protein is found in tumors of the brain and meninges, meningitis, and multiple sclerosis.

## NORMAL VALUES

IgG: Less than 8.3 mg/dL.
IgM: Absent.

## COST

Low.

## ADDITIONAL TESTS TO ORDER

See Myelin Basic Protein, Cerebrospinal Fluid.

# PROTHROMBIN CONSUMPTION TEST (SERUM PROTHROMBIN TIME)

## DECREASED

Ask the following questions:

1. What is the platelet count? If the platelet count is decreased, look for idiopathic and secondary thrombocytopenic purpura (such as found in hypersplenism and aplastic anemia).
2. What is the PTT? A prolonged PTT suggests that the cause of the decreased prothrombin consumption is hemophilia and circulating anticoagulants.

## NORMAL VALUES

15 seconds or more.

## COST

Low.

## ADDITIONAL TESTS TO ORDER

CBC, platelet count, ANA, coagulation profile, PTT, bleeding time, thrombin time, fibrin split products, liver–spleen scan, bone marrow examination, and hematology consult.

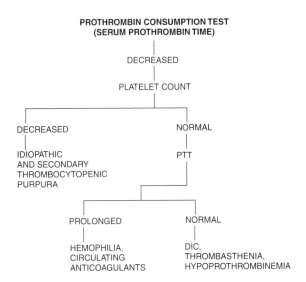

**PROTHROMBIN CONSUMPTION TEST
(SERUM PROTHROMBIN TIME)**

DECREASED

PLATELET COUNT

DECREASED

IDIOPATHIC
AND SECONDARY
THROMBOCYTOPENIC
PURPURA

NORMAL

PTT

PROLONGED

HEMOPHILIA,
CIRCULATING
ANTICOAGULANTS

NORMAL

DIC,
THROMBASTHENIA,
HYPOPROTHROMBINEMIA

# PROTHROMBIN TIME

## PROLONGED

Ask the following questions:

1. Is there a history of drug ingestion? If this is true, look for salicylate intoxication and the ingestion of dicumarol derivatives.
2. Are the liver function tests abnormal? Abnormal liver function tests suggest alcoholism, cirrhosis, and biliary obstruction.
3. Is the thrombin time also prolonged? If that is the case, look for disseminated intravascular coagulation and circulatory anticoagulants.

## NORMAL VALUES

11–14 seconds (check with your laboratory).

## COST

Low.

## ADDITIONAL TESTS TO ORDER

CBC, platelet count, bleeding time, PTT, capillary fragility test, thrombin time, fibrin split products, fibrinogen, liver function tests, and hematology consult.

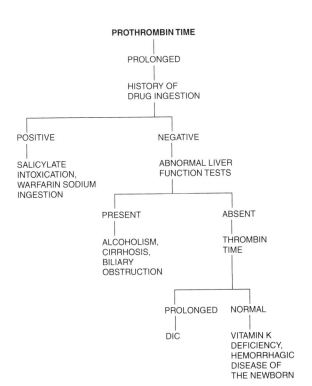

**PROTHROMBIN TIME**

PROLONGED

HISTORY OF
DRUG INGESTION

POSITIVE

SALICYLATE
INTOXICATION,
WARFARIN SODIUM
INGESTION

NEGATIVE

ABNORMAL LIVER
FUNCTION TESTS

PRESENT

ALCOHOLISM,
CIRRHOSIS,
BILIARY
OBSTRUCTION

ABSENT

THROMBIN
TIME

PROLONGED

DIC

NORMAL

VITAMIN K
DEFICIENCY,
HEMORRHAGIC
DISEASE OF
THE NEWBORN

# PULMONARY CAPILLARY WEDGE PRESSURE

## DEFINITION

This is the pressure in the pulmonary capillaries obtained by threading a catheter from the jugular or subclavian vein through the right side of the heart and into the pulmonary artery and ultimately into the pulmonary capillaries.

## INCREASED

The pulmonary capillary wedge pressure is increased in congestive heart failure, hypervolemia, and mitral stenosis and regurgitation. It is also increased in left-to-right shunts.

## DECREASED

The pulmonary capillary wedge pressure is decreased in vasomotor and hypovolemic shock, liver disease, hypoproteinemia, burns, and adult respiratory distress syndrome.

## NORMAL VALUES

8–12 mm Hg.

## COST

Medium.

## ADDITIONAL TESTS TO ORDER

CBC, urinalysis, chemistry panel, drug screen, arterial blood gas analysis, serum and urine osmolality, blood volume studies, chest radiograph, ECG, echocardiography, venous pressure and circulation time, angiocardiography, CT scan of the chest, cardiology consult, and pulmonary consult.

# PULMONARY FUNCTION STUDIES

## FORCED VITAL CAPACITY (FVC)

### Decreased

This is decreased in both *obstructive* and *restrictive lung disease.* To differentiate these two groups of conditions further, a 1-second forced expiratory volume (FEV$_1$) should be obtained. If this is decreased, the patient has *obstructive disease.* If it is normal or only slightly decreased, the patient probably has *restrictive disease.*

### Administering a Bronchodilator

If the patient with obstructive disease improves after using a bronchodilator such as albuterol or epinephrine, then *asthma* is the most likely diagnosis. If little or no improvement is seen, emphysema is the most likely diagnosis.

### Carbon Monoxide Diffusing Capacity (D$_{LCO}$)

If this is decreased, the patient has sarcoidosis, pulmonary fibrosis, scleroderma, pneumoconiosis, or other collagen diseases. If this is normal, the patient probably has kyphoscoliosis, neuromuscular disease, ankylosing spondylitis, or other diseases of the chest wall, CNS, or spine.

### Normal Values

FVC: 4000–4800 mL (check with local laboratory).
FEV$_1$: 81–83% of FVC.

## Cost

Low.

## FUNCTIONAL RESIDUAL CAPACITY (FRC)

### Decreased

An FRC of less than 75% indicates restrictive lung disease and is found in pulmonary fibrosis, sarcoidosis, pneumoconiosis, and drug- or radiation-induced interstitial fibrosis.

### Increased

FRC is increased to over 125% in obstructive disease such as asthma and emphysema.

### Normal Values

2400–3000 mL, based on age, sex, height, and weight.

### Cost

Low.

## VITAL CAPACITY (VC)

### Definition

This is the maximum volume of air that can be exhaled after a maximum inspiration. There is no time limit.

### Decreased

The vital capacity is reduced in both obstructive and restrictive disease. These diseases include asthma, emphysema, pulmonary fibrosis, sarcoidosis, pneumoconiosis, scleroderma, neuromuscular disease, kyphoscoliosis, CNS disease, pleural effusion, and pneumothorax.

## Normal Values

4000–4800 mL, depending on age, sex, height, and weight.

## Cost

Low.

# RESIDUAL VOLUME (RV)

## Definition

This is the volume of gas remaining in the lungs after maximum exhalation.

## Increased

Residual volume is increased in obstructive disease such as asthma or emphysema.

## Decreased

Residual volume is decreased in restrictive disease such as pulmonary fibrosis, sarcoidosis, pneumoconiosis, pleural effusion, pneumothorax, and kyphoscoliosis or neuromuscular disease.

## Normal Values

1200–1500 mL, based on age, sex, height, and weight.

## Cost

Low.

# FLOW VOLUME LOOPS (FV LOOPS)

## Definition

In this test, the flow rates on maximum inspiratory and expiratory effort are plotted on a graph. The patient inhales and exhales fully as rapidly as possible.

## Decreased Volume, Decreased Flow Rate

This is found in obstructive disease such as asthma and emphysema.

## Decreased Volume, Normal Flow Rate

This is found in restrictive disease such as pulmonary fibrosis, sarcoidosis and pneumoconiosis.

## Normal Values

Smooth-steep curves on both sides of the loop.

## Cost

Medium.

# CARBON MONOXIDE DIFFUSING CAPACITY (DLco)

## Definition

This test measures the ability of the alveolar capillary membranes to extract a known quantity of carbon monoxide from inspired air.

## Decreased

The diffusing capacity is decreased in pulmonary fibrosis, sarcoidosis, and other restrictive diseases. It can also be reduced in ventilation perfusion mismatch such as in certain patients with pulmonary emphysema. Patients with multiple pulmonary emboli may also have a decreased diffusing capacity.

## Normal Values

25 mL/torr per minute.

## Cost

Medium.

# PEAK INSPIRATORY FLOW RATE (PIFR)

## Definition

This is the maximum flow rate on forced inspiration.

## Decreased

The peak inspiratory flow rate is decreased in upper airway obstruction such as laryngitis, laryngeal obstruction or paralysis, and chest wall disease such as ankylosing spondylitis and neuromuscular disorders.

## Normal Values

300 L/min.

## Cost

Low.

# PEAK EXPIRATORY FLOW RATE (PEFR)

## Definition

This is the maximum flow rate on forced expiration.

## Decreased

This test is decreased in obstructive disease (e.g., emphysema). It is normal in restrictive disease (e.g., pulmonary fibrosis).

## Normal Values

450 L/min.

## Cost

Low.

# MAXIMUM MIDEXPIRATORY FLOW RATE (MMFR)

## Definition

This is the expiratory flow rate between the first 25% and 75% of forced expiration. Normally, the flow rate is highest during this period of the $FEV_1$ test.

## Decreased

This is decreased in obstructive disease (e.g., asthma, emphysema), especially small airway disease in smokers. It is the first test to become positive in obstructive disease. It is normal in restrictive disease.

## Normal Values

Check with the local laboratory.

## Cost

Low.

## MAXIMUM VOLUNTARY VENTILATION (MVV)

### Definition

This is the maximum amount of air a person can inhale and exhale in a given period of time, usually 10–15 seconds.

### Decreased

Like the $FEV_1$, this test is decreased in obstructive disease (e.g., asthma, emphysema). It may also be decreased in combined obstructive and restrictive disease.

### Normal Values

170 L/min.

### Cost

Low.

## ADDITIONAL TESTS TO ORDER

CBC, urinalysis, chemistry panel, ECG, sedimentation rate, arterial blood gas analysis, serial electrolytes, ventilation perfusion scan, pulmonary angiography, bronchoscopy, chest radiograph, MRI of the lungs, lung biopsy, carbon dioxide diffusing capacity, exercise pulmonary function test, alpha$_1$-antitrypsin, sputum analysis and culture, sputum for eosinophils, and pulmonary consult.

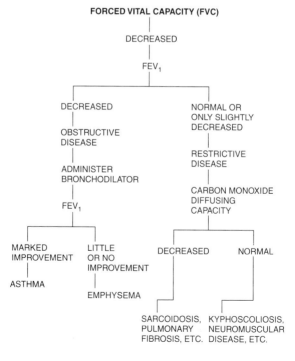

**FORCED VITAL CAPACITY (FVC)**

DECREASED

FEV$_1$

DECREASED

OBSTRUCTIVE DISEASE

ADMINISTER BRONCHODILATOR

FEV$_1$

MARKED IMPROVEMENT

ASTHMA

LITTLE OR NO IMPROVEMENT

EMPHYSEMA

NORMAL OR ONLY SLIGHTLY DECREASED

RESTRICTIVE DISEASE

CARBON MONOXIDE DIFFUSING CAPACITY

DECREASED

NORMAL

SARCOIDOSIS, PULMONARY FIBROSIS, ETC.

KYPHOSCOLIOSIS, NEUROMUSCULAR DISEASE, ETC.

# PYRUVATE KINASE

## DECREASED

Congenital nonspherocytic anemia, drug toxicity, and metabolic liver disease.

## NORMAL VALUES

2.0–8.8 U/g Hb.

## COST

Low.

## ADDITIONAL TESTS TO ORDER

See page 487.

# RADIOACTIVE IODINE (RAI) FIBRINOGEN VENOGRAM

## POSITIVE

This scan is positive in deep vein thrombosis of the lower extremities.

## NORMAL VALUES

No areas of focal increased uptake.

## COST

Medium.

## ADDITIONAL TESTS TO ORDER

Plethysmography, venous ultrasonography, phlebography, and cardiology consult.

# RADIOACTIVE IODINE (RAI) TOTAL BODY SCAN

## POSITIVE

This test is positive when thyroid tissue exists in other areas of the body such as ovary (struma ovarii), substernal thyroid, and sublingual thyroid.

## NORMAL VALUES

No extra thyroid tissue.

## COST

Medium to high.

## ADDITIONAL TESTS TO ORDER

See page 482.

# RADIOACTIVE IODINE (RAI) UPTAKE AND SCAN (SEE ALGORITHM)

## INCREASED UPTAKE

This is found in toxic adenoma and Graves' disease.

## DECREASED UPTAKE

This is found in thyroid cysts, nonfunctioning adenomas, nontoxic nodular goiter, Riedel's struma, hypothyroidism, Hashimoto's disease, and malignant diseases.

## NORMAL VALUES

Homogeneous uptake, normal-sized thyroid gland.

## COST

Medium.

## ADDITIONAL TESTS TO ORDER

CBC, urinalysis, sedimentation rate, free $T_4$, TSH, thyroid ultrasound, CT scan of thyroid, needle aspiration, and consultation with an endocrinologist.

**RADIOACTIVE IODINE UPTAKE AND SCAN**

```
                    RADIOACTIVE IODINE UPTAKE AND SCAN
                                     |
          ┌──────────────────────────┴──────────────────────────┐
     INCREASED                                              DECREASED
      UPTAKE                                                 UPTAKE
   ┌──────┴──────┐                              ┌───────────────┴───────────────┐
 FOCAL        DIFFUSE                        FOCAL                           DIFFUSE
   |             |                             |                               |
 TOXIC        GRAVES'                        CYST,                      HYPOTHYROIDISM,
ADENOMA       DISEASE                   NONFUNCTIONING                  HASHIMOTO'S
                                           ADENOMA,                       DISEASE
                                           NONTOXIC
                                           NODULAR
                                           GOITER,
                                           RIEDEL'S
                                           STRUMA,
                                        MALIGNANCIES
```

# RADIOACTIVE IODINE (RAI) UPTAKE STIMULATION TEST

## DEFINITION

In this test, RAI uptake is measured after the administration of TSH or TRH.

1. No response to TSH: This is found in primary hypothyroidism and Hashimoto's thyroiditis.
2. Response to TSH: This is found in hypopituitarism and hypothalamic disorders.
3. No response to TRH: This is found in hypopituitarism.
4. Response to TRH: A good response to TRH suggests that the hypothyroidism is secondary to a hypothalamic disorder.

## NORMAL VALUES

Increased RAI uptake after TSH and TRH.

## COST

Medium to high.

## ADDITIONAL TESTS TO ORDER

Thyroid scans, sedimentation rate, thyroid antibody titer, free $T_4$, TSH, ultrasonography of the thyroid, MRI of the thyroid, MRI of the brain, and endocrinology consult.

# RADIOALLERGOSORBENT TESTS (RAST)

## POSITIVE

These tests are positive when a patient is hypersensitive or allergic to a specific allergen such as trees, grass, molds, venom, weeds, house dust, animal hair, and foods. These tests can be used to screen for allergens in hay fever, asthma, and allergic dermatitis.

## NORMAL VALUES

Negative.

## COST

Medium.

## ADDITIONAL TESTS TO ORDER

Patch tests, scratch tests, intradermal sensitivity tests, eosinophil count, sputum or nasal smear for eosinophils, chest radiograph, spirometry, therapeutic trial of antihistamines or corticosteroids, and consultation with an allergist.

# RED BLOOD CELL COUNT (RBC)

## INCREASED

The RBC is increased in primary and secondary poly-cythemia and hemoconcentration (such as dehydration). To differentiate between secondary polycythemia caused by pulmonary disease and other forms of polycythemia, the clinician should order an arterial blood oxygen saturation test. If the $Po_2$ is decreased, chronic pulmonary disease is likely.

## DECREASED

If the RBC is decreased, one should look at the WBC and platelet count. If the WBC is increased but the platelet count is normal, one should consider hemorrhage, hemolytic anemia, and chronic infectious disease to be likely. If the WBC is increased but the platelet count is decreased, leukemia or myeloid metaplasia is a possibility. If both the WBC and platelet count are decreased, one should consider hypersplenism, aplastic anemia, myelophthisic anemia, sideroblastic anemia, and megaloblastic anemia in the differential diagnosis. The clinician should look for a significantly enlarged spleen. If present, the patient may well have hypersplenism as the cause of the pancytopenia. A normal WBC in the presence of a decreased RBC may mean hemodilution, iron-deficiency anemia, anemia of chronic blood loss, or anemia of chronic disease.

## NORMAL VALUES

Men: 4.2–5.4 million/mm$^3$.
Women: 3.6–5.0 million/mm$^3$.

## COST

Low.

## ADDITIONAL TESTS TO ORDER

CBC, platelet count, sedimentation rate, red cell indices, blood smear, serum iron and IBC, serum $B_{12}$ and folic acid, serum haptoglobins, reticulocyte count, bone marrow examination, liver–spleen scan, CT scans, therapeutic trial stool for occult blood, and hematology consult.

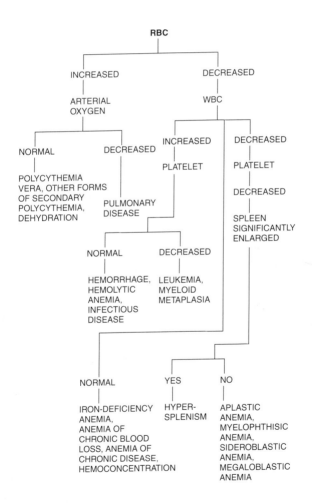

# RED CELL CASTS

## PRESENT

The presence of red cell casts in the urine indicates acute inflammatory or vascular disorders of the glomerulus. To differentiate these disorders, the following tests are indicated:

1. *ASO titer:* An increased ASO titer suggests acute glomerulonephritis.
2. *ANA:* A positive ANA suggests a collagen disease.
3. *Blood culture:* A positive blood culture suggests subacute bacterial endocarditis.
4. If these tests are *negative,* one should look for renal infarction, renal vein thrombosis, polycystic kidneys, and lower nephron nephrosis.

## NORMAL VALUES

0–1 per high-power field.

## COST

Low.

## ADDITIONAL TESTS TO ORDER

CBC, urinalysis, Addis count, 24-hour urine protein, ASO titer, ANA, VDRL, chemistry panel, blood cultures, urine cultures, renal biopsy, and nephrology consult.

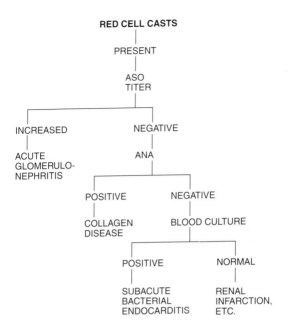

# RED CELL FRAGILITY

## INCREASED

The red cell fragility is increased in autoimmune hemolytic anemia, hereditary spherocytosis, drug toxicity, chemical poisoning, and burns. A direct Coombs' test should be ordered to differentiate auto-immune hemolytic anemia from the other conditions.

## DECREASED

Red cell fragility is decreased in polycythemia vera, obstructive jaundice, thalassemia, sickle cell anemia, and iron-deficiency anemia. The MCV further differentiates these conditions. It is decreased in thalassemia, sickle cell anemia, and iron-deficiency anemia. It is normal in polycythemia vera and obstructive jaundice.

## NORMAL VALUES

Hemolysis begins at 0.45–0.39% saline and ends at 0.33–0.30% saline.

## COST

Low.

## ADDITIONAL TESTS TO ORDER

CBC, red cell survival, Coombs' test, serum iron and iron-binding capacity, hemoglobin electrophoresis, sickle cell preparation, chemistry panel, and hematology consult.

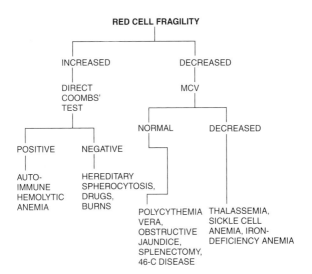

**RED CELL FRAGILITY**

INCREASED

DIRECT COOMBS' TEST

POSITIVE

AUTO-IMMUNE HEMOLYTIC ANEMIA

NEGATIVE

HEREDITARY SPHEROCYTOSIS, DRUGS, BURNS

DECREASED

MCV

NORMAL

POLYCYTHEMIA VERA, OBSTRUCTIVE JAUNDICE, SPLENECTOMY, 46-C DISEASE

DECREASED

THALASSEMIA, SICKLE CELL ANEMIA, IRON-DEFICIENCY ANEMIA

# RED CELL SIZE DISTRIBUTION WIDTH (RDW)

## INCREASED

RDW is increased in *iron-deficiency anemia*. It is also increased in folic acid deficiency, pernicious anemia, hemolytic anemia, sideroblastic anemia, transfusion, HbH, and alcohol abuse. RDW is normal in thalassemia and chronic simple anemia, thus helping in the differentiation of these conditions from iron-deficiency anemia.

## NORMAL VALUES

8.5–11.5.

## COST

Low.

## ADDITIONAL TESTS TO ORDER

CBC, platelet count, sedimentation rate, blood smear, serum iron and ferritin, serum $B_{12}$ and folic acid, red cell survival, hemoglobin electrophoresis, and hematology consult.

# RED CELL SURVIVAL TIME

## DECREASED

Survival time of red cells is decreased in most hemolytic anemias. To differentiate these further, a direct *Coombs' test* is indicated. A positive Coombs' test makes one suspect autoimmune hemolytic anemia and chronic lymphatic leukemia. If the Coombs' test is negative, one should perform a *red cell fragility test. Increased* red cell fragility suggests hereditary spherocytosis. Decreased red cell fragility with decreased red cell survival time suggests sickle cell anemia. A normal red cell fragility test and negative Coombs' test should prompt one to look for pernicious anemia, uremia, paroxysmal nocturnal hemoglobinuria, and other disorders.

## NORMAL OR INCREASED

Red cell survival may be normal or increased in certain hemolytic anemias, including thalassemia minor, hemoglobin C trait, sickle cell trait, and elliptocytosis.

## NORMAL VALUES

25–35 days (may vary, so check with your local laboratory).

## COST

Medium.

## ADDITIONAL TESTS TO ORDER

CBC, blood smear, urinalysis, chemistry panel, serum $B_{12}$, ANA, VDRL, Ham test, hemoglobin electrophoresis, sickle cell preparation, bone marrow examination, and hematology consult.

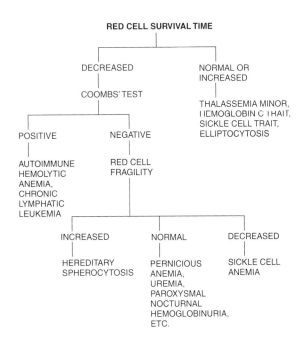

RED CELL SURVIVAL TIME

DECREASED

COOMBS' TEST

NORMAL OR INCREASED

THALASSEMIA MINOR, HEMOGLOBIN C TRAIT, SICKLE CELL TRAIT, ELLIPTOCYTOSIS

POSITIVE

AUTOIMMUNE HEMOLYTIC ANEMIA, CHRONIC LYMPHATIC LEUKEMIA

NEGATIVE

RED CELL FRAGILITY

INCREASED

HEREDITARY SPHEROCYTOSIS

NORMAL

PERNICIOUS ANEMIA, UREMIA, PAROXYSMAL NOCTURNAL HEMOGLOBINURIA, ETC.

DECREASED

SICKLE CELL ANEMIA

# RENAL
# ULTRASONOGRAPHY

## POSITIVE

This test is positive in renal cysts, tumors, hydronephrosis, chronic glomerulonephritis, polycystic kidney, and perinephric abscess. It also may be used to
diagnose a perirenal hematoma. It is especially useful
to differentiate a cyst from a neoplasm. It can also
determine the pathologic features of a nonfunctioning kidney. In patients with acute renal failure, ultrasonography often demonstrates postrenal causes
such as bilateral hydronephrosis at no risk to the patient.

## NORMAL VALUES

Normal size, shape, and position of the kidney with
homogeneous parenchyma.

## COST

Medium.

## ADDITIONAL TESTS TO ORDER

CBC, urinalysis, chemistry panel, sedimentation rate,
urine culture, IVP, CT scan of abdomen and pelvis,
cystoscopy and retrograde pyelography, nuclear scan
of the kidney, renal biopsy, nephrology consult, and
urology consult.

# RENIN

## INCREASED

Plasma renin is increased in Bartter's syndrome, renal hypertension, secondary aldosteronism, and Addison's disease. Addison's disease can be separated from this group by obtaining a serum or urine aldosterone determination. This hormone is decreased in Addison's disease.

## DECREASED

Plasma renin is decreased in primary aldosteronism, corticosteroid therapy, and ADH therapy. To differentiate these further, a serum or urine aldosterone determination is indicated. This hormone is increased in primary aldosteronism.

## NORMAL VALUES

0.2–5 ng/mL per hour. Values vary with age and sodium depletion.

## COST

Low.

## ADDITIONAL TESTS TO ORDER

Serial electrolytes, renin suppression tests, plasma cortisol, serum aldosterone, urinary aldosterone, flat plate of abdomen, CT scan of abdomen, IVP, renal angiography, endocrinology consult, and nephrology consult.

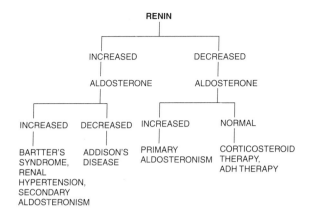

# RENOGRAM

## POSITIVE

This scan is positive in renal artery stenosis (delayed appearance of uptake in ischemic kidney), obstructive uropathy, unilateral renal disease, and infarction. It can be used to evaluate renal disease in renal failure and azotemia when an IVP is contraindicated. It is also useful in patients who are allergic to iodine.

## NORMAL VALUES

Equal flow and homogeneous simultaneous uptake in both kidneys. Normal size and shape of both kidneys.

## COST

Medium to high.

## ADDITIONAL TESTS TO ORDER

Hypertensive IVP, cystoscopy and retrograde pyelography, CT scan of abdomen, renal ultrasonography, renal angiography, and urology and nephrology consult.

# RESIDUAL VOLUME, URINE

## INCREASED

Residual volume of urine is increased in the bladder
in bladder neck obstruction from median bar hypertrophy, interureteral bar hypertrophy, and prostatic
hypertrophy. It is also increased in prostatitis, prostatic carcinoma, urethral stricture, and neurogenic
bladder.

## NORMAL VALUE

< 60 cc of urine.

## COST

Low.

## ADDITIONAL TESTS TO ORDER

Urinalysis, urine culture and colony count, cystogram, ultrasonography of the urinary bladder, cystoscopy, PSA, prostatic biopsy, CT scan of pelvis, urology consult, and gynecology consult.

# RETICULOCYTE COUNT

## INCREASED

The reticulocyte count is increased in hemolytic anemia, after treatment of anemias, and in neoplastic infiltration of the bone marrow such as leukemia. To differentiate these conditions further, a *serum haptoglobin* determination should be obtained. If it is decreased, hemolytic anemia is the cause of the reticulocytosis. If it is normal, then the reticulocytosis is due to metastatic carcinoma, leukemia, treatment of anemia, or hemorrhage.

## DECREASED

A decrease in reticulocyte count may be due to aplastic anemia, pernicious anemia, iron-deficiency anemia, or chronic infection. To differentiate these conditions, one should investigate the *WBC* and *platelet count.* If either or both of these is decreased, then the patient may have aplastic anemia or pernicious anemia. Red cell morphology distinguishes between these two conditions.

## NORMAL VALUES

Adults: 0.5–2.5%.
Children: 0.5–4.0%.
Infants: 2–5%.

## COST

Low.

## ADDITIONAL TESTS TO ORDER

CBC, chemistry panel, serum haptoglobins, blood smear for morphology, serum $B_{12}$ and folic acid, stool for occult blood, platelet count, bone marrow examination, and hematology consult.

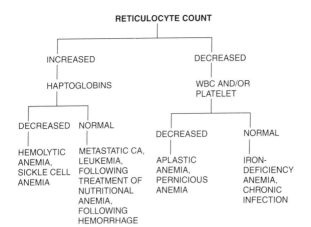

**RETICULOCYTE COUNT**

- INCREASED
  - HAPTOGLOBINS
    - DECREASED
      - HEMOLYTIC ANEMIA, SICKLE CELL ANEMIA
    - NORMAL
      - METASTATIC CA, LEUKEMIA, FOLLOWING TREATMENT OF NUTRITIONAL ANEMIA, FOLLOWING HEMORRHAGE
- DECREASED
  - WBC AND/OR PLATELET
    - DECREASED
      - APLASTIC ANEMIA, PERNICIOUS ANEMIA
    - NORMAL
      - IRON-DEFICIENCY ANEMIA, CHRONIC INFECTION

**Reticulocyte Count    501**

# RETROGRADE PYELOGRAPHY

## POSITIVE

This test is positive in obstructing lesions of the ureters and renal pelvis (such as stones, stricture, neoplasms, and congenital anomalies) and in renal tuberculosis, renal neoplasms, and chronic renal disease. It is indicated in unexplained hematuria, to determine the cause of hydronephrosis found on IVP and to examine the urinary tract when an elevated BUN, allergic history, and other findings suggest that an IVP is unwise. It also is useful in defining a renal mass, but ultrasonography and CT scan are more valuable in this regard.

## NORMAL VALUES

Normal size, shape, and position of kidneys, ureters, and bladder. No filling defects or obstruction.

## COST

Medium.

## ADDITIONAL TESTS TO ORDER

CBC, sedimentation rate, urinalysis, urine culture and colony count, AFB culture, chemistry panel, cystoscopy, ultrasonography, CT scan of abdomen and pelvis, PSA, voiding cystogram, renal scan, and urology consult.

# RETROPERITONEAL ULTRASONOGRAPHY

## POSITIVE

This test shows the enlarged retroperitoneal lymph nodes of retroperitoneal sarcoma, lymphoma, and metastatic carcinoma. The procedure is also useful in determining the response of these nodes to therapy.

## NORMAL VALUES

Retroperitoneal lymph nodes not visualized.

## COST

Medium.

## ADDITIONAL TESTS TO ORDER

CT scan of abdomen, lymphangiography, exploratory laparotomy, and oncology consult.

# RHEUMATOID FACTOR

## POSITIVE

Ask the following questions:

1. What is the anti-DNA test? If this is positive, the patient probably has lupus erythematosus.
2. What is the Sjögren's antibody titer? If this is positive, the patient probably has Sjögren's disease.

If the foregoing test results are negative, the patient probably has *rheumatoid arthritis,* although other collagen diseases, malignant disease, thyroid disorders, infection, and myocardial infarction may cause a positive test. In addition, elderly patients may have a false-positive test result.

## NORMAL VALUES

Negative.

## COST

Low.

## ADDITIONAL TESTS TO ORDER

CBC, sedimentation rate, chemistry panel, ANA, radiograph of joints, bone scan, synovianalysis, synovial biopsy, and rheumatology consult.

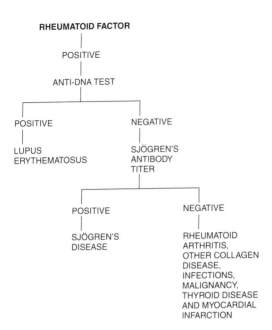

**RHEUMATOID FACTOR**
|
POSITIVE
|
ANTI-DNA TEST

POSITIVE

LUPUS
ERYTHEMATOSUS

NEGATIVE
|
SJÖGREN'S
ANTIBODY
TITER

POSITIVE
|
SJÖGREN'S
DISEASE

NEGATIVE
|
RHEUMATOID
ARTHRITIS,
OTHER COLLAGEN
DISEASE,
INFECTIONS,
MALIGNANCY,
THYROID DISEASE
AND MYOCARDIAL
INFARCTION

# ROCKY MOUNTAIN SPOTTED FEVER ANTIBODIES

## INCREASED

These antibodies are increased in Rocky Mountain spotted fever, as the name implies.

## NORMAL VALUES

Negative or no significant rise in titer between specimens.

## COST

Low.

## ADDITIONAL TESTS TO ORDER

Weil–Felix reaction, skin biopsy, CBC, LDH and chemistry panel, and consultation with an infectious disease specialist.

# RUBELLA ANTIBODY TESTS

## INCREASED

These antibodies are increased in patients who have or have had rubella. Active disease is diagnosed by testing a second specimen drawn 3 weeks after the first. A fourfold rise in titer indicates active infection. This test is important in establishing whether a pregnant woman is susceptible to rubella so she can be adequately immunized and protected from producing a child with a congenital anomaly. $\gamma$-Globulin is administered to pregnant women who are seronegative. If it can be established that a woman is not pregnant, the rubella vaccine may be administered. This vaccine must not be given to pregnant women.

## NORMAL VALUES

Less than 1:10 titer indicates that the patient is susceptible to rubella.

## COST

Low.

## ADDITIONAL TESTS TO ORDER

Viral isolation.

# SALIVARY GLAND SCAN

## FOCAL INCREASED UPTAKE

This is associated with Warthin's tumor, oncocytoma, or mucoepidermoid tumor.

## FOCAL DECREASED UPTAKE

This is associated with benign tumors, cysts, and adenocarcinoma.

## NORMAL VALUES

Uniform uptake throughout the glands.

## COST

Medium.

## ADDITIONAL TESTS TO ORDER

MRI, sialography, and consultation with an oral surgeon.

# SCHILLING TEST

## POSITIVE

A positive test (less than 8% excretion of cobalt-tagged $B_{12}$ in the urine) indicates either pernicious anemia or malabsorption syndrome. To differentiate these two disorders, the test should be repeated with intrinsic factor. If the urinary excretion of cobalt-tagged $B_{12}$ rises to normal, the patient probably has pernicious anemia. If the test remains positive, the patient probably has malabsorption syndrome. Remember, renal insufficiency and inadequate urine collection can yield a false-positive test result.

## NORMAL VALUES

Greater than 8% excretion of cobalt-tagged $B_{12}$ in the urine.

## COST

Medium.

## ADDITIONAL TESTS TO ORDER

CBC, chemistry panel, serum $B_{12}$ and folic acid, gastric analysis, D-xylose absorption test, bone marrow examination, small bowel biopsy, hematology consult, and gastroenterology consult.

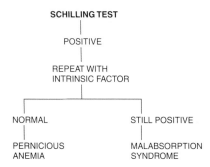

**SCHILLING TEST**
|
POSITIVE
|
REPEAT WITH
INTRINSIC FACTOR
|
NORMAL               STILL POSITIVE
|                          |
PERNICIOUS       MALABSORPTION
ANEMIA             SYNDROME

# SEDIMENTATION RATE

## INCREASED

The sedimentation rate is increased in infectious disease (particularly pelvic inflammatory disease and abscess formation), collagen disease, neoplasm, toxemia, nephritis, heavy metal poisoning, tissue necrosis such as myocardial infarction, multiple myeloma, and macroglobulinemia. Infectious disease can be distinguished by the elevated *WBC*. An *RBC* should be done to separate those conditions associated with anemia such as collagen disease, multiple myeloma, and macroglobulinemia.

## DECREASED

A decreased sedimentation rate is found in polycythemia vera, sickle cell anemia, spherocytosis, congestive heart failure, hypofibrinogenemia, Cushing's disease, and corticosteroid therapy. An RBC can be used to differentiate these disorders further. It is elevated in polycythemia vera and is decreased in sickle cell anemia and spherocytosis.

## NORMAL VALUES

Westergren, men: 0–15 mm/hour.
Westergren, women: 0–20 mm/hour.
Westergren, children: 0–10 mm/hour.

## COST

Low.

## ADDITIONAL TESTS TO ORDER

CBC, urinalysis, blood smear, serum protein electrophoresis, ANA, blood cultures, culture of other body fluids, chemistry panel, CRP, ASO titer, serologic tests, biopsy of tissue, bone scan, gallium scan, plain radiographs, MRI, CT scans, and consultation with an infectious disease expert or rheumatologist.

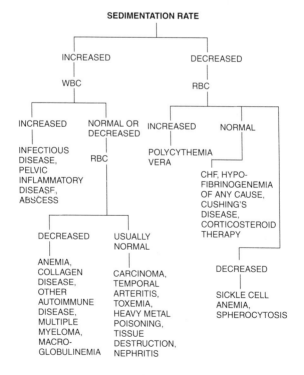

# SEMEN ANALYSIS

## ABNORMAL

An abnormal test is a count below 40 million/mL, more than 20% sperm deformity, and less than 60% motile sperm in a specimen. Abnormal results are found in male infertility, Klinefelter's syndrome, hypothalamic lesions, after vasectomy, and elevated prolactin.

## NORMAL VALUES

More than 70 million sperm/mL.
More than 60% active.
More than 80% normal forms.

## COST

Low.

## ADDITIONAL TESTS TO ORDER

Consultation with a urologist who specializes in male infertility.

# SHAKE TEST

## POSITIVE

A positive test on amniotic fluid indicates fetal maturity and, consequently, less susceptibility to hyaline membrane disease. Pulmonary surfactant in the amniotic fluid forms bubbles or foam in the presence of 95% ethyl alcohol. Dilutions can be made to determine the exact stage of immaturity.

## NORMAL VALUES

A positive result indicates fetal maturity. When the test is negative, the fetus is immature and susceptible to hyaline membrane disease.

## COST

Low.

## ADDITIONAL TESTS TO ORDER

Lecithin/sphingomyelin ratio, amniotic fluid creatinine, amniotic fluid cytology, pelvic ultrasonography, and gynecology consult.

# SICKLE CELL TEST

## POSITIVE

A positive test is found in sickle cell anemia and sickle cell trait. False-positive results occur for up to 4 months after a transfusion.

## NORMAL VALUES

Negative.

## COST

Low.

## ADDITIONAL TESTS TO ORDER

CBC, platelet count, sedimentation rate, hemoglobin electrophoresis, red cell fragility, red cell survival time, liver–spleen scan, and hematology consult.

# SIGMOIDOSCOPY AND ANOSCOPY

## POSITIVE

These tests are positive in carcinoma of the rectum and sigmoid colon, polyps, the various forms of colitis, diverticulitis, hemorrhoids, anal fistulas, anal fissures, and rectal strictures. Biopsies are often taken. They are both indicated in the workup of rectal bleeding. Remember, the anoscope must be used to diagnose rectal fissures and most hemorrhoids.

## NORMAL VALUES

Normal mucosa, no mass or obstructing lesions. No bleeding.

## COST

Medium.

## ADDITIONAL TESTS TO ORDER

CBC, urinalysis, chemistry panel, coagulation profile, stool for occult blood, culture, ova and parasites times three, *Giardia* antigen, barium enema, colonoscopy, gastroenterology consult, and proctology consult.

# SJÖGREN'S ANTIBODY TEST

## INCREASED

These antibodies are increased in primary Sjögren's disease. If the patient has combined rheumatoid arthritis and Sjögren's disease, these antibodies will not be present.

## NORMAL VALUES

Negative.

## COST

Low.

## ADDITIONAL TESTS TO ORDER

Schirmer test, thyroglobulin antibody titer, Epstein–Barr virus antibody titer, sedimentation rate, RA test, thyroid peroxidase antibody titer, biopsy of salivary gland, and rheumatology consult.

# SMALL BOWEL SERIES

## POSITIVE

Abnormalities that may be detected with a small bowel series include regional enteritis, Meckel's diverticulum, intussusception, malabsorption syndrome, malrotation, adhesions, neoplasms, small bowel ulcers, tuberculosis, intra-abdominal hernias, and parasites (e.g., ascariasis). Water-soluble material may be used to evaluate obstructing lesions.

## NORMAL VALUES

Normal size, shape, and position of small intestine without filing defects, obstruction, or mass.

## COST

Medium.

## ADDITIONAL TESTS TO ORDER

CBC, urinalysis, urine 5-HIAA, sedimentation rate, chemistry panel, stool for occult blood, culture and ova and parasites, stool for fat and trypsin, CT scan of abdomen, D-xylose absorption, lactose tolerance test, biopsy, exploratory laparotomy, and gastroenterology consult.

# SMEARS AND MICROSCOPIC EXAMINATION OF BODY FLUIDS

## SPUTUM SMEAR

The sputum smear is extremely useful in patients with pneumonia. It demonstrates leukocytes, clear evidence that an adequate specimen of sputum was obtained for culture. It also can be used immediately to identify the organism (e.g., *Streptococcus pneumoniae*). The next logical step is a sputum culture for common pathogens. If this is negative and the diagnosis of pneumonia is still entertained, cold agglutinin, MG streptococcal agglutinins, and *Legionella* cultures should be obtained to rule out *Mycoplasma pneumoniae* and legionnaire's disease. If these are negative, AFB smear and cultures, guinea pig inoculation, and fungal cultures and skin test are obtained. Finally, consideration of viral pneumonia is made, and acute- and convalescent-phase sera are ordered. Antibiotic treatment should not be withheld until all these studies are completed. In addition to bacterial pneumonia, sputum smears are used in diagnosing anthrax, bubonic plague, histoplasmosis, actinomycosis, nocardiosis, coccidiomycosis, blastomycosis, ascariasis, echinococcosis, and infection with *Paragonimus westermani*.

## Cost

Low.

## Additional Tests to Order

CBC, sedimentation rate, chemistry panel, tuberculin skin tests, serologic studies for suspected organisms, fungal skin tests, Kveim test, chest radiograph, CT scan or MRI of chest, ECG, echocardiogram, and pulmonary consult for bronchoscopy or bronchography.

## BLOOD SMEARS

Blood smears are most often ordered to diagnose parasitic illnesses such as malaria, trypanosomiasis, and filariasis. They can also be used to diagnose many spirochetal diseases such as syphilis, infection with *Borrelia recurrentis,* and Weil's disease.

### Cost

Low.

### Additional Tests to Order

CBC, urine, chemistry panel, sedimentation rate, serologic tests, blood cultures, bone marrow biopsy, animal inoculation, dark field examination, and consultation with an infectious disease specialist.

## URINE SMEAR

At the same time a clean catch urine is obtained for culture, it is wise to examine the unspun urine under high dry microscopy for motile bacteria. A few organisms per HPF are good laboratory evidence of a urinary tract infection, and antibiotic therapy can be started immediately. The urine smear can also be used to diagnose tuberculosis, Weil's disease, histoplasmosis, echinococcosis, and schistosomiasis. A clinical pathologist should be consulted for assistance.

## Cost

Low.

## Additional Tests to Order

Urine culture, urinalysis, CBC, blood cultures, blood smears, serologic tests, IVP, cystoscopy and retrograde pyelogram, CT scan of abdomen and pelvis, tuberculin test, other skin tests, liver biopsy, spinal fluid examination, and consultation with an infectious disease specialist.

## URETHRAL SMEAR

A urethral smear has classically been used to diagnose gonorrhea. The gram-negative diplococci are distinct, especially if they are intracellular. A urethral smear is also useful after prostatic massage to determine the presence of bacterial prostatitis. A certain number of leukocytes per HPF is typical. Urethral smears are of little value in diagnosing nongonococcal urethritis caused by *Chlamydia trachomatis.* This infection is better diagnosed by cultures and serologic techniques.

## Cost

Low.

## Additional Tests to Order

CBC, urinalysis, sedimentation rate, chemistry panel, cultures of exudate, vaginal smear and culture, serologic tests for *Neisseria gonorrhoeae* and *Chlamydia trachomatis,* cystoscopy, culture of material obtained after prostatic massage, and urology consult.

## SMEARS OF PENILE LESIONS

These are useful in diagnosing chancroid, granuloma inguinale, and syphilis (dark-field examination), but not lymphogranuloma venereum. A clinical pathologist should be consulted for assistance.

### Cost

Low.

### Additional Tests to Order

See page 206.

## SMEARS OF SKIN LESIONS

Smears of exudates from carbuncles, abscesses, and furuncles only rarely assist in identifying the responsible organism, so this test is rarely used. Skin smears are useful in the diagnosis of bubonic plague (Giemsa stain), leprosy, glanders, anthrax (Gram stain), pinta, syphilis, rat bite fever, yaws, tetanus, actinomycosis, blastomycosis, smallpox, herpes zoster (Tzanck preparation), herpes simplex (Tzanck preparation), and scabies (KOH preparation). A clinical pathologist should be consulted for assistance.

### Cosl

Low.

### Additional Tests to Order

CBC, sedimentation rate, chemistry panel, routine cultures of exudates, fungal cultures, serologic tests, skin tests, therapeutic trial, skin biopsy, animal inoculation, and consultation with an infectious disease specialist.

## CEREBROSPINAL FLUID SMEAR

This technique is useful for the rapid diagnosis of bacterial meningitis, and it may demonstrate pneumococci, meningococci, or *Haemophilus influenzae* bacilli using a Gram stain technique. Other organisms that may be diagnosed by this method are *Cryptococcus* (India ink preparation), *Gonococcus,* and *Mycobacterium tuberculosis.*

### Cost

Low.

### Additional Tests to Order

CSF analysis and culture, routine fungi, AFB, serologic tests, guinea pig inoculation, CT scan or MRI of brain, nose and throat culture, blood cultures, sputum cultures, VDRL, and neurology consult.

## STOOL SMEAR

Stool smears may be stained with methylene blue to show leukocytes, which are almost diagnostic of bacillary dysentery (*Shigella, Salmonella,* turista). Stool smears are also useful in detecting ova and parasites, especially the agents of *Entamoeba, Giardia, Ascaris, Taenia solium* and *T. saginata, Diphyllobothrium latum, Enterobius* (Scotch tape preparation), hookworm, *Paragonimus westermani, Schistosoma, Strongyloides,* and *Trichuris.*

### Cost

Low.

### Additional Tests to Order

Stool cultures, stool for occult blood, serologic tests and skin test, stool for *Giardia* antigen, sigmoidoscopy and barium enema, colonoscopy and rectal biopsy, liver biopsy, and gastroenterology consult.

# SODIUM

## INCREASED

The serum sodium is increased in any condition that causes a loss of water without corresponding loss of salt. This occurs in dehydration, diabetes insipidus, heat exhaustion, Cushing's syndrome, and aldosteronism. To differentiate these conditions further, one should look at the chloride. If it is increased, then the patient most likely has dehydration, diabetes insipidus, or heat exhaustion. If it is decreased, one should consider Cushing's syndrome and aldosteronism.

## DECREASED

Ask the following questions:

1. What is the chloride? An increased chloride points to Addison's disease, diabetic acidosis, renal tubular acidosis, nephritis, and certain diuretics as the cause. A decreased chloride prompts consideration of congestive heart failure, SIADH, pyloric obstruction, vomiting, malabsorption, and diuretics as the cause.
2. What is the blood sugar? A marked increase in the blood sugar suggests diabetic acidosis.
3. What is the plasma cortisol? If the plasma cortisol is decreased, consider Addison's disease. Decreased sodium, increased chloride but normal blood sugar and plasma cortisol should prompt consideration of renal tubular acidosis, nephritis, and certain diuretics as the cause.
4. What is the blood volume? The blood volume is increased in congestive heart failure and SIADH.

## NORMAL VALUES

135–145 mEq/L.

## COST

Low.

## ADDITIONAL TESTS TO ORDER

CBC, urinalysis, chemistry panel, serial electrolytes, plasma cortisol, serum ADH, plasma renin, 24-hour urine aldosterone, arterial blood gases, withholding of all drugs, if possible, and consultations with an endocrinologist and nephrologist.

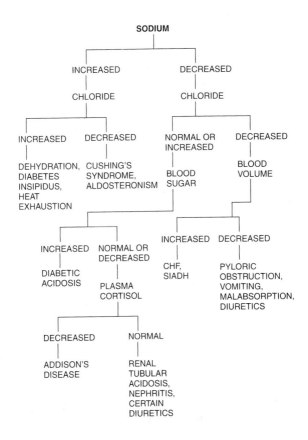

# SODIUM, URINE

## INCREASED

Ask the following question: What is the urine volume? If the *urine* volume is *increased* in the face of an *increased sodium* concentration, think of diabetic acidosis, diuretic use, chronic renal failure, and salicylate toxicity. If the *urine* volume is *decreased* but the *sodium* concentration is *increased,* think of dehydration, starvation, Addison's disease, SIADH, and acute tubular necrosis.

## DECREASED

Ask the following question: What is the urine volume? A *decreased sodium* concentration with an *increased* urine *volume* suggests aldosteronism, Cushing's disease, pulmonary emphysema, malabsorption syndrome, and diabetes insipidus. A *decreased* urine *sodium* concentration with a *decreased* urine *volume* suggests pyloric obstruction, prolonged vomiting or diarrhea, congestive heart failure, acute renal failure, and diaphoresis.

## NORMAL VALUES

Child: 40–180 mmol/day.
Adult: 40–210 mmol/day.

## COST

Low.

## ADDITIONAL TESTS TO ORDER

CBC, chemistry panel, urinalysis, serum and urine osmolality, repeated serum electrolytes, urine culture, Fishberg concentration test, serum ADH assay, plasma cortisol, blood volume, plasma renin, 24-hour urine aldosterone, nephrology consult, and endocrinology consult.

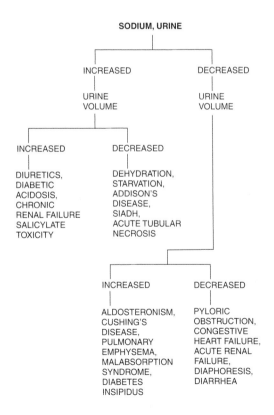

SODIUM, URINE

INCREASED

URINE VOLUME

INCREASED

DIURETICS, DIABETIC ACIDOSIS, CHRONIC RENAL FAILURE SALICYLATE TOXICITY

DECREASED

DEHYDRATION, STARVATION, ADDISON'S DISEASE, SIADH, ACUTE TUBULAR NECROSIS

DECREASED

URINE VOLUME

INCREASED

ALDOSTERONISM, CUSHING'S DISEASE, PULMONARY EMPHYSEMA, MALABSORPTION SYNDROME, DIABETES INSIPIDUS

DECREASED

PYLORIC OBSTRUCTION, CONGESTIVE HEART FAILURE, ACUTE RENAL FAILURE, DIAPHORESIS, DIARRHEA

# SOMATOMEDIN C

## INCREASED

Suggestive of acromegaly.

## DECREASED

This indicates hypopituitarism or pituitary dwarfism. It can also be decreased in cirrhosis, hypothyroidism, and malnutrition. A decrease of somatomedin C is also found in end organ resistance to growth hormone (Laron dwarfism).

## NORMAL VALUES

Check with local laboratory.

## COST

Medium.

## ADDITIONAL TESTS TO ORDER

FSH, LH, free $T_4$, TSH, prolactin, plasma cortisol and testosterone, plasma estrogen, CT scan of brain and pituitary gland, and endocrinology consult.

# SPECIFIC GRAVITY, URINE

## INCREASED

The urine specific gravity is increased in dehydration, prolonged vomiting or diarrhea, diabetes mellitus, nephrosis, and SIADH.

## DECREASED

Ask the following questions:

1. Is the BUN increased? This suggests nephritis (glomerulonephritis and chronic pyelonephritis).
2. Does the specific gravity increase after antidiuretic hormone administration? This suggests pituitary diabetes insipidus. If there is no response to ADH administration, the patient probably has renal diabetes insipidus, provided the BUN is normal.

## NORMAL VALUES

1.015–1.025 on normal fluid intake and diet.

## COST

Low.

## ADDITIONAL TESTS TO ORDER

CBC, chemistry panel, sedimentation rate, urinalysis, Fishberg concentration test, serum osmolality, creatinine clearance, Hickey–Hare test, urine culture, plasma antidiuretic hormone assay, CT scan of brain and pituitary gland, IVP, and nephrology consult.

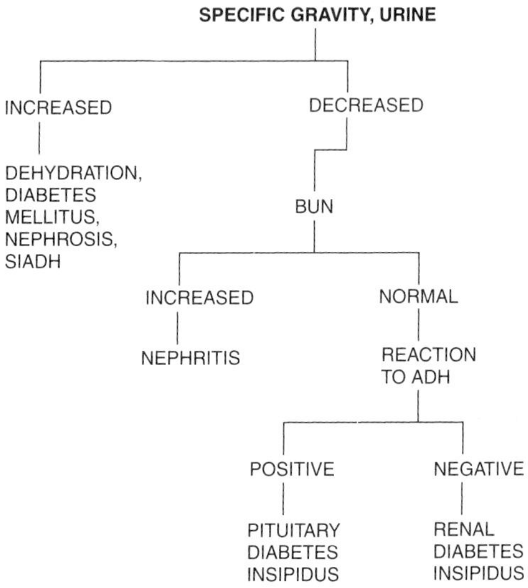

**SPECIFIC GRAVITY, URINE**

INCREASED

DEHYDRATION,
DIABETES
MELLITUS,
NEPHROSIS,
SIADH

DECREASED

BUN

INCREASED

NEPHRITIS

NORMAL

REACTION
TO ADH

POSITIVE

PITUITARY
DIABETES
INSIPIDUS

NEGATIVE

RENAL
DIABETES
INSIPIDUS

# SPLEEN SCAN

## POSITIVE

This scan is positive in Hodgkin's disease, metastatic neoplasms, trauma, and splenic infarct. It can be useful to evaluate spleen size in liver and hematologic disorders and to assist in determining the need for splenectomy. It is also helpful in locating accessory spleens.

## NORMAL VALUES

Uniform uptake, normal shape and size.

## COST

Medium.

## ADDITIONAL TESTS TO ORDER

CBC, urinalysis, sedimentation rate, chemistry panel, bone marrow examination, ANA, CT scan of abdomen, liver scan, and hematology consult.

# SPLEEN ULTRASONOGRAPHY

## POSITIVE

This test is positive in hematoma, cysts, and metastatic neoplasms of the spleen. It is also used to determine the size of the spleen in hemolytic anemias and thrombocytopenic purpura when a splenectomy is contemplated. The spleen also has a characteristic echo pattern in long-standing sickle cell disease.

## NORMAL VALUES

Normal size, shape and position of the spleen with a homogeneous echo pattern.

## COST

Medium.

## ADDITIONAL TESTS TO ORDER

CBC, urinalysis, chemistry panel, sedimentation rate, serum haptoglobins, liver–spleen scan, red cell survival time, CT scan of abdomen, splenic angiography, bone marrow biopsy, and hematology consult.

# SPUTUM CULTURE, ROUTINE

## POSITIVE

A positive sputum culture is found in many different disorders, including pneumonia, abscess, bronchitis, bronchiectasis, and empyema. A *chest radiograph* identifies an infiltrate in most cases of *pneumonia,* distinguishing this disorder from other members of this group. If the chest radiograph is negative, one should consider repeat cultures to rule out contamination, bronchoscopy, bronchography, and a pulmonary consult.

## NEGATIVE

If the culture is negative and an infectious disease is strongly suspected, one should perform AFB smear and culture, anaerobic culture and fungal cultures, or skin tests. It may be necessary to do cultures for Eaton agent pneumonia and legionnaires' disease. A pulmonary consult is valuable in this instance also.

## NORMAL VALUES

Negative.

## COST

Low.

## ADDITIONAL TESTS TO ORDER

CBC, sputum smear, chest radiograph, sedimentation rate, thoracentesis, lung biopsy, cold agglutinins, MG Streptococcus agglutinin, guinea pig inoculation, serologic tests, and pulmonary consult.

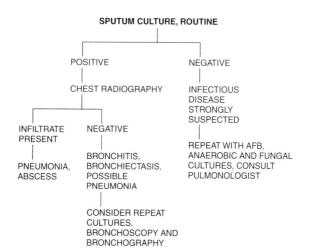

**SPUTUM CULTURE, ROUTINE**

POSITIVE

CHEST RADIOGRAPHY

INFILTRATE PRESENT

PNEUMONIA, ABSCESS

NEGATIVE

BRONCHITIS, BRONCHIECTASIS, POSSIBLE PNEUMONIA

CONSIDER REPEAT CULTURES, BRONCHOSCOPY AND BRONCHOGRAPHY

NEGATIVE

INFECTIOUS DISEASE STRONGLY SUSPECTED

REPEAT WITH AFB, ANAEROBIC AND FUNGAL CULTURES, CONSULT PULMONOLOGIST

# STOOL ANALYSIS

## BLOOD

Bright red blood may signify rectal carcinoma, polyp, hemorrhoids, or anal fissure. Darker blood or blood mixed with stool often signifies carcinoma of the colon, ulcerative colitis, amebic colitis, bacillary dysentery, diverticulitis, or upper GI bleeding with rapid transit. Dark or black stools that are Hemoccult-positive suggest bleeding peptic ulcer or other upper GI bleeding source. Normal-looking stools that are Hemoccult-positive can indicate bleeding anywhere in the entire GI tract.

## WBC

Significant leukocytes in the stool usually indicate infection with *Salmonella*, bacillary dysentery, or cholera.

## COLOR

*Black* stools signify upper GI bleeding, iron, certain foods and Pepto-Bismol. *Clay color* stools suggest obstructive jaundice. *Yellow to green* stools may appear in diarrhea, regardless of the cause. The green stools are usually indicative of severe diarrhea.

## FAT

Increased fat in the stool indicates malabsorption syndrome of many causes. A stool quantitative fat analysis should be done.

## MUCUS

Increased mucus is present in irritable bowel syndrome, ulcerative colitis, bacillary dysentery, and carcinoma. When mixed with blood, it is more suggestive of ulcerative colitis and carcinoma.

## NORMAL VALUES

Consult your laboratory.

## COST

Low.

## ADDITIONAL TESTS TO ORDER

Sigmoidoscopy, colonoscopy, esophagoscopy, gastroscopy, barium enema, upper GI series, small bowel series, CT scan of abdomen, gastrointestinal bleeding scan, stool cultures, stool for ova and parasites, quantitative stool fat, liver function tests, and gastroenterology consult.

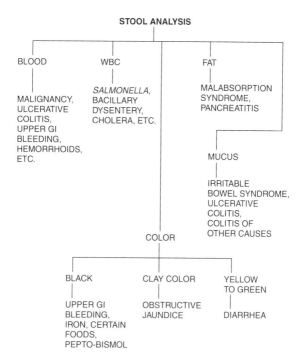

# STREPTOCOCCAL ANTIBODY TESTS (ASO, ADB, STREPTOZYME)

## INCREASED

These antibody titers are increased in streptococcal pharyngitis, rheumatic fever, glomerulonephritis, and pyoderma. ASO are often high in rheumatic fever and glomerulonephritis, whereas the ADB titer is highest in pyoderma.

## NORMAL VALUES

### ASO Titer

Less than 166 Todd U.

### ADB Titer

Less than 340 U in adults.
Less than 480 U in children.
Less than 170 U in children younger than 4 years old.

### Streptozyme

Negative.

## COST

Low.

## ADDITIONAL TESTS TO ORDER

CBC, sedimentation rate, CRP, chemistry panel, throat culture, ECG, urinalysis, Addis count, renal biopsy, echocardiography, and consultation with a cardiologist or nephrologist.

# SULFHEMOGLOBIN

## INCREASED

Sulfhemoglobin is increased in toxicity from acetanilid, aniline dyes, phenacetin, sulfides, sulfonamides, benzene chemicals, nitrates, and nitrites.

## NORMAL VALUES

Less than 1% of total hemoglobin.

## COST

Low.

## ADDITIONAL TESTS TO ORDER

Methemoglobin, CBC, blood smear, red cell survival, blood gas analysis, urine drug screen, sedimentation rate, chemistry panel, and toxicology consult.

# SWEAT TEST

## POSITIVE

An increased concentration of sodium and chloride in sweat is typical of cystic fibrosis. False-positive results can occur in Addison's disease, congenital adrenocortical hyperplasia, ectodermal dysplasia, diabetes insipidus, and G6PD, among other conditions.

## NORMAL VALUES

Under 14 years of age: Less than 40 mEq/L sodium and chloride in the sweat.

## COST

Low.

## ADDITIONAL TESTS TO ORDER

DNA analysis, pulmonary function testing, and consultation with a pulmonologist.

# SYNOVIAL FLUID ANALYSIS

Ask the following questions:

1. What is the WBC? If this is markedly increased and a culture is positive, the patient probably has septic arthritis or tuberculosis.
2. If the WBC is markedly increased, what is the RA factor or mucin clot test? If these are positive, consider the possibility of rheumatoid arthritis. If these are negative, the patient may have lupus erythematosus, Reiter's disease, or rheumatic fever.
3. If the WBC is normal or slightly increased, what is the RBC? If the RBC is increased, the patient may have traumatic arthritis.
4. If the WBC is normal or slightly increased, are crystals present? The presence of crystals indicates gout or pseudogout. In pseudogout, the crystals are weakly positive birefringent to polarized light. Uric acid crystals are strongly negative birefringent.
5. If the WBC is normal or slightly increased and no significant RBCs or crystals are present, the patient probably has osteoarthritis. However, septic arthritis and other forms of arthritis may still be possible.

## NORMAL VALUES

Fluid is transparent, light yellow, and contains fewer than 2000 WBCs/mm$^3$. No crystals seen. Good mucin clot formation.

## COST

Medium.

## ADDITIONAL TESTS TO ORDER

CBC, urine, chemistry panel, sedimentation rate, blood cultures, RA factor, ANA, radiograph of joints, bone scan, MRI of joint, arthrography, arthroscopy, orthopedic consult, and rheumatology consult.

**SYNOVIAL FLUID ANALYSIS**

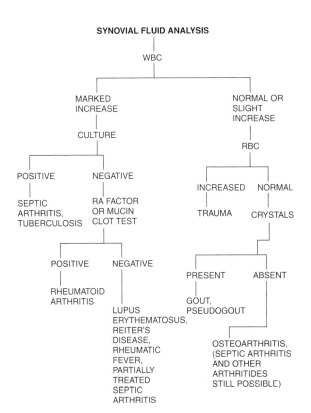

# T AND B LYMPHOCYTES

## T CELLS INCREASED

An increase of T cells occurs in Graves' disease.

## T CELLS DECREASED

T cells are decreased in thymic dysplasia, ataxia–telangiectasia, severe combined immunodeficiency disorders, Wiskott–Aldrich syndrome, Hodgkin's disease, and chronic lymphatic leukemia. To differentiate these conditions further, a B-cell count should be obtained. The B-cell count is *increased* in thymic dysplasia and ataxia–telangiectasia, whereas it is *decreased* in severe combined immunodeficiency disorder and in some cases of Wiskott–Aldrich syndrome. It is normal in Hodgkin's disease and chronic lymphocytic leukemia.

In patients with HIV infections, the progress of the disease can be monitored by performing counts of subpopulations of T lymphocytes. The CD4 T-cell determination is useful in this regard. Three CD4 categories have been established:

Category I: More than 500 CD4 cells/mm$^3$
Category II: 200–499 CD4 cells/mm$^3$
Category III: Fewer than 200 CD4 cells/mm$^3$

Category I is the mildest form of this disease, whereas category III is the most severe.

## NORMAL VALUES

B cells: 10–30% of total lymphocytes.
T cells: 70–90% of total lymphocytes.

## COST

Medium.

## ADDITIONAL TESTS TO ORDER

Lymphocyte mitogen study, CBC, sedimentation rate, chemistry panel, HIV antibody titer, serum protein electrophoresis, ANA, bone marrow examination, lymph node biopsy, and hematology consult.

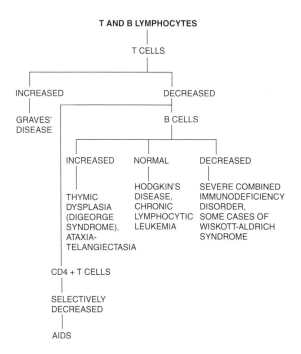

# TECHNETIUM-99M RESTING HEART SCAN

## INCREASED UPTAKE

Areas of increased uptake of technetium-99m stannous pyrophosphate may signify a recent myocardial infarction. This scan can be used to diagnose a myocardial infarction when cardiac enzymes and serial ECGs are equivocal.

## DECREASED UPTAKE

Areas of decreased uptake may indicate an old myocardial infarction.

## NORMAL VALUES

Uniform uptake.

## COST

Medium.

## ADDITIONAL TESTS TO ORDER

Serial cardiac enzymes, serial ECGs, cardiac catheterization and coronary angiography, and cardiac consult.

# TEICHOIC ACID ANTIBODY TITER

## INCREASED

This antibody is increased in infections with *Staphylococcus aureus.* It is helpful in differentiating between skin contamination and a genuine staphylococcal infection.

## NORMAL VALUES

Titer of less than 1:8.

## COST

Low.

## ADDITIONAL TESTS TO ORDER

CBC, urinalysis, chemistry panel, sedimentation rate, CRP, repeated blood cultures, needle aspiration of abscess, echocardiography, and consultation with an infectious disease expert.

# TESTOSTERONE

## INCREASED

This hormone is increased in ovarian tumors, Leydig cell tumors, adrenal neoplasms, testosterone therapy, hyperthyroidism, ectopic FSH production, and Stein–Leventhal syndrome. To differentiate these conditions further, one should order a serum FSH. This value is increased in ectopic FSH production and Stein–Leventhal syndrome. It is normal or decreased in the other conditions in this group.

## DECREASED

This hormone is decreased in hypogonadism, Klinefelter's syndrome, orchiectomy, and pituitary insufficiency. These conditions can be further differentiated by a serum FSH. This value is decreased in pituitary insufficiency but is increased in the other conditions in this group.

## NORMAL VALUES

Men: 300–1200 ng/dL.
Women: 20–80 ng/dL.

## COST

Low.

## ADDITIONAL TESTS TO ORDER

Free testosterone, plasma cortisol, free $T_4$ and TSH, serum estradiol, FSH and LH, urine 17-ketosteroids, pelvic ultrasonography, CT scan of abdomen and pelvis, gynecology consult in women and urology consult in men, and endocrinology consult in both. A therapeutic trial of testosterone may be done in male hypogonadism.

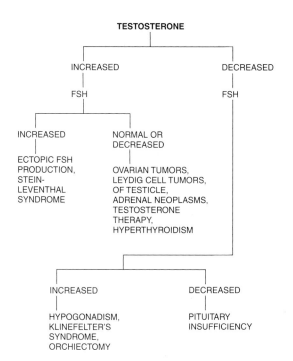

**TESTOSTERONE**

INCREASED

FSH

INCREASED

ECTOPIC FSH
PRODUCTION,
STEIN-
LEVENTHAL
SYNDROME

NORMAL OR
DECREASED

OVARIAN TUMORS,
LEYDIG CELL TUMORS,
OF TESTICLE,
ADRENAL NEOPLASMS,
TESTOSTERONE
THERAPY,
HYPERTHYROIDISM

DECREASED

FSH

INCREASED

HYPOGONADISM,
KLINEFELTER'S
SYNDROME,
ORCHIECTOMY

DECREASED

PITUITARY
INSUFFICIENCY

# THALLIUM GATED EQUILIBRIUM HEART SCAN

## DEFINITION

This test is similar to a thallium stress scan, except multiple images of the myocardium are made during an exercise tolerance test in synchrony with various ECG recordings. It therefore allows the cardiologist to determine the ejection fraction, ejection velocity, and left ventricular wall motion. By repeating the test with nitroglycerin, one can determine the value of this medical therapy.

## NORMAL VALUES

Uniform uptake of thallium-201 in all images taken.

## COST

High.

## ADDITIONAL TESTS TO ORDER

ECG, chest radiograph, exercise tolerance test, coronary angiography, and cardiac consult.

# THALLIUM STRESS SCAN

## DECREASED UPTAKE

When thallium-201 is injected intravenously at the time of maximum stress during an exercise tolerance test, ischemic areas show decreased uptake. Areas of myocardial infarction and damage also show decreased uptake.

## NORMAL VALUES

Uniform uptake of thallium-201.

## COST

High.

## ADDITIONAL TESTS TO ORDER

ECG, chest radiograph, exercise tolerance test, coronary angiography, and cardiac consult.

# THERAPEUTIC DRUG MONITORING

## DEFINITION

Therapeutic drug levels are monitored to allow better clinical management in various diseases. The following is a list of the most important drugs that may be monitored and their therapeutic range.

Anticonvulsants
  Phenytoin: 10–20 $\mu$g/mL
  Carbamazepine: 4–12 $\mu$g/mL
  Phenobarbital: 15–40 $\mu$g/mL
  Valproic acid: 50–100 $\mu$g/mL
  Ethosuximide: 40–100 $\mu$g/mL
Antibiotics
  Amikacin: 10–30 $\mu$g/mL
  Gentamicin: 4–10 $\mu$g/mL
  Tobramycin: 4–10 $\mu$g/mL
  Chloramphenicol: 10–20 $\mu$g/mL
Cardiac drugs
  Digoxin: 0.5–2.0 ng/mL
  Quinidine: 2.0–5.0 $\mu$g/mL
  Procainamide: 4.0–8.0 $\mu$g/mL
Pulmonary drugs
  Theophylline: 10–20 $\mu$g/mL
Psychiatric drugs
  Lithium: 0.6–1.2 mmol/L
  Amitriptyline: 75–250 ng/mL
  Nortriptyline: 50–150 ng/mL

Whenever a patient must be on a drug for a long time, the local laboratory should be consulted about possible monitoring of the therapeutic drug level.

## COST

Low to medium.

# THROAT CULTURE, ROUTINE

## POSITIVE

The most common organism detected by routine throat culture is β-hemolytic *Streptococcus*. If this culture is positive, the infection should be treated, and an ASO titer should be done to detect rheumatic fever and acute glomerulonephritis. If the throat culture is positive for *Staphylococcus aureus* or *Neisseria meningitidis,* this may identify a carrier of these diseases.

## NEGATIVE

A negative routine throat culture is found in diphtheria, viral pharyngitis, and infectious mononucleosis. If the sore throat or exudate continues, one should repeat the routine culture and also use special media to detect *Corynebacterium diphtheriae.* A streptozyme test or ASO titer helps to identify streptococcal pharyngitis. A Monospot test helps to identify infectious mononucleosis. If these tests are negative, one should repeat the routine culture.

## NORMAL VALUES

Negative.

## COST

Low.

## ADDITIONAL TESTS TO ORDER

Streptozyme test, ASO titer, Monospot test, CBC, sedimentation rate, culture on Loeffler's medium, acute- and convalescent-phase serum for viral studies, and infectious disease consult.

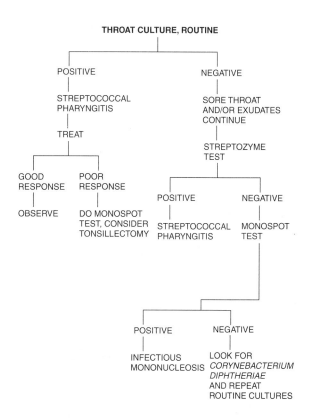

**THROAT CULTURE, ROUTINE**

POSITIVE

STREPTOCOCCAL
PHARYNGITIS

TREAT

GOOD
RESPONSE

OBSERVE

POOR
RESPONSE

DO MONOSPOT
TEST, CONSIDER
TONSILLECTOMY

NEGATIVE

SORE THROAT
AND/OR EXUDATES
CONTINUE

STREPTOZYME
TEST

POSITIVE

STREPTOCOCCAL
PHARYNGITIS

NEGATIVE

MONOSPOT
TEST

POSITIVE

INFECTIOUS
MONONUCLEOSIS

NEGATIVE

LOOK FOR
*CORYNEBACTERIUM
DIPHTHERIAE*
AND REPEAT
ROUTINE CULTURES

# THROMBIN TIME

## INCREASED

This is increased in afibrinogenemia, hypofibrinogenemia, heparin therapy, disseminated intravascular coagulation, liver disease, and dysproteinemia such as multiple myeloma. To differentiate these conditions further, one should order a PTT. The PTT is increased in heparin therapy and disseminated intravascular coagulation, whereas it is normal in hypofibrinogenemia, whatever the cause, and the dysproteinemias.

## NORMAL VALUES

24–35 seconds (values vary greatly by laboratory).

## COST

Low.

## ADDITIONAL TESTS TO ORDER

CBC, platelet count, PTT, prothrombin time, fibrin split products, bleeding time, protein electrophoresis, chemistry panel, bone marrow examination, and hematology consult.

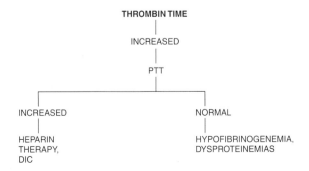

# THYROGLOBULIN

## INCREASED

This substance is increased in untreated and metastatic differentiated carcinoma of the thyroid. It is used to follow the course of these tumors. It is also increased in hyperthyroidism, subacute thyroiditis, benign adenoma, and nontoxic nodular goiter. The thyroglobulin is normal in medullary carcinoma of the thyroid. This test is limited by the fact that the assay is unreliable in the presence of antithyroglobulin antibodies, which occur in many patients with thyroid carcinoma.

## NORMAL VALUES

50 ng/mL or less.

## COST

Low.

## ADDITIONAL TESTS TO ORDER

Free $T_4$, calcitonin, RAI uptake and scan, antithyroglobulin antibodies, sedimentation rate, whole-body radionuclide scan, thyroid ultrasound, CT scan or MRI, and endocrinology consult.

# THYROID ANTIBODIES

## INCREASED

Thyroid antibodies (antimicrosomal or antithyro-globulin) are found in Graves' disease, Hashimoto's disease, lymphadenoid goiter, and other thyroid disorders. Extremely high titers are found in *Hashimoto's disease.* False-positive results occur in lupus erythematosus, rheumatoid arthritis, and Sjögren's syndrome.

## NORMAL VALUES

Values vary by laboratory.

## COST

Low.

## ADDITIONAL TESTS TO ORDER

CBC, urinalysis, chemistry panel, ANA, sedimentation rate, free $T_4$, TSH, needle biopsy of thyroid, CT scan, and endocrinology consult.

# THYROID ULTRASONOGRAPHY

## POSITIVE

This test is positive in thyroid cysts, adenomas, and carcinomas. It is most useful in differentiating a cyst from a tumor. If a cold nodule is found on a thyroid scan, this is the next procedure to order, to determine whether the cold nodule is a cyst or a tumor.

## NORMAL VALUES

The thyroid is normal in size and position and has a homogeneous echo pattern (moderately echogenic throughout).

## COST

Medium.

## ADDITIONAL TESTS TO ORDER

CBC, urinalysis, chemistry panel, free $T_4$, TSH, thyroid antibodies, RAI uptake and scan, CT scan of the thyroid, fine needle aspiration, surgical consult, and endocrinology consult.

# THYROID-STIMULATING HORMONE (TSH)–SENSITIVE ASSAY

## INCREASED

The TSH-sensitive assay is increased in primary hypothyroidism.

## DECREASED

A decreased TSH-sensitive assay is found in hyperthyroidism, hypopituitarism, and tertiary hypothyroidism. To differentiate these three, first one must obtain a free $T_4$. If this is elevated, hyperthyroidism is confirmed. Next, one should perform a TRH stimulation test. If there is no response, the patient has hypopituitarism. If a response is seen, the patient has tertiary (hypothalamic) hypothyroidism.

## NORMAL VALUES

A response.

## COST

Low.

## ADDITIONAL TESTS TO ORDER

Free $T_3$, RAI uptake and scan, thyroid ultrasound, thyroid antibodies, TBG, sedimentation rate, therapeutic trial, and endocrinology consult.

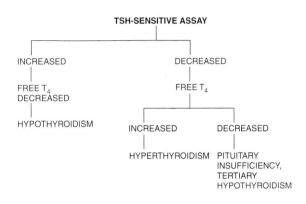

# THYROTROPIN-RELEASING HORMONE (TRH) STIMULATION TEST

## GOOD RESPONSE

A good response is found in the normal state and primary hypothyroidism. This helps to differentiate myxedema from the other causes of hypothyroidism.

## LITTLE OR NO RESPONSE

This is seen in pituitary insufficiency and hyperthyroidism.

## DELAYED RESPONSE

A delayed response of elevation of the TSH is seen in tertiary (hypothalamic) hypothyroidism.

## NORMAL VALUES

An increase of TSH to twice baseline levels after TRH administration.

## COST

Medium.

## ADDITIONAL TESTS TO ORDER

CBC, urinalysis, chemistry panel, sedimentation rate, free $T_4$, RAI uptake and scan, therapeutic trial, and endocrinology consult.

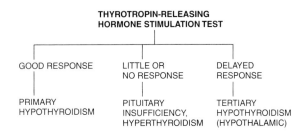

**THYROTROPIN-RELEASING
HORMONE STIMULATION TEST**

| GOOD RESPONSE | LITTLE OR NO RESPONSE | DELAYED RESPONSE |
|---|---|---|
| PRIMARY HYPOTHYROIDISM | PITUITARY INSUFFICIENCY, HYPERTHYROIDISM | TERTIARY HYPOTHYROIDISM (HYPOTHALAMIC) |

# THYROXINE-BINDING GLOBULIN (TBG)

## INCREASED

This protein is increased in therapy with certain drugs, hypothyroidism, pregnancy, porphyria, and congenital TBG increase. To differentiate these conditions further, one should obtain a drug history and discontinue the drug. If the drug history is negative, a *free T$_4$* is indicated. This distinguishes *hypothyroidism* from the rest of the conditions in the group. The free T$_4$ is *normal* in *congenital TBG increase.*

## DECREASED

TBG is decreased in nephrotic syndrome, liver disease, acidosis, acromegaly, androgen and other drug therapy, and congenital TBG deficiency. To distinguish nephrotic syndrome and liver disease, one should obtain a serum albumin determination. This value is decreased in those two conditions, but it is normal in the rest of the disorders in this group.

## NORMAL VALUES

15–25 $\mu$g/dL.

## COST

Low.

## ADDITIONAL TESTS TO ORDER

Urine porphobilinogen and porphyrins, pregnancy test, 24-hour urine protein, liver function tests, growth hormone, arterial blood gases, and endocrinology consult.

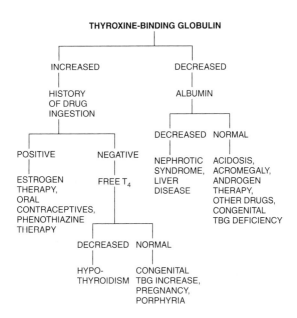

THYROXINE-BINDING GLOBULIN

INCREASED

HISTORY
OF DRUG
INGESTION

POSITIVE

ESTROGEN
THERAPY,
ORAL
CONTRACEPTIVES,
PHENOTHIAZINE
THERAPY

NEGATIVE

FREE T$_4$

DECREASED

HYPO-
THYROIDISM

NORMAL

CONGENITAL
TBG INCREASE,
PREGNANCY,
PORPHYRIA

DECREASED

ALBUMIN

DECREASED

NEPHROTIC
SYNDROME,
LIVER
DISEASE

NORMAL

ACIDOSIS,
ACROMEGALY,
ANDROGEN
THERAPY,
OTHER DRUGS,
CONGENITAL
TBG DEFICIENCY

# TORCH TEST

## INDICATIONS

This is a combination of serologic tests for *Toxoplasma*, rubella, cytomegalovirus, and herpes simplex that is performed on mothers and newborn infants to determine whether they have been exposed to these organisms. Positive tests are more of prognostic significance than the basis for treatment because treatment is useless in all but toxoplasmosis.

## NORMAL VALUES

Negative.

## COST

Low to medium.

## ADDITIONAL TESTS TO ORDER

Repeat titers, viral isolation, tissue cultures, CSF antibody studies, and consultation with a neonatologist.

# TOTAL PROTEIN

## INCREASED

Total protein is increased in hemoconcentration, as occurs in dehydration, vomiting and diarrhea, diabetes insipidus, and in states in which one or more proteins are increased, such as multiple myeloma, sarcoidosis, or collagen disease. To differentiate these two groups, one should look at the serum albumin. It is increased in dehydration, vomiting and diarrhea, and diabetes insipidus. It is decreased in multiple myeloma, sarcoidosis, and collagen disease.

## DECREASED

Ask the following questions:

1. What is the globulin? If the globulin is *increased*, look for nephrosis, eclampsia, cirrhosis, chronic hepatitis, monoclonal gammopathies (e.g., multiple myeloma), and exfoliative dermatitis. If the globulin is decreased, look for disorders that cause hemodilution such as congestive heart failure, excessive IV fluids, acute renal failure, and SIADH or disorders that restrict protein production such as starvation and malabsorption syndrome. Also in this group are burns and hypogammaglobulinemia.
2. What is the BUN? Decreased globulin with an increased BUN is often associated with nephrosis or eclampsia. A normal or decreased BUN is found in cirrhosis, chronic hepatitis, exfoliative dermatitis, and multiple myeloma.
3. Are the liver function tests abnormal? This distinguishes cirrhosis and chronic hepatitis from the rest of the group.

## NORMAL VALUES

Total protein: 6–8 g/dL.

## COST

Low.

## ADDITIONAL TESTS TO ORDER

CBC, urinalysis, sedimentation rate, chemistry panel, serum protein electrophoresis, ANA, blood volume, RA test, Kveim test, lymph node biopsy, 24-hour urine protein, liver function tests, liver biopsy, renal biopsy, immunoelectrophoresis, spirometry, D-xylose absorption test, plasma ADH, and oncology consult.

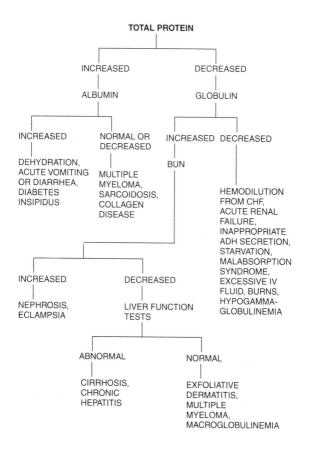

# TOTAL THYROXINE (T₄)

## INCREASED

An increased total $T_4$ is found in hyperthyroidism, subacute thyroiditis, estrogen therapy, oral contraceptive use, and pregnancy. To distinguish hyperthyroidism and subacute thyroiditis from the rest of the conditions in this group, one should order a $T_3$ uptake. The *$T_3$ uptake* is *increased* in hyperthyroidism and subacute thyroiditis, but it is decreased in estrogen therapy, oral contraceptive use, and pregnancy.

## DECREASED

The *total $T_4$* is *decreased* in androgen therapy, steroid therapy, nephrotic syndrome, severe liver disease, hypopituitarism, and primary hypothyroidism. Once again, the disorders in this group can be differentiated further by ordering a $T_3$ uptake. The *$T_3$ uptake* is *decreased* in primary hypothyroidism and pituitary insufficiency, whereas it is *increased* in patients who are receiving androgen or corticosteroid therapy or who have nephrotic syndrome or severe liver disease.

## NORMAL VALUES

Total $T_4$: 5–12.5 μg/dL.
$T_3$ uptake: 25–35%.

## COST

Low.

## ADDITIONAL TESTS TO ORDER

Free $T_4$, sensitive assay-TSH, RAI uptake and scan, sedimentation rate, chemistry panel, pregnancy test, TRH stimulation test, 24-hour urine protein, and endocrinology consult.

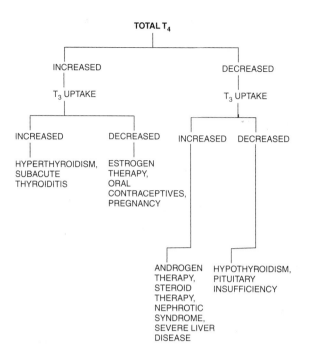

TOTAL T$_4$

INCREASED

T$_3$ UPTAKE

INCREASED

HYPERTHYROIDISM, SUBACUTE THYROIDITIS

DECREASED

ESTROGEN THERAPY, ORAL CONTRACEPTIVES, PREGNANCY

DECREASED

T$_3$ UPTAKE

INCREASED   DECREASED

ANDROGEN THERAPY, STEROID THERAPY, NEPHROTIC SYNDROME, SEVERE LIVER DISEASE

HYPOTHYROIDISM, PITUITARY INSUFFICIENCY

**Total Thyroxine (T$_4$)     567**

# TOXOPLASMOSIS ANTIBODY TESTS

## POSITIVE

A titer of 1:256 or higher strongly suggests toxoplasmosis. However, a rising titer is much more significant. IgM antibodies are also more suggestive of active disease. They appear within 1 week of infection and disappear in 4 months. False-positive test results occur in collagen disease and rheumatoid arthritis. False-negative results occur in newborn infants and immunocompromised hosts.

## NORMAL VALUES

Negative.

## COST

Low.

## ADDITIONAL TESTS TO ORDER

Tissue culture, animal inoculation, tissue biopsy, chemistry panel, and consultation with an infectious disease specialist.

# TOXOPLASMOSIS
# SKIN TEST

## POSITIVE

A positive test indicates the patient has at some time been infected with *Toxoplasma gondii*.

## NORMAL VALUES

Negative.

## COST

Low.

## ADDITIONAL TESTS TO ORDER

Serologic tests, ophthalmology consult, culture of organisms in the peritoneal cavity of mice, and neurology consult.

# *TRICHINELLA* SKIN TEST

## POSITIVE

A positive reaction occurs within 15–20 minutes of inoculation and indicates trichinosis.

## NORMAL VALUES

Negative.

## COST

Low.

## ADDITIONAL TESTS TO ORDER

Eosinophil count, chemistry panel, serum IgE, serologic tests (bentonite flocculation test), muscle biopsy, and consultation with an infectious disease specialist or parasitologist.

# TRIGLYCERIDE

The triglyceride is most useful in distinguishing among the various types of lipoproteinemia.

## MARKEDLY INCREASED

Ask the following questions:

1. Are the chylomicrons increased? If these are increased along with the increased triglycerides, look for type V and type I lipoproteinemias. Normal chylomicrons suggest type III lipoproteinemia.
2. What is the cholesterol? An increased cholesterol with both increased chylomicrons and triglyceride identifies type V lipoproteinemia. A normal cholesterol with both increased triglyceride and chylomicrons identifies type I lipoproteinemia. An increased cholesterol with increased triglyceride but normal chylomicrons identifies type III lipoproteinemia.

## MILDLY TO MODERATELY INCREASED

Ask the following question: What is the cholesterol? If the cholesterol is increased in this group, the patient has type IIb lipoproteinemia. If the cholesterol is normal or only slightly increased, the patient has type IV lipoproteinemia.

## NORMAL

A normal triglyceride with an elevated cholesterol (usually marked increase) is typical of type IIa lipoproteinemia.

## SECONDARY LIPOPROTEINEMIAS

Triglyceride is increased in nephrotic syndrome, hypothyroidism, diabetes mellitus, glycogen storage disease, and insulinoma.

## DECREASED

Triglyceride is decreased in malnutrition, malabsorption syndrome, advanced cirrhosis, and congenital $\alpha$-$\beta$-lipoproteinemia.

## NORMAL VALUES

50–150 mg/dL.

## COST

Low.

## ADDITIONAL TESTS TO ORDER

CBC, urinalysis, chemistry panel, free $T_4$, 24-hour urine protein, lipoprotein electrophoresis, renal biopsy, liver biopsy, and consultation with a metabolic disease specialist.

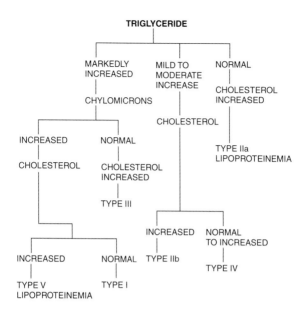

TRIGLYCERIDE

MARKEDLY INCREASED — CHYLOMICRONS

- INCREASED CHOLESTEROL
  - INCREASED — TYPE V LIPOPROTEINEMIA
  - NORMAL — TYPE I
- NORMAL — CHOLESTEROL INCREASED — TYPE III

MILD TO MODERATE INCREASE — CHOLESTEROL

- INCREASED — TYPE IIb
- NORMAL TO INCREASED — TYPE IV

NORMAL — CHOLESTEROL INCREASED — TYPE IIa LIPOPROTEINEMIA

# TRYPSIN, STOOL

## ABSENT

Absence of trypsin in the stools suggests pancreatic insufficiency.

## NORMAL VALUES

Positive.

## COST

Low.

## ADDITIONAL TESTS TO ORDER

Quantitative stool fat, duodenal analysis, secretin test, serum amylase and lipase, CT scan of abdomen, and gastroenterology consult.

# TUBERCULIN TEST

## POSITIVE

A *positive* reaction to this test means that the patient has or had tuberculosis or has been inoculated against tuberculosis. To distinguish between active and dormant tuberculosis, one should order sputum for AFB smear and culture, chest radiographs, and guinea pig inoculation of sputum or other body fluids (e.g., CSF). A patient who is clinically ill probably has tuberculosis. A positive test in a healthy patient probably signifies healed tuberculosis or infection with a different type of mycobacteria.

## NEGATIVE

A *negative* tuberculin test does not rule out tuberculosis. The patient may have miliary tuberculosis or pleural effusion. A negative tuberculin test is also found in sarcoidosis. A negative test to the intermediate tuberculin test (1:1000) in a person highly suspected of harboring the disease should prompt consideration of the stronger (1:100) tuberculin test.

## COST

Low.

# TYROSINE, URINE

## INCREASED

Tyrosine is increased in the urine in hypertyrosinemia, hyperthyroidism, Hartnup's disease, galactosemia, hepatic failure, and during the first trimester of pregnancy.

## NORMAL VALUES

Consult your local laboratory.

## COST

Low.

## ADDITIONAL TESTS TO ORDER

CBC, urinalysis, chemistry panel, urine amino acids, free $T_4$, pregnancy test, serum galactose, liver function tests, and consultation with an expert in metabolic disease.

# UPPER GASTROINTESTINAL SERIES AND ESOPHAGOGRAM

## POSITIVE

Positive findings are gastric and duodenal ulcers, carcinoma of the stomach and esophagus, hiatal hernia, achalasia of the esophagus, reflux esophagitis, diffuse esophageal spasm, stomal ulcers, and benign tumors of the upper GI tract. Esophageal and duodenal diverticula may be found. Endoscopy is a more definitive procedure, but it is more expensive and invasive. This test is indicated in the workup of melena. Water-soluble material may be used to evaluate obstructing lesions.

## NORMAL VALUES

Normal size, shape, and position of the esophagus, stomach and duodenum without filling defects, mass, or obstruction.

## COST

Medium.

## ADDITIONAL TESTS TO ORDER

CBC, chemistry panel, gastric analysis, stool for occult blood, serum gastrin, endoscopy (EGD), CT scan of abdomen, esophageal manometry, Bernstein test, and gastroenterology consult.

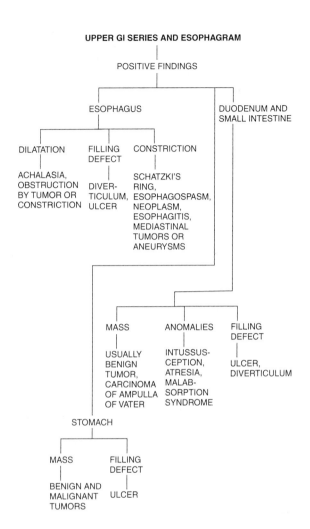

UPPER GI SERIES AND ESOPHAGRAM

POSITIVE FINDINGS

ESOPHAGUS

DUODENUM AND SMALL INTESTINE

DILATATION

ACHALASIA, OBSTRUCTION BY TUMOR OR CONSTRICTION

FILLING DEFECT

DIVERTICULUM, ULCER

CONSTRICTION

SCHATZKI'S RING, ESOPHAGOSPASM, NEOPLASM, ESOPHAGITIS, MEDIASTINAL TUMORS OR ANEURYSMS

MASS

USUALLY BENIGN TUMOR, CARCINOMA OF AMPULLA OF VATER

ANOMALIES

INTUSSUSCEPTION, ATRESIA, MALABSORPTION SYNDROME

FILLING DEFECT

ULCER, DIVERTICULUM

STOMACH

MASS

BENIGN AND MALIGNANT TUMORS

FILLING DEFECT

ULCER

# URIC ACID

## INCREASED

Ask the following questions:

1. Is the patient an infant or child? If the answer is yes, then the patient may have Lesch–Nyhan syndrome or Down's syndrome.
2. Is the BUN or urine protein increased? An increased BUN suggests renal disease, whereas increased urine protein suggests toxemia of pregnancy or myeloma.
3. Is there an associated increase in the white or red cell count? This may indicate polycythemia vera or leukemia.
4. If none of the foregoing questions can be answered positively, the patient probably has gout. However, other hematologic conditions (e.g., lymphoma, megaloblastic anemia) and the effect of drugs (e.g., thiazides, cytotoxics, and ethambutol) must be excluded.

## NORMAL VALUES

Adult males: 3.5–8.0 mg/dL.
Adult females: 2.5–6.2 mg/dL.
Children: 2.0–7.0 mg/dL.

## COST

Low.

## ADDITIONAL TESTS TO ORDER

CBC, urinalysis, chemistry panel, thyroid profile, arthrocentesis, chromosomal analysis, and hematology consult.

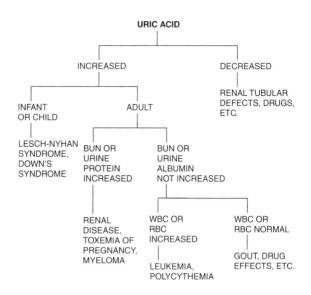

URIC ACID

INCREASED — DECREASED

DECREASED: RENAL TUBULAR DEFECTS, DRUGS, ETC.

INCREASED:
- INFANT OR CHILD: LESCH-NYHAN SYNDROME, DOWN'S SYNDROME
- ADULT:
  - BUN OR URINE PROTEIN INCREASED: RENAL DISEASE, TOXEMIA OF PREGNANCY, MYELOMA
  - BUN OR URINE ALBUMIN NOT INCREASED:
    - WBC OR RBC INCREASED: LEUKEMIA, POLYCYTHEMIA
    - WBC OR RBC NORMAL: GOUT, DRUG EFFECTS, ETC.

# URIC ACID, URINE

## INCREASED

Ask the following questions:

1. What is the serum uric acid? If both the urine and serum uric acid are increased, think of conditions with increased uric acid production such as lymphoma, leukemia, or gout. If the serum uric acid is decreased, consider Fanconi's syndrome, liver disease, drugs, starvation, and febrile illness.
2. What is the WBC? If the WBC is increased, consider leukemia or polycythemia vera. If it is normal, consider lymphoma, toxemia of pregnancy, or gout with increased uric acid production.

## DECREASED

The urine uric acid is decreased in renal disease such as nephritis and renal failure and in gout associated with decreased uric acid excretion.

## NORMAL VALUES

0.4–1.0 q/24 hours.

## COST

Low.

## ADDITIONAL TESTS TO ORDER

CBC, chemistry panel, urinalysis, bone marrow examination, serum haptoglobins, free $T_4$, pregnancy test, synovianalysis, radiographs of joints, cystoscopy and retrograde pyelography, serum copper and ceruloplasmin, renal biopsy, rheumatology consult, and nephrology consult.

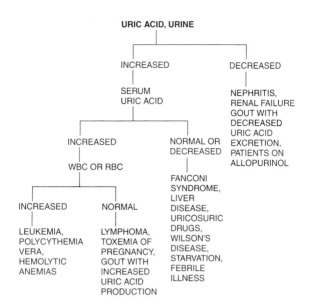

**URIC ACID, URINE**

- INCREASED
  - SERUM URIC ACID
    - INCREASED
      - WBC OR RBC
        - INCREASED
          - LEUKEMIA, POLYCYTHEMIA VERA, HEMOLYTIC ANEMIAS
        - NORMAL
          - LYMPHOMA, TOXEMIA OF PREGNANCY, GOUT WITH INCREASED URIC ACID PRODUCTION
    - NORMAL OR DECREASED
      - FANCONI SYNDROME, LIVER DISEASE, URICOSURIC DRUGS, WILSON'S DISEASE, STARVATION, FEBRILE ILLNESS
- DECREASED
  - NEPHRITIS, RENAL FAILURE GOUT WITH DECREASED URIC ACID EXCRETION, PATIENTS ON ALLOPURINOL

# URINARY BLADDER ULTRASONOGRAPHY

## POSITIVE

This test is positive in bladder tumors, large bladder stones, and bladder neck obstruction. It is most useful in determining residual urine volume after voiding. Therefore, it avoids the use of a catheter and, consequently, the risk of infection.

## NORMAL VALUES

Normal thickness of bladder walls and no masses, less than 100 mL of residual volume.

## COST

Medium.

## ADDITIONAL TESTS TO ORDER

CBC, urinalysis, urine culture, PSA, catheterization for residual urine, IVP, cystoscopy and retrograde pyelography, CT scan of pelvis, and urology consult.

# URINE CULTURE

## POSITIVE

1. Do a colony count. If colony count shows over 100,000 colonies/mL, a diagnosis of urinary tract infection is confirmed.
2. To differentiate between cystitis and pyelonephritis, examine the urine for white cell casts or clumps. Pyelonephritis is the most likely diagnosis if these are present.

## NEGATIVE

1. If the colony count is below 10,000 and a urinary tract infection is strongly suspected, repeat the urine culture, being sure to obtain an anaerobic culture, as well. If this is negative and the patient is a woman, obtain a culture for *Chlamydia* and *Gonococcus.* Finally, perform an IVP, culture for AFB, and consult a urologist.
2. Remember, interstitial nephritis can cause pyuria, and the urine cultures are repeatedly negative.

## COST

Low.

## NEITHER DEFINITELY POSITIVE NOR DEFINITELY NEGATIVE

Patients with colony counts between 10,000 and 100,000 should be treated depending on the clinical picture.

## NORMAL VALUES

Negative.

## ADDITIONAL TESTS TO ORDER

CBC, urinalysis, chemistry panel, serum protein electrophoresis, urine culture, colony count, AFB culture, anaerobic culture, IVP, cystoscopy and retrograde pyelography, pelvic ultrasound, urethral smear after prostatic massage, voiding cystogram, gynecology consult, urology consult, and nephrology consult.

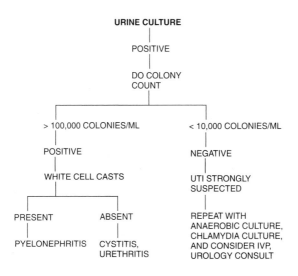

**URINE CULTURE**

POSITIVE

DO COLONY COUNT

> 100,000 COLONIES/ML

POSITIVE

WHITE CELL CASTS

PRESENT

PYELONEPHRITIS

ABSENT

CYSTITIS, URETHRITIS

< 10,000 COLONIES/ML

NEGATIVE

UTI STRONGLY SUSPECTED

REPEAT WITH ANAEROBIC CULTURE, CHLAMYDIA CULTURE, AND CONSIDER IVP, UROLOGY CONSULT

# UROBILINOGEN, STOOL

## INCREASED

Urobilinogen is increased in the stool in hemolytic anemias, but false-positive results occur in porphyria. To distinguish between the two disorders, one should perform a Watson–Schwartz test on the urine. This test is positive in the intermittent abdominal form of porphyria.

## DECREASED

Urobilinogen is absent or decreased in the stool in obstructive jaundice, severe liver disease, aplastic anemia, and oral antibiotic therapy. To differentiate these conditions further, one should order a serum bilirubin.

## NORMAL VALUES

130–250 Ehrlich units/100 g of stool.

## COST

Low.

## ADDITIONAL TESTS TO ORDER

CBC, liver function tests, CT scan of abdomen, hematology consult, and gastroenterology consult.

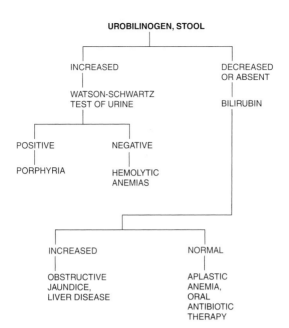

**UROBILINOGEN, STOOL**

INCREASED

WATSON-SCHWARTZ
TEST OF URINE

POSITIVE

PORPHYRIA

NEGATIVE

HEMOLYTIC
ANEMIAS

DECREASED
OR ABSENT

BILIRUBIN

INCREASED

OBSTRUCTIVE
JAUNDICE,
LIVER DISEASE

NORMAL

APLASTIC
ANEMIA,
ORAL
ANTIBIOTIC
THERAPY

# UROBILINOGEN, URINE

## INCREASED

Urobilinogen is increased in the urine in liver disease and hemolytic anemia. To differentiate these two, one should look for bilirubin in the urine. The presence of bilirubin in the urine suggests liver disease, whereas its absence points to hemolytic anemia. A positive response to Ehrlich's reagent may also mean that porphobilinogen is present. Consequently, a Watson–Schwartz test should be done to rule out porphyria.

## ABSENT

Patients with obstructive jaundice have no urobilinogen in the urine, especially if the obstruction is complete. The one exception is ascending cholangitis, because bacteria in the bile ducts can convert the bilirubin to urobilinogen.

## NORMAL VALUES

0.1–1 Ehrlich unit/dL.

## COST

Low.

## ADDITIONAL TESTS TO ORDER

Liver function tests, CBC, serum haptoglobins, hepatitis profile, gallbladder ultrasound, HIDA scan, CT scan of abdomen, and gastroenterology consult.

**UROBILINOGEN, URINE**

```
UROBILINOGEN, URINE
        |
   ┌────┴────────────────────┐
INCREASED                  ABSENT
   |                          |
BILIRUBIN                 BILIRUBIN
   |                          |
┌──┴──────┐               PRESENT
PRESENT  ABSENT              |
   |       |             OBSTRUCTIVE
LIVER   WATSON-SCHWARTZ  JAUNDICE
DISEASE  TEST
           |
      ┌────┴────┐
   POSITIVE  NEGATIVE
      |         |
  PORPHYRIA  HEMOLYTIC
             ANEMIA
```

# VANILLYLMANDELIC ACID (VMA) AND CATECHOLAMINES

## INCREASED

The 24-hour urine VMA and catecholamines are increased in tumors of the adrenal medulla, such as pheochromocytomas, neuroblastomas, ganglioneuromas, and ganglioblastomas. These levels may also be increased in progressive muscular dystrophy and myasthenia gravis. False-positive results may result from certain foods (e.g., tea, coffee, bananas, chocolate), certain drugs (e.g., aspirin, chlorpromazine, penicillin), and starvation.

## NORMAL VALUES

VMA: 9 mg or less/24 hours.
Catecholamines: 100 $\mu$g or less/24 hours.

## COST

Low.

## ADDITIONAL TESTS TO ORDER

CT scan of abdomen, plasma catecholamines, arteriography, metiodobenzylguanidine scan, and endocrinology consult.

# VENEREAL DISEASE RESEARCH LABORATORY (VDRL) AND RAPID PLASMA REAGIN (RPR)

## POSITIVE

A positive result usually means that the patient has syphilis. After proper treatment, the test becomes negative in 6 to 18 months in most patients with primary or secondary syphilis. Several conditions cause a false-positive reaction, including malaria, lupus erythematosus, and various gammopathies. A negative VDRL of the CSF does not rule out CNS syphilis.

## NORMAL VALUES

Negative.

## COST

Low.

## ADDITIONAL TESTS TO ORDER

FTA–ABS (fluorescent treponemal antibody absorption test), dark-field examination of specimens, MRI of brain, TPI, CSF analysis and FTA–ABS, and consultation with a neurologist or infectious disease specialist.

# VENOGRAPHY

## POSITIVE

This test is most commonly used to diagnose deep vein thrombosis of the lower extremities. It may also be helpful in evaluating varicose veins before surgery and in diagnosing the cause of edema of the extremities.

## NORMAL VALUES

No dilatation or constriction of veins. No intraluminal thrombus or other obstruction.

## COST

Medium.

## ADDITIONAL TESTS TO ORDER

CBC, coagulation profile, blood viscosity, iodine-135 fibrinogen scan, impedance phlebography, Doppler study of the veins, cardiology consult, and consultation with a vascular surgeon.

# VENTILATION-PERFUSION SCAN

## DEFINITION

This test involves the use of two radioactive substances, one to show the distribution of the blood supply to various parts of the lung and the other to show the distribution of the air supply to various parts of the lung. Technetium-labeled macroaggregated albumin is injected IV to show the pulmonary vasculature, whereas krypton-81m or xenon-33I is breathed into the lung to show the adequacy of the ventilation in various parts of the lung.

## DECREASED PERFUSION

Single or multiple areas of decreased perfusion usually signify *pulmonary emboli.* However, false-positive results occur in pulmonary emphysema, lung cancer, and congenital anomalies.

## DECREASED VENTILATION

Abnormalities on the ventilation scan may be found in pneumonia, emphysema, atelectasis, tumors, and cysts. The ventilation scan usually is normal in *pulmonary embolism.* On the other hand, the perfusion scan usually is normal in pneumonia, atelectasis, and tumors.

## NORMAL VALUES

Perfusion scan: uniform uptake.
Ventilation scan: uniform uptake.

## COST

High.


## ADDITIONAL TESTS TO ORDER

CBC, chemistry panel, arterial blood gas analysis, chest radiograph, ECG, pulmonary angiography, sputum culture and analysis, cytology of sputum, bronchoscopy, pulmonary consult, and cardiology consult.

# VIRAL ISOLATION AND ANTIBODY TESTS

## INDICATIONS

These tests are ordered to establish the diagnosis of many viral infections such as lymphocytic chorio-meningitis, viral encephalitis, herpes simplex, mumps, measles, influenza and varicella zoster virus infections. Acute- and convalescent-phase blood specimens are required.

## NORMAL VALUES

Negative or no rise in titer between acute- and conva-lescent-phase specimen.

## COST

Low to medium.

## ADDITIONAL TESTS TO ORDER

CBC, urinalysis, sedimentation rate, chemistry panel, CSF analysis, skin tests, biopsy, cultures and sero-logic tests to rule out bacterial infection, and consul-tation with an infectious disease specialist.

# VISCOSITY, BLOOD

## INCREASED

Increased viscosity is associated with polycythemia, hyperproteinemia, and certain anemias in which the red cell configuration contributes to the increased viscosity. To differentiate these conditions, one should order an *RBC*. If it is *increased,* one should suspect polycythemia vera or secondary polycythemia. If it is normal or decreased, a *serum protein* is indicated. If the serum protein is increased, one should suspect multiple myeloma or macroglobulinemia. If it is normal, sickle cell anemia, hereditary spherocytosis, and other congenital anemias are possibilities.

## NORMAL VALUES

1.4–2.0 times the viscosity of water.

## COST

Low.

## ADDITIONAL TESTS TO ORDER

CBC, platelet count, blood smear for morphology, sedimentation rate, chemistry panel, protein electrophoresis, immunoelectrophoresis, bone marrow examination, and oncology consult.

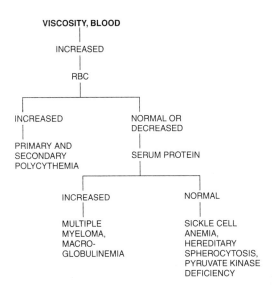

**VISCOSITY, BLOOD**
|
INCREASED
|
RBC

INCREASED
|
PRIMARY AND
SECONDARY
POLYCYTHEMIA

NORMAL OR
DECREASED
|
SERUM PROTEIN

INCREASED
|
MULTIPLE
MYELOMA,
MACRO-
GLOBULINEMIA

NORMAL
|
SICKLE CELL
ANEMIA,
HEREDITARY
SPHEROCYTOSIS,
PYRUVATE KINASE
DEFICIENCY

# VITAMIN B$_{12}$

## INCREASED

Vitamin B$_{12}$ is increased in leukemia, polycythemia vera, liver disease, and anemia. It may also be increased during oral contraceptive use. To differentiate these conditions, one should order a CBC, BUN, and liver function tests.

## DECREASED

Vitamin B$_{12}$ is decreased in pernicious anemia, hypothyroidism, gastric atrophy, gastric carcinoma, and malabsorption syndrome. To differentiate malabsorption syndrome from the other conditions in this group, a folic acid level should be determined. This value is decreased in malabsorption.

## NORMAL VALUES

200–800 pg/mL.

## COST

Low.

## ADDITIONAL TESTS TO ORDER

CBC, urinalysis, chemistry panel, sedimentation rate, Schilling test, D-xylose absorption test, urine 5-HIAA, mucosal biopsy, liver function tests, free T$_4$, upper GI series and small bowel follow through, therapeutic trial, and gastroenterology consult.

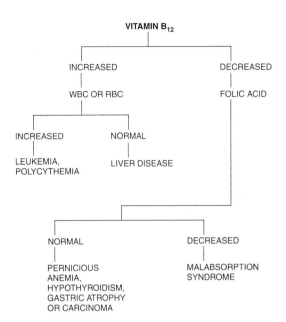

**VITAMIN B₁₂**

INCREASED

WBC OR RBC

INCREASED

LEUKEMIA,
POLYCYTHEMIA

NORMAL

LIVER DISEASE

DECREASED

FOLIC ACID

NORMAL

PERNICIOUS
ANEMIA,
HYPOTHYROIDISM,
GASTRIC ATROPHY
OR CARCINOMA

DECREASED

MALABSORPTION
SYNDROME

# VITAMIN D METABOLITES (25-HYDROXYCALCIFEROL)

## DECREASED

This metabolite of vitamin D is decreased in malabsorption syndrome, anticonvulsant therapy, liver disease, hyperthyroidism, diet, lack of sunlight, rheumatoid arthritis, and nephrotic syndrome. To distinguish between malabsorption syndrome and the rest of the group, one should order a D-xylose absorption test or serum carotene. These are decreased in malabsorption syndrome. To distinguish between liver disease and the rest of the group, liver function tests are indicated. To rule out nephrotic syndrome, one should order a 24-hour urine protein, renal function tests, or a renal biopsy. To rule out hyperthyroidism, a free $T_4$ assay is indicated.

## NORMAL VALUES

10–55 ng/mL.

## COST

Medium.

## ADDITIONAL TESTS TO ORDER

CBC, urinalysis, chemistry panel, PTH assay, liver function tests, serum folic acid, serum carotene, urine 5-HIAA, 24-hour urine protein, mucosal biopsy, renal biopsy, free $T_4$, RA test, ANA, 1,25-$(OH)_2$ $D_3$, gastroenterology consult, nephrology consult, and endocrinology consult.

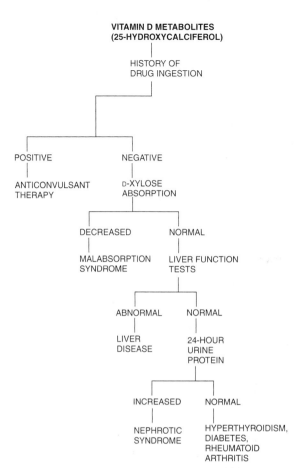

**VITAMIN D METABOLITES
(25-HYDROXYCALCIFEROL)**

HISTORY OF
DRUG INGESTION

POSITIVE

ANTICONVULSANT
THERAPY

NEGATIVE

D-XYLOSE
ABSORPTION

DECREASED

MALABSORPTION
SYNDROME

NORMAL

LIVER FUNCTION
TESTS

ABNORMAL

LIVER
DISEASE

NORMAL

24-HOUR
URINE
PROTEIN

INCREASED

NEPHROTIC
SYNDROME

NORMAL

HYPERTHYROIDISM,
DIABETES,
RHEUMATOID
ARTHRITIS

**Vitamin D Metabolites    601**

# VITAMINS, MISCELLANEOUS

## VITAMIN A, BLOOD

This substance is *decreased* in vitamin A deficiency, Crohn's disease, and malabsorption syndrome and *increased* in hypervitaminosis A syndrome, diabetes mellitus, chronic nephritis, and hypothyroidism.

### Normal Values

30–95 $\mu$g/dL.

### Cost

Low.

### Additional Tests to Order

CBC, chemistry panel, D-xylose absorption test, stool for fat and trypsin, therapeutic trial, and GI consult.

## VITAMIN $B_6$, BLOOD

This substance is *decreased* in chronic alcoholism, malnutrition, malabsorption syndrome, pregnancy, and the use of certain drugs.

### Normal Values

5–24 ng/mL.

## Cost

Low.

## Additional Tests to Order

CBC, urinalysis, sedimentation rate, chemistry panel, NCV studies, D-xylose absorption test, therapeutic trial, and neurology consult.

## VITAMIN C, PLASMA

This substance is *decreased* in vitamin C deficiency. Smoking, obesity, stress, alcohol, and infection increase the demand for vitamin C.

## Normal Values

0.2–2.0 mg/dL.

## Cost

Low.

## Additional Tests to Order

CBC, capillary fragility, platelet count, radiograph of long bones, chemistry panel, consultation with a metabolic disease expert, and therapeutic trial.

## VITAMIN E, BLOOD

This substance is *decreased* in malabsorption syndrome, premature infants, and $\beta$-lipoproteinemia and *increased* in hyperlipemia associated with obstructive liver disease.

## Normal Values

Adults: 0.5–1.8 mg/dL.
Premature infants: 0.31 ± 0.06 mg/dL.


## Cost

Low.


## Additional Tests to Order

CBC, urine, chemistry panel, lipid profile, liver function tests, therapeutic trial, D-xylose absorption test, and consultations with a hematologist and hepatologist.


## VITAMIN K

This vitamin is *decreased* in malnutrition, chronic pancreatitis, cystic fibrosis, malabsorption syndrome, and liver disorders. In infants, it is associated with hemorrhagic disease of the newborn.


## Normal Values

0.13–1.19 ng/mL.


## Cost

Low.


## Additional Tests to Order

CBC, urinalysis, prothrombin time, PTT, coagulation profile, hematology consult, and therapeutic trial.

# WHITE BLOOD CELL COUNT (WBC), CEREBROSPINAL FLUID

## INCREASED

An increase in WBCs in the CSF is most often due to an infectious process, but it may also be related to leukemia or lymphoma. A predominance of mononuclear cells usually means a viral origin, whereas the predominance of neutrophils usually signifies a bacterial process. However, because of an overlap here, one should look at the CSF glucose. If it is decreased, one should consider bacterial, tuberculous, or fungal meningitis as the most likely cause. If it is normal, a viral cause, multiple sclerosis, syphilis, malignant disease, or leukemia is probably the cause, although the glucose level can be reduced in severe leukemic infiltration.

## NORMAL VALUES

0–5 cells/mm$^3$.

## COST

Low.

## ADDITIONAL TESTS TO ORDER

CBC, chemistry panel, sedimentation rate, blood cultures, CSF analysis, CSF smear and cultures, CT scan, MRI, bone marrow examination, and neurology consult.

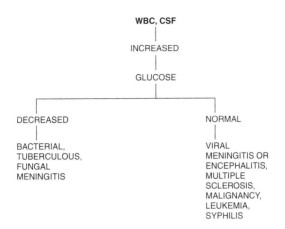

WBC, CSF

INCREASED

GLUCOSE

DECREASED

BACTERIAL,
TUBERCULOUS,
FUNGAL
MENINGITIS

NORMAL

VIRAL
MENINGITIS OR
ENCEPHALITIS,
MULTIPLE
SCLEROSIS,
MALIGNANCY,
LEUKEMIA,
SYPHILIS

# WHITE BLOOD CELL COUNT (WBC), DIFFERENTIAL

1. Increased neutrophils: This finding is usually a sign of bacterial infections, but it may occur in hemorrhage, trauma, corticosteroid therapy, and tissue necrosis.
2. Increased lymphocytes: This finding is a sign of a viral infection, infectious mononucleosis, and lymphatic leukemia.
3. Increased monocytes: An increased percentage of monocytes is found in severe infections and monocytic leukemia. The atypical lymphs in infectious mononucleosis may be confused with monocytes.
4. Increased eosinophils: Allergic disorders and parasitic diseases are usually the cause of eosinophilia, but periarteritis nodosa may be the cause.
5. Increased basophils: This finding is associated with chronic myelogenous leukemia and certain blood dyscrasias.

## NORMAL VALUES

Neutrophils: 60–70%.
Lymphocytes: 20–40%
Monocytes: 2–6%.
Eosinophils: 1–4%.
Basophils: 0.5–1%.

## COST

Low.

## ADDITIONAL TESTS TO ORDER

CBC, urinalysis, platelet count, reticulocyte count, sedimentation rate, total eosinophil count, stool for ova and parasites, blood cultures, urine cultures, immunologic studies, chemistry panel, Monospot test, ANA, bone marrow examination, and hematology consult.

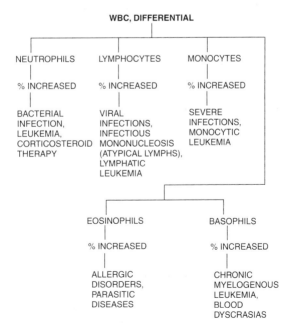

# WHITE BLOOD CELL COUNT (WBC), TOTAL

Ask the following questions:

1. Is the WBC increased? An increased WBC suggests infectious disease (particularly bacterial), leukemia, myelofibrosis, hemorrhage, trauma, tissue necrosis, hemolytic anemia, and polycythemia.
2. If the WBC is increased, what is the RBC? An increased RBC along with an elevated WBC suggests primary and secondary polycythemia. A decreased RBC in association with an increased WBC suggests hemolytic anemia, leukemia, myelofibrosis, certain infectious diseases, and hemorrhage. Further differentiation can be made by looking at the platelet count. If this is decreased, leukemia and myelofibrosis are more likely.
3. Is the WBC decreased? A decreased WBC by itself suggests viral disease or agranulocytosis. If it is accompanied by a drop in the RBC and platelet count, consider hypersplenism, aplastic anemia, aleukemic leukemia, myelophthisic anemia, megaloblastic anemia, and paroxysmal nocturnal hemoglobinuria.
4. Is the spleen significantly enlarged? In the presence of pancytopenia, this suggests hypersplenism which, of course, has many causes.

## NORMAL VALUES

$5,000-10,000/mm^3$.

## COST

Low.

## ADDITIONAL TESTS TO ORDER

CBC, platelet count, urinalysis, reticulocyte count, sedimentation rate, serum haptoglobins, serum $B_{12}$

and folic acid, chemistry panel, blood cultures, cultures of exudates and fluids from other body compartments, bone marrow examination, liver–spleen scan, CT scans, Donath–Landsteiner test, stool for occult blood, red cell survival, Coombs' test, and hematology consult.

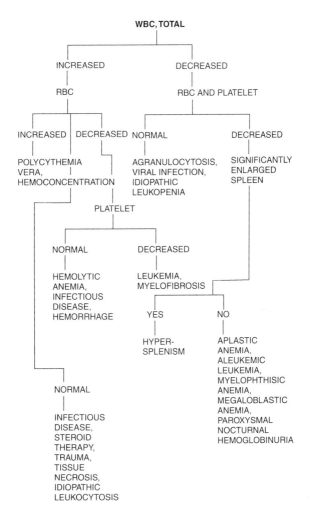

# WHITE BLOOD CELL COUNT (WBC), URINE

## INCREASED

Increased WBCs in the urine usually means a urinary tract infection. However, when there is a significant increase in RBCs, one should suspect glomerulonephritis, tuberculosis, polycystic kidney, collagen disease, and other disorders. To differentiate cystitis and tuberculosis, one should order a routine and AFB culture. If the number of RBCs in the urine is normal, then urinary tract infection is strongly suspected. If one also sees WBC casts or clumps of WBCs, then pyelonephritis or interstitial nephritis is suspected.

## NORMAL VALUES

0–4/high-powered field.

## COST

Low.

## ADDITIONAL TESTS TO ORDER

Urinalysis, sedimentation rate, AFB smear and culture, tuberculin skin test, routine urine culture and colony count, vaginal smear and culture, IVP, cystoscopy, ANA, ASO titer, renal biopsy, chemistry panel, and urology consult.

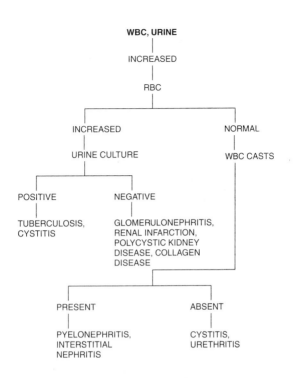

**WBC, URINE**

INCREASED

RBC

INCREASED — NORMAL

URINE CULTURE — WBC CASTS

POSITIVE — NEGATIVE

TUBERCULOSIS, CYSTITIS

GLOMERULONEPHRITIS, RENAL INFARCTION, POLYCYSTIC KIDNEY DISEASE, COLLAGEN DISEASE

PRESENT — ABSENT

PYELONEPHRITIS, INTERSTITIAL NEPHRITIS

CYSTITIS, URETHRITIS

# D-XYLOSE ABSORPTION

## DECREASED

D-Xylose absorption is decreased in malabsorption syndromes resulting from intestinal wall disease and intestinal bacterial overgrowth. It is normal in steatorrhea resulting from pancreatic insufficiency.

## NORMAL VALUES

Urine: 1.2 g or more in a 5-hour collection.

## COST

Medium.

## ADDITIONAL TESTS TO ORDER

Urine 5-HIAA, mucosal biopsy, quantitative stool fat, small bowel series, bile acid breath tests, secretin test, secretin cholecystokinin test, bentiromide test, and gastroenterology consult.

# ZINC PROTOPORPHYRINS

## INCREASED

This substance is increased in the blood in lead poisoning, iron-deficiency anemia, anemia of chronic disease, and porphyria erythropoietica.

## NORMAL VALUES

$< 35\ \mu$g/dL.

## COST

Low.

## ADDITIONAL TESTS TO ORDER

CBC, urinalysis, chemistry panel, urine porphobilinogen and porphyrins, liver function tests, blood lead level, serum iron and IBC, and consultation with a metabolic disease specialist.

# PART II

## DIAGNOSTIC TEST SELECTION

# SECTION A

## SELECTION OF DIAGNOSTIC TESTS IN THE WORKUP OF SYMPTOMS AND SIGNS

(Note: As much as possible, tests are divided into groups according to the sequence in which they are usually ordered and their cost-effectiveness.)

1. **Abdominal pain, acute:**
   A. CBC, urinalysis, chemistry panel, sedimentation rate, serum amylase and lipase, pregnancy test, flat plate of abdomen and upright, chest radiograph, and ECG.
   B. Consultation with a surgeon or gastroenterologist, gallbladder ultrasonography, IVP, HIDA scan, CT scan of abdomen with contrast, lateral decubitus films, serial cardiac enzymes, peritoneal tap, and double enema.
   C. Gastroscopy, colonoscopy, laparoscopy, and gallium scan.

2. **Abdominal pain, chronic recurrent:**
   A. CBC, sedimentation rate, chemistry panel, urine culture and colony count, serum amylase and lipase, pregnancy test, stool for occult blood, ova, and parasites, chest radiograph, plain abdominal films, and ECG.
   B. Esophagogram, upper GI series, small bowel series, barium enema and sigmoidoscopy, gallbladder ultrasound, and IVP.
   C. Gastroenterology consult, EGD, colonoscopy, CT scan of abdomen and pelvis, gallium or indium scan, renal and pelvic ultrasonography, mesenteric angiography, lymphangiography, and exploratory laparotomy.

3. **Abdominal swelling, focal:**
   A. CBC, sedimentation rate, urinalysis, chemistry panel, amylase and lipase, stool for occult blood times three, ECG, chest radiograph, and plain abdominal films.

B. Gastroenterology consult, urine culture, blood cultures, esophagogram, upper GI series, small bowel series, barium enema, IVP, gallbladder series, and peritoneal tap.

C. Abdominal and pelvic ultrasonography, CT scan of abdomen, gastroscopy, colonoscopy, ERCP, laparoscopy, gallium or indium scan, lymphangiography, and exploratory laparotomy.

4. **Abdominal swelling, generalized:**

   A. CBC, sedimentation rate, chemistry panel, flat plate of abdomen and upright, ultrasonography, peritoneal tap and peritoneal fluid analysis and culture, and tuberculin test.

   B. Gastroenterology consult, CT scan of abdomen.

   C. Upper GI series, EGD, colonoscopy, barium enema, small bowel series, laparoscopy, and exploratory laparotomy.

5. **Absent or diminished pulse:**

   Radiographs of the extremity involved, Doppler ultrasound, digital subtraction angiography, ankle–brachial index, conventional angiography; if acute onset, serial ECGs, serial cardiac enzymes, and blood cultures to rule out bacterial endocarditis; cardiology consult, consultation with a vascular surgeon.

6. **Alopecia:**

   Smear and culture of scrapings for bacteria and fungi, skin biopsy, thyroid profile, ANA, VDRL, serum iron and IBC, and dermatology consult.

7. **Amenorrhea:**

   Pregnancy test, trial of cyclic progesterone, gynecology consult, serum prolactin, CT scan of brain, FSH, LH, serum estradiol, buccal smear for sex chromogens, serum cortisol, and referral to an endocrinologist.

8. **Amnesia:**

   Drug screen, IV thiamine, neurology consult, psychiatric consult, CT scan or MRI of brain, EEG, psychometric testing, and blood studies as dictated by other symptoms.

9. **Ankle clonus:**

   Neurology consult, CT scan or MRI of brain and spinal cord, CSF analysis, CSF for myelin basic protein and γ-globulin and FTA–ABS, evoked potential studies, and blood studies to rule out systemic disorders (e.g., ANA).

10. **Anorexia:**
    A. CBC, sedimentation rate, urinalysis, chemistry panel, thyroid profile, chest radiograph, upper GI series, and gallbladder series.
    B. Gastroenterology consult, small bowel series, barium enema, and endoscopic procedures.
    C. CT scan of abdomen, bone scan, endocrinology consult, and psychiatric consult.

11. **Anosmia or unusual odor:**
    ENT consult, drug screen, neurology consult, CT scan of brain, EEG, psychometric testing, psychiatric consult, CBC, chemistry panel, thyroid profile, serum $B_{12}$ and folic acid, glucose tolerance test, and liver profile.

12. **Anuria, oliguria:**
    A. CBC, urinalysis, chemistry panel, flat plate of abdomen, and ultrasonography or catheterization for residual urine.
    B. Nephrology or urology consult dictated by findings of foregoing studies, mannitol infusion, high-dose furosemide, serum and urine osmolality, serum protein electrophoresis, ASO titer, CRP, ANA, ECG, chest radiograph, BUN, creatinine ratio, and Swan–Ganz catheter placement.
    C. CT scan of abdomen, serum haptoglobin and hemoglobin, eosinophil count, aortography and renal angiography, and renal biopsy.

13. **Anxiety:**
    Psychiatric consult, EEG, CT scan of brain, Holter monitoring, thyroid profile, 24-hour urine catecholamines, 24-hour EEG, and EEG with pharyngeal electrodes.

14. **Aphasia, apraxia, agnosia:**
    CBC, VDRL, CT scan of brain, neurology consult, MRI, spinal tap, EEG, carotid duplex scan, and four-vessel cerebral angiography.

15. **Ascites:**
    A. Peritoneal fluid analysis and culture, urinalysis, liver function tests, ECG, echocardiography, circulation time, chest radiograph,

pulmonary function test, and tuberculin test.
- B. Gastroenterology consult, cardiology consult, CT scan of abdomen and pelvis, abdominal ultrasound, GI series, barium enema, liver biopsy, peritoneal fluid for cytology, and guinea pig inoculation.
- C. Colonoscopy, gastroscopy, ERCP, laparoscopy, and MRI.

16. **Ataxia:**
Neurology consult, audiograms, calories, electronystagmography, CT scan of brain, otology consult, MRI, CSF analysis, evoked potential studies, nerve conduction studies, and four-vessel cerebral angiography.

17. **Athetosis:**
Neurology consult, CT scan or MRI of brain, spinal tap, serum copper and ceruloplasmin, CBC, and liver function tests.

18. **Axillary masses:**
Smear and culture of exudate or aspirated material, CBC, sedimentation rate, chemistry panel, chest radiograph, skin tests for tuberculosis and fungi, mammography, exploration, and biopsy.

19. **Babinski's sign:**
CBC, urinalysis, chemistry panel, VDRL, neurology consult, CT scan or MRI of brain or spinal cord, depending on level suspected, CSF analysis, evoked potential studies, carotid scans, echocardiography, blood cultures, ECG, and serial cardiac enzymes.

20. **Back pain:**
- A. CBC, urinalysis, urine culture, sedimentation rate, chemistry panel, and radiographs of thoracic or lumbar spine.
- B. Orthopedic or neurology consult, CT scan or MRI of spine, EMG, dermatomal somatosensory-evoked potential studies, and nerve conduction studies.
- C. Bone scan, PSA (in men), RA test, serum protein electrophoresis, HLA–B27 antigen, gynecology consult, pelvic ultrasonography, CT scan of abdomen, combined CT scan and myelography, discography, abdominal ultrasound, aortography, and exploratory surgery.

21. **Bleeding gums:**
    CBC, sedimentation rate, chemistry panel, coagulation profile, radiograph of teeth, plasma ascorbic acid, and VDRL or FTA–ABS.
22. **Blindness:**
    Ophthalmology consult, retinoscopy, tonometry, slit-lamp examination, visual fields, ocular plethysmography, carotid scans, digital subtraction angiography, neurology consult, CT scan or MRI of brain and orbits, spinal tap, evoked potential studies, and four-vessel cerebral angiography.
23. **Blurred vision:**
    Ophthalmology consult, tonometry, slit-lamp examination, visual acuity, visual field examination, neurology consult, CT scan or MRI of brain, carotid scans, spinal tap, visual evoked potentials, and angiography.
24. **Bone mass or swelling:**
    Plain radiograph of area involved, orthopedic consult, bone scan, CT scan of bone, CBC, sedimentation rate, chemistry panel, PSA, serum protein electrophoresis, arthritis panel if joint is involved, and needle biopsy or exploratory surgery.
25. **Bradycardia:**
    ECG, cardiac enzymes, drug screen, chest radiograph, cardiology consult, thyroid profile, Holter monitoring, echocardiography, and neurology consult.
26. **Breast discharge:**
    Surgical consult, mammography; if focal lesion, biopsy; otherwise, prolactin, CT scan of brain, and endocrinology workup for pituitary tumor.
27. **Breast mass:**
    Surgical consult, mammography, ultrasonography, biopsy, and surgery.
28. **Breast pain:**
    Mammography, ultrasonography, culture of discharge, surgical consult, pregnancy test, trial of cyclic estrogens and progesterone, and psychiatric consult.
29. **Cardiac arrhythmia:**
    Cardiology consult, ECG, CBC, chemistry panel, sedimentation rate, thyroid profile, chest radiograph, serial cardiac enzymes, circulation time,

arterial blood gases, spirometry, echocardiography, Holter monitoring, blood cultures, 24-hour urine catecholamines, exercise tolerance testing, cardiac catheterization, and angiocardiography.

30. **Cardiac murmurs:**

    Cardiology consult, ECG, chest radiograph, cardiac series, phonocardiography, echocardiography, cardiac catheterization, angiocardiography; for murmur of recent onset, CBC, sedimentation rate, ASO titer, CRP, chemistry panel, cardiac enzymes, ECG, blood cultures, venous pressure and circulation time, pulmonary capillary wedge pressure, pulmonary function studies, and thyroid profile.

31. **Cardiomegaly:**

    Cardiology consult, ECG, chest radiograph, cardiac series, echocardiography, venous pressure and circulation time, 24-hour blood pressure monitoring, cardiac catheterization, angiocardiography, arterial blood gases; for cardiomegaly of recent onset, ASO titer, CRP, CBC, chemistry panel, cardiac enzymes, serial ECGs, thyroid profile, ANA, VDRL, CT scan of chest, and serial blood cultures.

32. **Chest deformity:**

    Plain films of chest, thoracic spine and ribs, sputum culture, pleural fluid analysis and culture, CT scan, pulmonary consult, pulmonary function tests, and aortography.

33. **Chest pain:**

    A. CBC, sedimentation rate, CRP, chemistry panel, VDRL, serial ECGs, serial cardiac enzymes, chest radiograph, sputum smear and culture, and arterial blood gases.

    B. Cardiology consult, ventilation–perfusion scan, echocardiography, thallium-201 scan, and exercise tolerance testing.

    C. Pulmonary angiography, cardiac catheterization and coronary angiography, 24-hour Holter monitoring, gastroenterology consult for esophagoscopy and gastroscopy, and gallbladder ultrasonography.

34. **Chest tenderness:**

    Radiographs of chest and ribs, serial ECGs and cardiac enzymes, CBC, sedimentation rate, chemistry panel, bone scan, CT scan of chest and mediastinum, and trigger-point injections.

35. **Chills:**
    A. CBC, sedimentation rate, chemistry panel, urinalysis, urine culture, blood cultures, febrile agglutinins, chest radiograph, and flat plate of abdomen.
    B. Infectious disease consult, ASO titer, CRP, ANA, DNA antibodies, sputum culture, culture of all available body fluids, HIV antibody titer, and serologic tests dictated by rest of clinical picture.
    C. Skin testing for tuberculosis, fungal infection, and trichinosis, Kveim test, bone scan, CT scan of chest and abdomen, CSF analysis, gallium scan, bone marrow biopsy, lymph node biopsy, and echocardiography.

36. **Choreiform movements:**
    Neurology consult, sedimentation rate, ASO titer, ECG, serum copper and ceruloplasmin, ANA, CT scan or MRI of brain, and cerebral angiography.

37. **Clubbing of fingers:**
    Consultation with a pulmonologist, CBC, sedimentation rate, chemistry panel, arterial blood gases, chest radiograph, ECG, pulmonary function tests, sputum analysis and culture, tuberculin test, bronchoscopy, bronchography, cardiology consult, echocardiography, cardiac catheterization and angiocardiography, upper GI series, barium enema, and gastroenterology consult.

38. **Coma:**
    Neurology consult, CBC, chemistry panel, electrolytes, arterial blood gases, drug screen, blood ammonia, administration of IV dextrose, serum and urine osmolality, urinalysis, CT scan of brain, spinal tap, blood lead level, EEG, and IV thiamine.

39. **Constipation:**
    CBC, chemistry panel, plain abdominal films to rule out intestinal obstruction, stool for occult blood, ova, and parasites, sigmoidoscopy, barium enema, gastroenterology consult, colonoscopy, thyroid profile, PTH, glucose tolerance

test, endocrinology consult, pelvic ultrasonography, and psychiatric consult.

40. **Convulsions:**
    Neurology consult, stat EEG, CT scan or MRI of brain, ECG, drug screen, CSF analysis and culture, CBC, urinalysis, sedimentation rate, VDRL, chemistry panel, ANA, chest radiograph, evoked potential study, wake and sleep EEG, carotid duplex scans, and cerebral angiography.

41. **Cough:**
    A. Withdrawal of all medication, if possible, CBC, sedimentation rate, chemistry panel, sputum analysis and culture, AFB smear and culture, chest radiograph, cold agglutinins, and *Legionella* culture.
    B. Fungal skin tests and cultures, CT scan of chest, ECG, echocardiography, pulmonary function studies, Kveim test, bronchoscopy, bronchography, allergy skin testing, alpha$_1$-antitrypsin test, sputum for eosinophils, ANA, venous pressure, and circulation time.

42. **Cramps, menstrual:**
    Pelvic ultrasonography, FSH, LH and estradiol, and gynecology consult.

43. **Cramps, muscular:**
    CBC, sedimentation rate, chemistry panel, electrolytes, urinalysis, spot urine sodium, 24-hour urine aldosterone, plasma renin, 24-hour urine calcium and potassium, serum PTH, thyroid profile, Doppler studies of the extremities, ankle–brachial index, femoral angiography, cardiology consult, and endocrinology consult.

44. **Crepitus:**
    Radiographs of involved area, chest radiograph, culture of exudate, anaerobic and aerobic, tissue biopsy, and surgical consult.

45. **Cyanosis:**
    Chest radiograph, arterial blood gases, blood methemoglobin and sulfhemoglobin, ventilation–perfusion scan, pulmonary function tests, pulmonary consult, ECG, echocardiography, cardiology consult, sputum culture and analysis, pulmonary angiography, and bronchoscopy.

46. **Deafness:**
Audiometry, caloric testing, ENT consult, tympanography, electronystagmography, CT scan of skull and mastoids, neurology consult, MRI of brain, evoked potential study, CSF analysis, and four-vessel cerebral angiography.

47. **Delayed puberty:**
Endocrinology consult, CBC, chemistry panel, thyroid profile, FSH, LH, serum estradiol, testosterone, buccal smear for Barr bodies, CT scan of brain, pelvic ultrasonography, gynecology consult, and psychiatric consult.

48. **Delirium:**
Neurology consult, psychiatric consult, CBC, sedimentation rate, ANA, chemistry panel, electrolytes, VDRL, drug screen, blood alcohol level, CT scan of brain, administration of IV glucose, IV thiamine, blood cultures, CSF analysis and culture, arterial blood gases, and carboxyhemoglobin determination.

49. **Delusions:**
Blood alcohol level, drug screen, CT scan of brain, EEG, CSF analysis, and psychiatric consult.

50. **Dementia:**
Neurology consult, CBC, chemistry panel, sedimentation rate, VDRL, HIV antibody titer, ANA, blood alcohol level, drug screen, thyroid profile, serum $B_{12}$ and folic acid, CT scan of brain, EEG, CSF analysis, VDRL or FTA–ABS, MRI of brain, cisternography, arterial blood gases, and psychiatric consult.

51. **Depression:**
Psychiatric consult, neurology consult, CT scan of brain, CBC, sedimentation rate, chemistry panel, VDRL, thyroid profile, serum cortisol, FSH, serum estradiol, therapeutic trial of estrogen if menopause suspected, drug screen, and endocrinology consult.

52. **Diaphoresis:**
Withholding of all drugs, if possible, CBC, sedimentation rate, urinalysis, chemistry panel, electrolytes, thyroid profile, blood alcohol level, ECG, chest radiograph, serial ECGs and cardiac enzymes, 24-hour urine VMA, 72-hour fast, insulin tolerance test, serum C-peptide,

blood cultures, urine cultures, cultures of any suspicious body fluid, and consultation with an infectious disease specialist.

53. **Diarrhea, acute:**
Stool smear and culture, occult blood, ova, and parasites, *Giardia* antigen, sigmoidoscopy, gastroenterology consult, colonoscopy, barium enema, CBC, electrolytes, chemistry panel, and blood cultures.

54. **Diarrhea, chronic:**
A. CBC, sedimentation rate, chemistry panel, stool smear and culture, stool for occult blood, ova, and parasites, thyroid profile, sigmoidoscopy, and barium enema.
B. Gastroenterology consult, colonoscopy, *Giardia* antigen, lactose tolerance test, urine 5-HIAA, D-xylose absorption test, serum gastrin, stool for quantitative fat and trypsin, duodenal analysis, stool volume after fasting, upper GI series, small bowel series, CT scan of abdomen, neurology consult, and search for anal sphincter incompetence.

55. **Difficulty in urinating:**
CBC, urinalysis, urine culture, sedimentation rate, chemistry panel, VDRL, PSA, prostatic massage and smear of discharge, ultrasonography of urinary bladder, catheterization for residual urine, urology consult, cystoscopy, IVP, cystometric testing, and neurology consult.

56. **Diplopia:**
Radiographs of skull and orbits, ophthalmology consult, Tensilon test, acetylcholine receptor antibody titer, CT scan of brain, orbits and sinuses, glucose tolerance test, thyroid profile, neurology consult, MRI, evoked potentials, and CSF analysis.

57. **Dizziness:**
Neurology consult, ENT consult, audiograms, caloric testing, radiograph of skull, mastoids and petrous bones, CT scan of brain, electronystagmography, cardiology consult, echocardiography, ECG, Holter monitoring, carotid scans, EEG, evoked potential studies, CSF analysis, MRI of brain, four-vessel cerebral angiography,

24-hour blood pressure monitoring, hospitalization for continuous observation and video
monitoring, and psychiatric consult.

58. **Drop attacks:**
   A. CBC, sedimentation rate, chemistry panel,
      VDRL, chest radiograph, ECG, and arterial
      blood gas analysis.
   B. EEG, Holter monitoring, 24-hour blood pres-
      sure monitoring, and carotid duplex scan.
   C. Cardiology consult, neurology consult, CT
      scan or MRI of brain, echocardiography, 72-
      hour fast with glucose monitoring, and four-
      vessel cerebral angiography.

59. **Dwarfism:**
   A. CBC, sedimentation rate, urinalysis, chem-
      istry panel, thyroid profile, VDRL, quantita-
      tive stool fat, sweat test, and radiographs of
      skull and long bones.
   B. Endocrinology consult, orthopedic consult,
      buccal smear for Barr bodies, CT scan of
      brain, serum growth hormone, somatomedin
      C level, overnight dexamethasone-suppres-
      sion test, and 24-hour urine calcium.

60. **Dysarthria:**
   Blood alcohol level, drug screen, EEG, Tensilon
   test, carotid scan, CT scan of brain, brain scan
   with flow study, serum copper and ceruloplasmin, MRI of brain, CSF analysis, and four-vessel
   cerebral angiography.

61. **Dysmenorrhea:**
   CBC, urinalysis and culture, vaginal smear and
   culture for *Neisseria gonorrhoeae* and *Chlamydia,* abdominal ultrasound, pregnancy test,
   laparoscopy, fern test, basal body temperatures,
   course of cyclic hormones, gynecology consult,
   and D&C.

62. **Dyspareunia:**
   CBC, urinalysis, urine culture, vaginal smear
   and culture, Pap smear, pregnancy test, pelvic
   ultrasonography, cervical and vaginal biopsy,
   gynecology consult, and psychiatric consult.

63. **Dysphagia:**
   A. Barium swallow and upper GI series.
   B. Gastroenterology consult, esophagoscopy,
      gastroscopy, biopsy, Tensilon test or acetyl-

choline receptor antibody titer, CBC, and serum iron and IBC.

C. CT scan of chest and mediastinum, esophageal manometry, and psychiatric consult.

64. **Dyspnea:**
    A. CBC, chemistry panel, sedimentation rate, arterial blood gas analysis, chest radiograph, ECG, venous pressure and circulation time, and pulmonary function studies.
    B. Cardiology consult, serial ECGs, serial cardiac enzymes, sputum smear and culture and analysis, echocardiography, and ventilation–perfusion scan.
    C. CT scan of chest, sputum for eosinophils, pulmonary angiography, pulmonary consult, bronchoscopy, cardiac catheterization, and angiocardiography.

65. **Dysuria:**
    Urinalysis, urine culture and colony count, urethral smear, vaginal smear and culture, IVP, cystoscopy and retrograde pyelography, cultures for *Neisseria gonorrhoeae, Chlamydia,* and *Mycobacterium tuberculosis,* pelvic ultrasonography, prostatic massage and examination of exudate, urology consult, and gynecology consult.

66. **Earache:**
    CBC, sedimentation rate, culture and sensitivity of exudate, throat culture, radiographs of mastoids and petrous bones, audiogram, tympanogram, ENT consult, neurology consult, trial of anticonvulsants, CT scan of brain, and RISA study.

67. **Ear discharge:**
    Smear, culture and sensitivity of discharge, CBC, sedimentation rate, ASO titer, throat culture, ENT consult, audiogram, tympanogram, radiographs of mastoids and petrous bones, CT scan of brain, and RISA study.

68. **Edema, generalized:**
    CBC, sedimentation rate, chemistry panel, serum protein electrophoresis, urinalysis, serum and urine osmolality, liver function tests, Addis count, ANA, anti-DNA antibodies, 24-hour urine protein, ECG, chest radiograph, venous pressure and circulation time, cardiology consult, echocardiography, pulmonary function

studies, CT scan of chest, thyroid profile, CT scan of abdomen and pelvis, lymphangiography, and venography.

69. **Edema, localized:**
Plain radiographs of the extremity, venous ultrasonography, impedance plethysmography, contrast venography, CBC, sedimentation rate, chemistry panel, bone scan, blood cultures, CT scan of area involved, CT scan of abdomen and pelvis, lymphangiography, thyroid profile, chest radiograph, and CT scan of chest.

70. **Enuresis:**
Urinalysis, intravenous pyelography, voiding cystogram, urine culture and colony count, urology consult, cystometric studies, EEG, neurology consult, and psychiatric consult.

71. **Epiphora:**
Drug screen, ophthalmology consult, and psychiatric consult.

72. **Epistaxis:**
CBC, coagulation profile, nasal smear for eosinophils, radiographs of sinuses, nasopharyngoscopy, ENT consult, CT scan of sinuses, and 24-hour blood pressure monitoring.

73. **Euphoria:**
Drug screen, alcohol level, CT scan of brain, EEG, and psychiatric consult.

74. **Exophthalmos:**
Ophthalmology consult, thyroid profile, TSH, LATS, endocrinology consult, radiograph of orbits, CT scan of brain, ocular plethysmography, digital subtraction angiography, and carotid angiography.

75. **Extremity pain:**
CBC, sedimentation rate, chemistry panel, radiograph of extremity and joints, synovial fluid analysis and culture, bone scan, MRI of joint, venous Doppler study, impedance plethysmography, contrast venography, femoral angiography, CT scan or MRI of lumbar spine, nerve conduction studies, EMG, evoked potential studies, combined myelography, and CT scan.

76. **Extremity pain, upper extremity:**
CBC, sedimentation rate, chemistry panel, urinalysis, plain radiographs of the extremity, radiograph of the joints, synovial analysis, bone

scan, orthopedic consult, neurology consult, radiograph of cervical spine and shoulders, MRI of cervical spine, nerve conduction velocity studies, EMG, angiography, venography, exercise tolerance testing, stellate ganglion block, and trigger-point injections.

77. **Eye pain:**

Ophthalmology consult, tonometry, slit-lamp examination, fluorescein dye test of cornea for foreign body or corneal laceration, culture and sensitivity of exudate, and trial of sumatriptan.

78. **Face pain:**

Radiographs of sinuses, radiograph of teeth, CT scan of sinuses and brain, radiograph of temporomandibular joint, referral to dentist, ENT consult, histamine test, trial of sumatriptan, trial of anticonvulsants, and neurology or neurosurgical consult.

79. **Facial flushing:**

Urine 5-HIAA, drug screen, blood alcohol level, FSH and estradiol, 24-hour urine catecholamines or VMA, serum gastrin, skin biopsy, muscle biopsy, CBC, blood volume studies, arterial blood gas analysis, serum cortisol, and erythropoietin.

80. **Facial mass:**

Skin biopsy, smears and cultures of exudates, radiographs of teeth, skull, jaw and sinuses, CT scan of brain and sinuses, bone scan, ENT consult, and consultation with an oral surgeon.

81. **Facial paralysis:**

Radiographs of mastoids and petrous bones with tomography, audiogram, ENT consult, CT scan of brain, CSF analysis and cultures, culture of any discharge from the ear, carotid duplex scan, neurology consult, MRI of brain, glucose tolerance test, and blood lead level.

82. **Facial swelling:**

CBC, sedimentation rate, radiographs of teeth and sinuses, mumps skin test, mumps antibody titer, consultation with an oral surgeon, chemistry panel, urinalysis, streptozyme test, ASO titer, Addis count, chest radiograph, ECG, circulation time, spirometry, thyroid profile, serum cortisol, radiographs of skull and long bone, and bone scan.

83. **Failure to thrive:**
   A. CBC, sedimentation rate, chemistry panel, urinalysis, urine culture, thyroid profile, sweat test, stool for quantitative fat, chest radiograph, ECG, and skeletal survey for bone age.
   B. Endocrinology consult, pediatric consult, CT scan of brain, serum growth hormone, somatomedin C, overnight dexamethasone-suppression test, and bone scan.

84. **Fatigue:**
   A. Withhold all drugs, if possible, CBC, sedimentation rate, chemistry panel, VDRL, RA test, ANA, urinalysis, urine myoglobin, thyroid profile, serum cortisol, ACTH stimulation test, skull radiograph, and heterophil antibody titer.
   B. Consultations with an endocrinologist and an infectious disease specialist, febrile agglutinins, brucellin antibody titer, sputum and urine for acid-fast bacilli smear and culture, skin tests for fungi, serial blood cultures, renal function tests, liver function tests, stool quantitative fat, and D-xylose absorption.
   C. Chest radiograph, radiograph of skull and long bones, bone scan, upper GI series, barium enema, IVP, gallbladder series, nerve conduction studies, EMG, skin test for trichinosis, muscle biopsy, acetylcholine receptor antibody titer, and neurology consult.
   D. CT scan of chest and abdomen, oncology consult, gallium or indium scan, and exploratory laparotomy.

85. **Femoral mass or swelling:**
   Plain films of groin, small bowel series, ultrasonography, culture of exudates, tuberculin test, Doppler study, venography, bone scan, lymphangiography, lymph node biopsy, and exploratory surgery.

86. **Fever of unknown origin:**
   A. CBC, sedimentation rate, chemistry panel, VDRL, ANA, tuberculin skin test, serial blood cultures, sputum culture, nose and throat culture, urinalysis and culture, ASO

titer, chest radiograph, ECG, plain abdominal films, and febrile agglutinins.

B. Consultation with an infectious disease specialist, culture of all available body fluids, CSF analysis and culture, heterophil antibody titer, acute- and convalescent-phase serum for viral studies, skin tests for fungi, *Trichinella* skin test, Kveim test, blood smear for parasites, stool for ova and parasites, skeletal survey or bone scan, radiograph of teeth, and thyroid profile.

C. Consultation with an oncologist, IVP, gallbladder series, liver function tests, upper GI series, barium enema, pelvic ultrasonography, CT scan of abdomen and pelvis, echocardiography, repeat series of blood cultures, gallium or indium scans, fibrin test, urine for etiocholanolone, urine for porphobilinogen, and angiography.

D. Exploratory laparotomy.

87. **Flank mass:**
   A. Urology consult, CBC, chemistry panel, sedimentation rate, urinalysis, urine culture and colony count, IVP, catheterization for residual urine, cystoscopy, and retrograde pyelography.

   B. Abdominal ultrasonography, CT scan of abdomen, renal angiography, and urine for homovanillic acid.

88. **Flank pain:**
   A. CBC, sedimentation rate, chemistry panel, urinalysis, urine culture and colony count, IVP, radiographs of thoracic spine, and blood cultures.

   B. Urology consult, abdominal ultrasound, CT scan of abdomen, cystoscopy, and retrograde pyelography.

   C. Anesthesiology consult, nerve block, aortography, renal angiography, MRI of thoracic and lumbar spine, and exploratory surgery.

89. **Flatulence:**
   A. Stools for occult blood, upper GI series, esophagogram, cholecystogram, stools for ova and parasites, barium enema and sigmoidoscopy, quantitative stool fat analysis, lactose tolerance test, and stool for trypsin.

B. Gastroenterology consult, urine 5-HIAA, small bowel series, gastroscopy, colonoscopy, ERCP, CT scan of abdomen, and mesenteric angiography.

90. **Foot and toe pain:**
    A. Radiograph of foot, CBC, sedimentation rate, chemistry panel, VDRL, and arthritis panel.
    B. Orthopedic consult, bone scan, Doppler flow studies, neurology consult, nerve conduction studies, EMG, and radiographs of spine.
    C. CT scan, angiography, arthroscopy, venography, and MRI.

91. **Foot deformities:**
    Radiographs of feet, bone scan, consultation with an orthopedic surgeon or podiatrist, and neurology consult.

92. **Foot ulceration:**
    A. Radiograph of foot, CBC, sedimentation rate, chemistry panel, urinalysis, VDRL, culture and dark-field examination of material from ulcer, bone scan, skin test for tuberculosis and fungal infection, Doppler flow study, and orthopedic consult.
    B. Bone scan, nerve conduction studies, femoral angiography, and venography.

93. **Forehead enlargement:**
    Radiograph of skull, calcium, phosphorus, alkaline phosphatase, VDRL, sedimentation rate, serum growth hormone, CT scan of brain, and bone scan.

94. **Frequency of urination:**
    A. Urinalysis, urine culture and colony count, ultrasonography of urinary bladder or catheterization for for residual urine, 24-hour urine volume, and IVP.
    B. Urology consult, cystoscopy and retrograde pyelography, pelvic ultrasonography, cystometric studies, and repeat urine culture for aerobic and anaerobic organisms.
    C. Consultation with an endocrinologist, plasma ADH, Hickey–Hare test, CT scan of brain and abdomen, thyroid profile, serum PTH, and psychiatric consult.

95. **Frigidity:**
    Pelvic and rectal examination, pelvic ultrasound, vaginal smear and culture and KOH

preparations, gynecology consult, endocrinology consult, and psychiatric consult.

96. **Gait disturbances:**
    A. Radiographs of hip and extremities, CBC and chemistry panel, radiograph of lumbar spine, serum $B_{12}$ and folic acid, and VDRL.
    B. Orthopedic or neurology consult, MRI of brain or spine, nerve conduction studies, EMG, dermatomal somatosensory-evoked potentials, CSF analysis, and muscle biopsy.

97. **Gangrene:**
    CBC, sedimentation rate, chemistry panel, culture of gangrenous area, plain radiographs of area involved, Doppler studies, skin and tissue biopsy, ANA, bone scan, Sia water test, immunoelectrophoresis, bone scan, and angiography.

98. **Gigantism:**
    CT scan of brain, growth hormone, arginine-insulin stimulation test, FSH, LH, urinary hydroxyproline, echocardiography, urine homocystine, thyroid profile, serum testosterone, and serum dehydroepiandrosterone sulfate.

99. **Girdle pain:**
    A. Radiographs of chest, ribs and thoracic spine, CBC, chemistry panel, and VDRL.
    B. Neurology consult, MRI of thoracic spine, EMG, CSF analysis, FTA–ABS of CSF, thoracic myelogram, and nerve block.

100. **Gynecomastia:**
    A. Urine drug screen, thyroid profile, serum prolactin, liver function tests, and serum iron and IBC.
    B. Endocrinology consult, serum FSH, LH, hCG, estradiol, buccal smear for Barr bodies, serum cortisol, cortisol suppression test, rapid ACTH test, and $\beta$-hCG assay.

101. **Halitosis:**
    A. Consultation with a periodontist, culture exudate of gums, gum biopsy, radiograph of teeth, nose and throat culture, chest radiograph, ENT consult, and radiograph of sinuses.
    B. Upper GI series and esophagogram, gastroenterology consult, esophagoscopy, and gastroscopy.

    C. 24-hour sputum collection and analysis, pulmonary consult, bronchoscopy, bronchography, AFB culture, and guinea pig inoculation.

102. **Hallucinations:**
Drug screen, blood alcohol level, VDRL, psychiatric consult, CT scan or MRI of brain, wake and sleep EEG, CSF analysis, sleep study, and psychometric testing.

103. **Headache:**
    A. CBC, sedimentation rate, chemistry panel, VDRL, radiograph of sinuses, radiograph of cervical spine, tonometry, visual acuity examination, therapeutic test of sumatriptan during attack, and histamine test.
    B. Neurology consult, CT scan or MRI of brain, CSF analysis, ophthalmology consult, therapeutic trial, MR angiography, conventional four-vessel cerebral angiography, and psychiatric consult.

104. **Head mass or swelling:**
Skull radiograph, aspiration or biopsy, neurology consult, and bone scan or CT scan.

105. **Heartburn:**
    A. Upper GI series, esophagogram, stool for occult blood, radionuclide esophageal reflux study, Bernstein test, and therapeutic trial.
    B. Gastroenterology consult, esophagoscopy, gastroscopy, and biopsy.
    C. Gallbladder ultrasonography, exercise tolerance testing, thallium stress scan, and esophageal manometry or pH monitoring.

106. **Heel pain:**
Radiograph of foot, CBC, sedimentation rate, chemistry panel, arthritis panel, bone scan, response to trigger-point injection, referral to orthopedic surgeon or podiatrist, plain films of lumbar spine, nerve conduction studies, and CT scan or MRI of lumbar spine.

107. **Hematemesis:**
CBC, chemistry panel, coagulation profile, type and cross match for 4 units of blood, gastroenterology consult, esophagoscopy, gastroscopy, and duodenoscopy.

108. **Hematuria:**
    A. Urinalysis and microscopic examination of

urinary sediment, culture, and colony count.

B. CBC, sedimentation rate, serum haptoglobins, chemistry panel, ASO titer, ANA, serum and urine osmolality, IVP if BUN is acceptable, and renal scan or ultrasound if not.

C. Urology consult, cystoscopy and retrograde pyelography, renal ultrasonography, CT scan of kidneys, culture urine for anaerobic organisms and AFB, renal angiography and selective renal venography, and renal biopsy.

109. **Hemianopsia:**
Ophthalmology consult, neurology consult, CT scan or MRI of brain, carotid duplex scan, CSF analysis, MR angiography or four-vessel cerebral angiography, visual-evoked potential study, and CSF γ-globulin.

110. **Hemiparesis and hemiplegia:**
Neurology consult, CT scan or MRI of brain, carotid duplex scan, CSF analysis and culture, ECG, echocardiography (to identify source of possible emboli), blood cultures, ANA, HIV antibody testing, evoked potential studies, and four-vessel cerebral angiography.

111. **Hemoptysis:**
A. Sputum analysis and culture for routine organisms and AFB, chest radiograph, arterial blood gases (if acute onset) and ventilation–perfusion scan, and sputum cytology.

B. Pulmonary consult, CBC, coagulation profile, ECG, bronchoscopy, bronchography, pulmonary function studies, echocardiography, and cardiology consult.

C. CT scan of chest, MRI of chest, and needle biopsy of lesions.

112. **Hemorrhoids:**
Stool for occult blood, CBC, liver function tests, anoscopy, sigmoidoscopy, and barium enema.

113. **Hepatomegaly:**
A. CBC, sedimentation rate, chemistry panel, hepatitis profile, febrile agglutinins, heterophil antibody titer, chest radiograph, plain films of abdomen, ECG, and serum haptoglobin.

B. Gastroenterology consult, venous pressure and circulation time, CT scan of abdomen, liver scan, and serum iron and IBC.

C. Gallbladder ultrasound, ERCP, transhepatic cholangiography, MRI of abdomen, needle biopsy, and oncology consult.

114. **Hiccups:**

A. Upper GI series, esophagogram, and stool for occult blood.

B. CBC, sedimentation rate, chemistry panel, ECG, chest radiograph, tuberculin test, and sputum analysis and culture.

C. Esophagoscopy, gastroscopy, Bernstein test, radionuclide esophageal reflux scan, esophageal manometry, CT scan of abdomen, and psychiatric consult.

115. **Hip pain:**

A. Radiograph of hips, radiograph of lumbosacral spine, CBC, sedimentation rate, chemistry panel, urinalysis, trigger-point injection, and arthritis panel.

B. Orthopedic consult, neurology consult, bone scan, MRI of spine, serum protein electrophoresis, PSA, nerve conduction studies, and EMG.

116. **Hirsutism:**

A. Serum free testosterone, plasma cortisol, prolactin, skull radiograph, and urinary gonadotropin assay.

B. Referral to gynecologist or endocrinologist, CT scan of brain, pelvic ultrasonography, CT scan of abdomen and pelvis, and further endocrinology workup.

117. **Hoarseness:**

A. Throat culture, indirect laryngoscopy, CBC, sedimentation rate, sputum culture, and chest radiograph.

B. ENT consult, fiberoptic laryngoscopy, CT scans of chest and neck and mediastinum, AFB smear and culture, and sputum cytology.

C. Neurology consult, acetylcholine receptor antibody titer, Tensilon test, aortography, and mediastinoscopy.

118. **Horner's syndrome:**

A. Radiograph of chest, radiograph of cervical

spine, CBC, sedimentation rate, chemistry panel, and carotid duplex scan.

B. Neurology consult, pulmonary consult, MRI of cervical spine, CT scan or MRI of brain, CT scan of chest, nerve conduction studies, and EMG.

C. Aortography and mediastinography.

119. **Hyperactive reflexes:**
Neurology consult, MRI of brain or spinal cord, evoked potential studies, CSF analysis, CBC, sedimentation rate, chemistry panel, VDRL, ANA, serum $B_{12}$ and folic acid, carotid duplex scan, and four-vessel cerebral angiography.

120. **Hyperkinesis:**
A. Withholding of all drugs, if possible, CBC, sedimentation rate, ASO titer, CRP, chemistry panel, drug screen, thyroid profile, serum copper and ceruloplasmin, and VDRL.

B. Neurology consult, MRI of brain, EEG, CSF analysis, and psychiatric consult.

121. **Hyperpigmentation:**
Serum iron and IBC, thyroid profile, plasma cortisol, urine porphyrins and porphobilinogen, rapid ACTH stimulation test, serum $B_{12}$, urine $N$-methyl niacinamides, liver biopsy, and CT scan of abdomen.

122. **Hypersomnia:**
A. Withholding of all drugs, if possible, CBC, sedimentation rate, chemistry panel, VDRL, drug screen, blood alcohol, blood ammonia, and arterial blood gases.

B. Neurology consult, psychiatric consult, CT scan or MRI of brain, CSF analysis, EEG, and overnight sleep study.

123. **Hypertension:**
A. CBC, sedimentation rate, chemistry panel, serial electrolytes, urinalysis and microscopic urine culture and colony count, ANA, ECG, chest radiograph, and plain abdominal films.

B. Nephrology consult, hypertensive IVP or renal scan, 24-hour urine catecholamines, 24-hour urine aldosterone, plasma cortisol, and plasma renin.

C. Urology consult, cystoscopy and retrograde

pyelography, CT scan of abdomen, and renal angiography.

124. **Hypoactive reflexes:**
   A. Plain radiographs of spine, CBC, drug screen, urinalysis, chemistry panel, glucose tolerance test, serum $B_{12}$ and folic acid, VDRL, serial electrolytes, and CSF analysis.
   B. Neurology consult, CT scan or MRI of the lumbar, thoracic, or cervical spinal cord, nerve conduction studies, EMG, somatosensory-evoked potentials, radiograph of chest, and muscle biopsy.
   C. Combined myelography and CT scan and bone scan.

125. **Hypochondriasis:**
   A. CBC, sedimentation rate, chemistry panel, urinalysis, thyroid profile, ANA, ECG, chest radiograph, flat plate of abdomen, and heterophil antibody titer.
   B. Psychiatric consult, EEG, CT scan of brain, carotid scan, nerve conduction studies, and psychometric testing.

126. **Hypotension, chronic:**
   A. CBC, sedimentation rate, chemistry panel, thyroid panel, electrolytes, serum and urine osmolality, ECG, chest radiograph, blood volume, and arterial blood gas analysis.
   B. Cardiology consult, echocardiography, venous pressure and circulation time, CT scan of chest, and Holter monitoring.
   C. Endocrinology consult, CT scan of brain, serum cortisol, rapid ACTH stimulation test, FSH, LH, TSH, and 24-hour blood pressure monitoring.

127. **Hypothermia:**
   A. CBC, sedimentation rate, chemistry panel, urinalysis, thyroid panel, blood cultures, urine culture, drug screen, blood alcohol level, ECG, and chest radiograph.
   B. CT scan of brain, endocrinology consult, plasma cortisol, FSH, LH, growth hormone, C-peptide, glucose tolerance test, cardiology consult, and neurology consult.

128. **Impotence:**
   A. CBC, chemistry panel, urinalysis, urine culture and colony count, prostatic massage

and smear of exudate, VDRL, thyroid profile, and serum testosterone and gonadotropin assay.
- B. Urology consult, nocturnal tumescent study, penile blood pressure studies, cystoscopy, cystometric studies, and angiography.
- C. Neurology consult, nerve conduction studies, EMG, MRI of brain or spinal cord, and psychiatric consult.

129. **Incontinence of feces:**
- A. CBC, sedimentation rate, chemistry panel, VDRL, urinalysis and culture, radiograph of lumbar spine, anoscopy, sigmoidoscopy, cystometric studies, and PSA.
- B. Neurology consult, CT scans or MRI, nerve conduction studies, EMG, CSF analysis, evoked potential studies, and psychiatric consult.

130. **Incontinence of urine:**
- A. CBC, urinalysis and urine culture, chemistry panel, VDRL, PSA, IVP and cystogram, catheterization for residual urine, Q-Tip test for stress incontinence, and gynecology consult.
- B. Urology consult, pelvic ultrasound, cystoscopy, cystometrography, cystometric studies, and prostatic ultrasonography.
- C. Neurology consult, MRI of spinal cord or brain, CSF analysis, and evoked potential studies.

131. **Indigestion:**
- A. CBC, urinalysis, chemistry panel, sedimentation rate, serum $B_{12}$ and folic acid, upper GI series and esophagogram, stool for occult blood, and gallbladder ultrasonography.
- B. Gastroenterology consult, withholding of all drugs, alcohol, and caffeine, if possible, thyroid profile, stool for culture, ova, and parasites, panendoscopy of upper GI tract, esophageal manometry, Bernstein test, CT scan of abdomen, quantitative stool fat, and D-xylose absorption test.

132. **Infertility, female:**
Gynecology consult, obtaining of semen specimen from husband or partner, CBC, urinalysis, urine culture, vaginal smear, saline preparation,

KOH preparations and culture, basal body temperature charting, pelvic ultrasonography, tubal insufflation, hysterosalpingography, endometrial biopsy, serum FSH, LH and estradiol, cervical mucus for spinnbarkeit testing, laparoscopy, trial of clomiphene, and exploratory laparotomy.

133. **Infertility, male:**
   A. Determination of whether infertility is due to impotence, sperm count (two separate specimens), CBC, sedimentation rate, urinalysis, urine culture, chemistry panel, thyroid panel, and VDRL.
   B. Urologic consult, FSH, LH, testosterone, testicular biopsy, and ultrasonography of testicles.

134. **Inguinal swelling:**
   A. Transillumination, CBC, sedimentation rate, chemistry panel, VDRL, radiograph of hips and pelvis, small bowel series, ultrasonography, and needle aspiration.
   B. Bone scan, arteriography, venography, and exploratory surgery.

135. **Insomnia:**
   A. Drug screen, blood alcohol level, withholding of all drugs, caffeine, and alcohol, and psychiatric consult.
   B. CBC, sedimentation rate, urinalysis, chemistry panel, thyroid panel, VDRL, ECG, chest radiograph, and arterial blood gas analysis.
   C. Pulmonary consult, pulmonary function tests, circulation time, echocardiography, exercise tolerance testing, 24-hour Holter monitoring, 24-hour blood pressure monitoring, CT scan or MRI of brain, and sleep study.

136. **Intracranial or cervical bruit:**
   Cardiology or neurology consult, carotid duplex scan, CBC, thyroid profile, CT scan of brain, digital subtraction angiography, MR angiography, and four-vessel cerebral angiography.

137. **Jaundice:**
   A. CBC, sedimentation rate, reticulocyte count, serum haptoglobins, urinalysis, chemistry panel, liver panel, hepatitis profile, VDRL,

**641**

ECG, chest radiograph, flat plate of abdomen, and ultrasonography of gallbladder.

B. Febrile agglutinins, Monospot test, cytomegalovirus antibody titer, leptospirosis antibody titer, blood smear for parasites, ANA, and smooth muscle antibody titer.

C. Gastroenterology consult, CT scan of abdomen, ERCP, transhepatic cholangiography, serum iron and IBC, upper GI series, barium enema, peritoneoscopy, antimitochondrial antibody titer, and exploratory laparotomy.

138. **Jaw pain:**
Radiograph of teeth and jaw, radiograph of TM joints, radiograph of sinuses, dental consult, CBC, sedimentation rate, chemistry panel, and CT scan of TM joints.

139. **Jaw swelling:**
Radiograph of jaw and teeth, radiograph of skull and sinuses, dental consult, CBC, sedimentation rate, chemistry panel, urinalysis, growth hormone, PTH assay, CT scan of swelling, and biopsy or exploration.

140. **Joint pain:**
A. CBC, sedimentation rate, ASO titer, RA titer, CRP, ANA, chemistry panel, VDRL, urinalysis, radiograph of involved joints, and synovial fluid analysis and culture.

B. Orthopedic or rheumatology consult, CT scan or MRI of joint, bone scan, trial of therapy, arthroscopy, arthrography, gonococcal antibody titer, coagulation profile, serologic tests for Lyme disease, brucellin antibody titer, blood cultures, Monospot test, sickle cell preparation, urine for homogentisic acid, and HLA–B27 antigen.

141. **Joint swelling:**
A. Synovial analysis and culture and radiograph of joint.

B. Rheumatology or orthopedic consult, CBC, urinalysis, ASO titer, RA test, ANA, anti-DNA antibodies, sedimentation rate, chemistry panel, and trial of therapy.

C. MRI, arthroscopy, and arthrography.

142. **Kyphosis:**
A. CBC, sedimentation rate, urinalysis, chemistry panel, arthritis panel, chest radiograph,

radiograph of thoracic spine, sputum routine culture, and AFB smear and culture.
B. Muscle biopsy, FSH, LH, estradiol, bone scan, HLA−B27 antigen, and bone biopsy.

143. **Leg ulceration:**
Surgical consult, CBC, sedimentation rate, chemistry panel, VDRL, dark-field examination, culture of exudate, radiograph of involved area, bone scan, venography, arteriography, and biopsy.

144. **Lip pain:**
CBC, sedimentation rate, urinalysis, chemistry panel, VDRL, culture of exudates, serology for herpes zoster (varicella), Tzanck test, herpes simplex serology, therapeutic trial, and consultation with an oral surgeon or dermatologist.

145. **Lip swelling:**
CBC, sedimentation rate, urinalysis, chemistry panel, VDRL, smear and culture of exudate, nose and throat culture, radiograph of teeth, Tzanck test, serology for varicella and herpes simplex, therapeutic trial, and consultation with an oral surgeon or dermatologist.

146. **Lordosis:**
Radiograph of thoracic and lumbar spine, radiograph of hips, muscle biopsy, EMG, bone scan, and tuberculin test.

147. **Lymphadenopathy:**
A. CBC, sedimentation rate, nose and throat culture, culture of material from any area supplied by lymph nodes, chemistry panel, heterophil antibody titer, brucellin antibody titer, febrile agglutinins, VDRL, chest radiograph and flat plate of abdomen, and tuberculin test.
B. Consultation with an infectious disease expert or oncologist, radiograph of long bones, bone scan, radiograph of hands, bone marrow biopsy, lymph node biopsy, Kveim test, brucellergen skin test, skin test for fungal diseases, lymphangiogram, liver biopsy, and CT scans of abdomen and chest.

148. **Melena:**
A. Stool for occult blood, ova, and parasites, CBC, coagulation studies, upper GI series, and esophagogram.

B. Gastroenterology consult, esophagoscopy, gastroscopy, duodenoscopy, small bowel series, liver function tests, nuclear scan after intravenous chromium-tagged red cells, fluorescein string test, mesenteric angiography, splenic venography, and exploratory laparotomy.

149. **Memory loss:**
Drug screen, blood alcohol level, IV thiamine, neurology consult, CT scan or MRI of brain, EEG, CSF analysis, evoked potential studies, psychometric testing, cisternography, CBC, sedimentation rate, urinalysis, chemistry panel, ANA, serum $B_{12}$ and folic acid, VDRL, chest radiograph, and HIV testing.

150. **Menorrhagia:**
A. Pap smear, vaginal smear and culture, CBC, sedimentation rate, urinalysis, pregnancy test, chemistry panel, ANA, VDRL, coagulation profile, thyroid panel, and flat plate of abdomen.

B. Gynecology consult, pelvic ultrasonography, CT scan of abdomen and pelvis, laparoscopy, endometrial biopsy, trial of cyclic progesterone, D&C, and full endocrine workup.

151. **Mental retardation:**
Neurology consult, CBC, sedimentation rate, chemistry panel, serum galactose level, VDRL, thyroid panel, urine screen for carbohydrates, amino acids and organic acids, chromosomal analysis, skull radiograph, EEG, CT scan of brain, psychometric testing, and CSF analysis.

152. **Metrorrhagia:**
A. Pap smear, vaginal smear and culture, CBC, sedimentation rate, urinalysis, pregnancy test, chemistry panel, ANA, coagulation profile, thyroid panel, flat plate of abdomen, and serum iron and IBC.

B. Gynecology consult, pelvic ultrasonography, CT scan of abdomen and pelvis, laparoscopy, D&C, and full endocrine workup.

153. **Monoplegia:**
Neurology consult, CT scan or MRI of brain, MRI of cervical, thoracic, or lumbar spine, nerve

conduction studies, EMG, evoked potentials, carotid scans, CSF analysis, four-vessel cerebral angiography, echocardiography, ANA, VDRL, blood cultures, CBC, and chemistry panel.

154. **Mouth pigmentation:**
CBC, sedimentation rate, urinalysis, chemistry panel, VDRL, heavy metal screen, hair analysis for arsenic, serum cortisol, rapid ACTH test, GI series with small bowel follow-through, barium enema, and endoscopy.

155. **Muscular atrophy:**
A. CBC, sedimentation rate, urinalysis, chemistry panel, ANA, serum protein electrophoresis, VDRL, muscle enzymes, urine creatine and creatinine, and acetylcholine receptor antibody titer.
B. Neurology consult, EMG, nerve conduction studies, CT scan or MRI of appropriate levels of the spine, CSF analysis, and muscle biopsy.

156. **Musculoskeletal pain, generalized:**
A. CBC, sedimentation rate, urinalysis, chemistry panel, electrolytes, RA test, ANA, serum protein electrophoresis, febrile agglutinins, Epstein–Barr antibody titer, antibody titer for Lyme disease, chest radiograph, ECG, and rheumatology consult.
B. Neurology consult, muscle enzymes, including CPK, serum aldolase, 24-hour urine creatine and creatinine, *Trichinella* skin test or antibody titer, EMG, nerve conduction studies, muscle biopsy, urine porphyrins and porphobilinogen, 24-hour urine potassium, sodium and calcium, MRI of spine, and CSF analysis.

157. **Nail abnormalities:**
*Focal:* Smear, culture and sensitivity of nail scraping for bacteria and fungi, radiograph of the digits, CBC, sedimentation rate, glucose tolerance test, venous Doppler study, angiography, nerve conduction studies, EMG, skin or nail biopsy, and dermatology consult.
*Diffuse:* CBC, sedimentation rate, chemistry panel, VDRL, ANA, thyroid profile, PTH, chest radiograph, ECG, arterial blood gas analysis,

pulmonary function tests, serial blood cultures, *Trichinella* antibody titer, muscle biopsy, nerve conduction studies, and EMG.

158. **Nasal discharge:**
   A. Smear and culture and examination for eosinophils, CBC, sedimentation rate, chemistry panel, VDRL, ANA, serum IgE, therapeutic trial, radiograph of sinuses, and tuberculin test.
   B. Consultation with an allergist, RAST, skin testing, nasopharyngoscopy, CT scan of sinuses, bone scan, and cultures for mucormycosis.

159. **Nasal obstruction:**
   A. CBC, sedimentation rate, chemistry panel, VDRL, ANA, ANCA, nasal smear and culture for bacteria and fungi, radiographs of sinuses, nasal smear for eosinophils, and trial of antibiotics or antihistamines.
   B. Allergy consult, IgE, RAST, skin testing, ENT consult, nasopharyngoscopy, CT scan of sinuses, and bone scan.

160. **Nausea and vomiting:**
   A. CBC, sedimentation rate, urinalysis, drug screen, chemistry panel, electrolytes, serum amylase and lipase, gallbladder ultrasonography, chest radiograph, ECG, flat plate of abdomen, pregnancy test (for women of childbearing age), and stool for occult blood.
   B. Gastroenterology consult, upper GI series and esophagogram or esophagoscopy, gastroscopy, duodenoscopy, IVP, HIDA scan, small bowel series, and barium enema.
   C. CT scan of abdomen and pelvis, laparoscopy, and exploratory laparotomy.

161. **Neck pain:**
   A. CBC, sedimentation rate, chemistry panel, arthritis panel, plain films of cervical spine, and chest radiograph.
   B. Neurology consult, MRI of cervical spine, EMG, nerve conduction studies, dermatomal somatosensory-evoked potential studies, CT scan of the brain, CSF analysis, MRI of the neck, and RAI uptake and scan.

162. **Neck stiffness:**
   A. Radiograph of cervical spine, radiograph of

chest, CBC, sedimentation rate, urinalysis, chemistry panel, arthritis panel, CT scan of brain, and CSF analysis and culture.

B. Neurology consult, MRI of cervical spine, EMG, nerve conduction studies, evoked potential studies, and bone scan.

163. **Neck swelling:**

A. CBC, sedimentation rate, urinalysis, chemistry panel, thyroid panel, chest radiograph, radiograph of cervical spine, and ECG.

B. Surgical consult, endocrinology consult, RAI uptake and scan, MRI of neck, venous pressure and circulation time, ultrasonography, lymph node biopsy, angiography, esophagoscopy, and CT scan of mediastinum.

164. **Nightmares:**

CBC, sedimentation rate, chemistry panel, drug screen, blood alcohol level, EEG, trial of anticonvulsants, sleep study, psychiatric consult, neurology consult, and MRI of brain.

165. **Nocturia:**

A. CBC, sedimentation rate, chemistry panel, urinalysis, urine culture and colony count, quantitative 24-hour urine volume, IVP and voiding cystogram or renal and bladder ultrasound, and thyroid profile.

B. Urology consult, cystoscopy and retrograde pyelography, cardiology consult, venous pressure and circulation time, echocardiography, serum and urine osmolality, 24-hour urine protein, Addis count, nephrology consult, and renal biopsy.

166. **Nose, regurgitation of food through:**

Neurology consult, ENT consult, Tensilon test, acetylcholine receptor antibody titer, nasopharyngoscopy, MRI of brain, EMG, nerve conduction studies, CSF analysis, and evoked potential studies.

167. **Nystagmus:**

A. Audiogram, caloric testing, radiographs of skull, mastoids and petrous bones, and visual acuity.

B. Neurology or ENT consult, MRI or CT scan of brain, electronystagmography, CSF analysis, evoked potential studies, cisternography, myelography, tomography, and four-vessel cerebral angiography.

168. **Obesity:**
   A. CBC, urinalysis, chemistry panel, glucose tolerance test, and thyroid profile.
   B. Endocrinology consult, serum cortisol, dexamethasone-suppression test, 72-hour fast with glucose monitoring, C-peptide, pelvic ultrasonography, chromosomal analysis, and CT scan of brain or MRI.

169. **Odor:**
   CBC, urinalysis, sedimentation rate, chemistry panel, drug screen, blood alcohol level, urine amino acids, and culture of mouth, gums, nasopharynx, and sputum.

170. **Opisthotonos:**
   Neurology consult, CBC, sedimentation rate, urinalysis, chemistry panel, electrolytes, blood cultures, drug screen, VDRL, CSF analysis, smear and culture, and EEG.

171. **Orthopnea** (see Dyspnea).

172. **Palpitations:**
   A. Withholding of all drugs, alcohol, and caffeine, if possible, drug screen, CBC, urinalysis, sedimentation rate, chemistry panel, ASO titer, CRP, thyroid panel, ECG, and chest radiograph.
   B. Cardiology consult, Holter monitoring, echocardiography, circulation time, exercise stress testing, and angiography.
   C. Endocrinology consult, RAI uptake and scan, 24-hour urine catecholamines or VMA, arterial blood gases, and spirometry.

173. **Papilledema:**
   A. Neurology consult, CT scan or MRI of the brain, visual evoked potential studies and visual field examination for possible optic neuritis, CSF analysis for possible pseudotumor cerebri, and blood lead level.
   B. Nephrology consult for hypertensive workup (see page 683).

174. **Paresthesias of the lower extremity:**
   A. CBC, sedimentation rate, urinalysis, chemistry panel, arthritis panel, VDRL, and radiographs of lumbosacral spine and hips.
   B. Orthopedic or neurology consult, CT scan

or MRI of lumbar spine, EMG, nerve conduction studies, evoked potential studies, neuropathy workup, including serum $B_{12}$ and folic acid, blood lead level, glucose tolerance test, urine for porphobilinogen, CSF analysis, quantitative urine niacin, thiamine and pyridoxine after loading, ANA, anti-dsDNA, serum protein electrophoresis, blood viscosity, lymph node biopsy, Kveim test, HIV antibody titer, heavy metal screen, thyroid profile, muscle and nerve biopsy, red blood cell transketolase activity, and therapeutic trial.

175. **Paresthesias of the upper extremity:**
    A. CBC, sedimentation rate, chemistry panel, urinalysis, arthritis panel, and plain films of cervical spine and chest.
    B. Neurology consult, MRI of brain or cervical spine, MRI of neck, EMG, nerve conduction studies, dermatomal somatosensory-evoked potential studies, and neuropathy workup (see page 683).

176. **Pathologic reflexes:**
    A. Neurology consult, MRI of brain or spinal cord, evoked potential studies, EEG, CSF examination, carotid scans, and four-vessel cerebral angiography or MR angiography.
    B. Cardiology consult, ECG, chest radiograph, blood cultures, echocardiography, serum protein electrophoresis, ANA, serum $B_{12}$ and folic acid, and VDRL.

177. **Pelvic mass:**
    A. Urinalysis, urine culture and colony count, vaginal smear and culture, and Pap smear.
    B. Gynecology or urology consult, pelvic ultrasonography, CT scan of abdomen and pelvis, laparoscopy, and exploratory laparotomy.

178. **Pelvic pain:**
    A. CBC, urinalysis, sedimentation rate, pregnancy test, urine culture and colony count, chemistry panel, VDRL, Pap smear, vaginal smear and culture, *Chlamydia* antigens, *Chlamydia* enzyme assay and culture, flat plate of abdomen, and PSA.
    B. Gynecology consult, urology consult, pelvic ultrasound, prostatic ultrasound, and cystoscopy.

C. CT scan of abdomen, laparoscopy, and exploratory laparotomy.

179. **Penile pain:**
A. Urinalysis, urine culture and colony count, prostatic massage and smear and culture of prostatic fluid, IVP, catheterization for residual urine or ultrasonography of bladder, and PSA.
B. Urology consult, cystoscopy and retrograde pyelography, and prostatic ultrasonography.

180. **Penile sores:**
Routine smear and culture, dark-field examination, VDRL, Frei test, biopsy of lesion, lymph node biopsy, Tzanck test, serologic tests for lymphogranuloma venereum, HIV antibody titer, urology consult, and dermatology consult.

181. **Perineal pain:**
CBC, sedimentation test, urinalysis and culture, chemistry panel, pregnancy test, vaginal smear and culture, prostatic massage and smear and culture of exudate, PSA, anoscopy, proctoscopy, pelvic ultrasound, gynecology consult, urology consult, and CT scan of pelvis.

182. **Periorbital edema:**
A. CBC, sedimentation rate, urinalysis, chemistry panel, thyroid panel, ANA, ASO titer, VDRL, chest radiograph, and radiographs of sinuses and orbits.
B. Neurology consult, nephrology consult, Addis count, serum complement, renal function tests, nose and throat culture, blood cultures, CT scan of brain, venous pressure and circulation time, *Trichinella* antibody titer, and CT scan of chest and mediastinum.

183. **Peristalsis, visible:**
CBC, urinalysis, sedimentation rate, chemistry panel, electrolytes, plain abdominal films, and surgical consult.

184. **Photophobia:**
CBC, sedimentation rate, urinalysis, tonometry, slit-lamp examination, ophthalmology consult, neurology consult, trial of $\beta$ blockers, CT scan of brain, CSF analysis, and histamine test.

185. **Polydipsia:**
A. CBC, sedimentation rate, urinalysis, chemistry panel, serum and urine osmolality, 24-

hour urine volume, glucose tolerance test, thyroid panel, chest radiograph, skeletal survey, and PTH assay.
   B. Endocrinology consult, serum ADH, Hickey–Hare test, intake and output before and after vasopressin, FSH, LH, ACTH, TSH, CT scan of brain, serum growth hormone, and psychiatric consult.

186. **Polyuria:**
   A. CBC, sedimentation rate, urinalysis, urine culture and colony count, chemistry panel, thyroid panel, 24-hour urine volume, serum and urine osmolality, spot urine sodium, skeletal survey, ECG, and chest radiograph.
   B. Endocrinology consult, glucose tolerance test, CT scan of brain, PTH assay, serum growth hormone, FSH, LH, ADH assay, intake and output before and after Pitressin, Addis count, and nephrology consult.

187. **Popliteal swelling:**
   A. CBC, sedimentation rate, chemistry panel, and radiographs of both knees.
   B. Orthopedic consult, MRI or CT scan of knee, aspiration of swelling or joint, bone scan, ultrasonography, angiography, and venography.

188. **Precocious puberty:**
   A. CBC, sedimentation rate, urinalysis, chemistry panel, VDRL, serum free testosterone, dihydrotestosterone, dehydroepiandrosterone, flat plate of abdomen, rapid ACTH test, serum cortisol, and urine pregnanetriol and pregnanediol.
   B. Endocrinology consult, CT scan of abdomen and pelvis, CT scan of the brain, ultrasonography of the testicle, ovarian biopsy, testicular biopsy, and laparoscopy.

189. **Priapism:**
   Urology consult, CBC, sedimentation rate, chemistry panel, urine culture and colony count, PSA, sickle cell preparation, coagulation profile, serum protein electrophoresis, Sia water test, blood viscosity, MRI of brain or spinal cord, and cystoscopy.

190. **Pruritus, generalized:**
   A. Smear, culture, KOH preparation of skin ex-

udate or scrapings, Wood's lamp examination for fungi, skin biopsy, patch tests, and dermatology consult.

B. CBC, sedimentation rate, urinalysis, chemistry panel, ANA, thyroid panel, serum protein electrophoresis, bone marrow examination, lymph node biopsy, liver scan or CT scan of abdomen, and bone scan.

191. **Pruritus ani:**
Anoscopy and sigmoidoscopy, stool for culture, ova, and parasites, scrapings of perianal area for KOH preparation, Scotch tape test for pinworm eggs, therapeutic preparation of vaginal fluid, culture for fungi, gynecology consult, and proctology consult.

192. **Pruritus vulvae:**
Saline and KOH preparation of vaginal discharge, culture for bacteria and fungi, biopsy of lesions, FSH and serum estradiol, gynecology consult, and dermatology consult.

193. **Ptosis:**
A. Ophthalmology consult, smear and culture of exudate, slit-lamp examination, tonometry, radiograph of orbits, and sedimentation rate.

B. Neurology consult, CT scan or MRI of brain, carotid angiography, Tensilon test, acetylcholine receptor antibody titer, and intravenous thiamine administration.

C. Radiograph of sinuses, ANA, VDRL, CBC, urinalysis, chemistry panel, glucose tolerance test, CSF examination, 24-hour urine creatine and creatinine, and muscle biopsy.

194. **Ptyalism:**
Heavy metal screen, blood alcohol level, drug screen, dental or oral surgery consult, neurology consult, CT scan or MRI of brain, nerve conduction studies, EMG, Tensilon test, and CSF analysis.

195. **Pulsatile swelling:**
Aortic ultrasonography, CT scan of abdomen or MRI, aortography, and angiography.

196. **Pulse irregularity:**
A. CBC, sedimentation rate, urinalysis, chemistry panel, thyroid panel, serial ECGs, serial

cardiac enzymes, chest radiograph, and cardiac series.
B. Cardiology consult, Holter monitoring, echocardiography, exercise tolerance testing, ASO titer, ANA, blood cultures, hospitalization for telemetry, and MRI or CT scan of heart.
C. Cardiac catheterization and angiocardiography or coronary angiography.

197. **Pulses, unequal:**
*Acute onset:* Doppler flow study, angiography, and consultation with a cardiovascular surgeon.
*Gradual onset:* Doppler flow study, ankle–brachial index, serial ECGs, cardiac enzymes, blood cultures, and angiography.

198. **Pupil abnormalities:**
A. Drug screen, blood alcohol level, CBC, sedimentation rate, VDRL, and chemistry panel.
B. Neurology consult, CT scan or MRI of brain, EEG, CSF examination, ophthalmology consult, slit-lamp examination, tonometry, and four-vessel cerebral angiography.

199. **Purpura and abnormal bleeding:**
A. CBC, sedimentation rate, chemistry panel, blood cultures, urinalysis, coagulation profile, ANA, serum protein electrophoresis, and platelet count.
B. Hematology consult, ECG, chest radiograph, bone scan, fibrinogen, fibrin split products, bone marrow examination, scan of liver and spleen, and skin, muscle, and kidney biopsy.

200. **Rales:**
A. CBC, sedimentation rate, urinalysis, chemistry panel, sputum analysis and culture for routine bacteria, AFB and fungi, tuberculin test, chest radiograph, ECG, and skin tests for fungi.
B. Pulmonary consult, sputum for eosinophils, spirometry, arterial blood gas analysis, ventilation–perfusion scan, pulmonary angiography, echocardiography, cardiology consult, pulmonary capillary wedge pressure, bronchoscopy, CT scan of chest, and bronchography.

201. **Rash:**

Smear and culture for routine bacteria and fungi, KOH preparation for fungi and scabies, Wood's lamp examination, dermatology consult, skin biopsy, CBC, sedimentation rate, urinalysis, chemistry panel, ANA, VDRL, blood cultures, Rocky Mountain spotted fever antibody titer, dark-field examination of lesions or blood, patch tests, intradermal allergy testing, RAST, GI series, barium enema, and gastroenterology consult.

202. **Raynaud's phenomena:**

A. Ice water test, CBC, sedimentation rate, urinalysis, chemistry panel, ANA, VDRL, serum protein electrophoresis, chest radiograph, radiograph of cervical spine, and EEG.

B. Hematology and rheumatology consult, Sia water test, immunoelectrophoresis, blood viscosity, cold agglutinins, sickle cell preparation, muscle biopsy, antisclerodermal antibody titer, and esophageal manometry.

C. Doppler flow study, digital subtraction angiography, and contrast angiography.

203. **Rectal bleeding:**

A. Anoscopy, sigmoidoscopy, barium enema, stool for occult blood, and stool for culture, ova, and parasites.

B. Gastroenterology consult, colonoscopy, coagulation profile, biopsy, and mesenteric angiography.

204. **Rectal discharge:**

A. Anoscopy, sigmoidoscopy, stool for occult blood, ova, and parasites, and culture.

B. Proctology consult, Frei test, barium enema, colonoscopy, IVP, CT scan of pelvis, and cystoscopy.

205. **Rectal mass:**

A. Sigmoidoscopy, anoscopy, smear and culture of any rectal or vaginal discharge, stool for occult blood, and urinalysis.

B. Urology consult, gynecology consult, proctology consult, pelvic ultrasound, PSA, prostatic ultrasound, and CT scan of pelvis.

206. **Rectal pain:**

A. Anoscopy, sigmoidoscopy, stool for occult

blood, smear and culture of rectal or vaginal
discharge, and urine culture.
B. Proctology consult, gynecology consult,
urology consult, pelvic ultrasound, pregnancy test, cystoscopy, PSA, and CT scan
of pelvis.

207. **Regurgitation, esophageal:**
A. Upper GI series, esophagogram, and stool
for occult blood.
B. Gastroenterology consult, esophagoscopy,
gastroscopy, gastric analysis, Bernstein test,
radionuclide esophageal reflux study, and
esophageal manometry.
C. CBC, serum iron, serum ferritin, ANA, antisclerodermal antibody titer, CT scan of mediastinum, and angiography.

208. **Respiration abnormalities:**
A. CBC, sedimentation rate, urinalysis, chemistry panel, thyroid panel, ECG, chest radiograph, drug screen, blood alcohol level, and
blood ammonia level.
B. Pulmonary consult, arterial blood gas analysis, pulmonary function studies, ventilation–perfusion scan, CT scan of chest, and
sleep study.
C. Neurology consult, CT scan of brain, and
CSF analysis.

209. **Restless leg syndrome:**
A. CBC, urinalysis, sedimentation rate, chemistry panel, electrolytes, drug screen, glucose tolerance test, arterial blood gases, and
pregnancy test.
B. Neurology consult, nerve conduction studies, EMG, evoked potential studies, Doppler
flow studies for peripheral vascular disease,
ankle–brachial index, and therapeutic trial
of a combination of levodopa and carbidopa.

210. **Scalp tenderness:**
Smear and cultures of exudates, KOH preparations, skin biopsy, skull radiograph, sedimentation rate, psychiatric consult, and CT scan of
brain.

211. **Scoliosis:**
Radiograph of spine, CBC, sedimentation rate,
urinalysis, chemistry panel, arthritis panel,
ANA, HLA–B27 antigen, tuberculin test, bone

scan, orthopedic consult, neurology consult, EMG, nerve conduction studies, and CT scans or MRI.

212. **Scotoma:**
Ophthalmology or neurology consult, visual field examination, slit-lamp examination, tonometry, histamine test, trial of $\beta$ blockers, CT scan or MRI of brain, visual evoked potential studies, carotid duplex scan, ocular plethysmography, carotid angiography, and CSF examination.

213. **Scrotal swelling:**
A. CBC, sedimentation rate, urinalysis and culture, smear and culture of prostatic fluid, PSA, and chemistry panel.
B. Urology consult, radionuclide scan of testicle, ultrasound of testicle, flat plate of abdomen, and testicular biopsy.

214. **Sensory loss:**
A. CBC, sedimentation rate, urinalysis, chemistry panel, ANA, serum protein electrophoresis, VDRL, chest radiograph, and radiograph of spine.
B. Neurology consult, CT scan or MRI of brain or spinal cord, EMG, nerve conduction studies, evoked potential studies, CSF analysis, carotid scans, digital subtraction angiography, and four-vessel cerebral angiography.
C. Neuropathy workup (see page 683).
D. Wake and sleep EEG to rule out complex partial seizure.

215. **Shoulder pain:**
A. Radiograph of shoulder, CBC, sedimentation rate, urinalysis, chemistry panel, arthritis panel, chest radiograph, and ECG.
B. Trigger-point injection, corticosteroid injection of bursae or joints, radiograph of cervical spine, nerve conduction velocity studies, and EMG.
C. Neurology consult, MRI of cervical spine, orthopedic consult, MRI of shoulder, digital subtraction angiography, brachial angiography, gallbladder ultrasound, upper GI series, and exercise tolerance test.

216. **Skin thickening:**
Free $T_4$, TSH, ANA, antisclerodermal antibody

titer, sedimentation rate, esophageal motility study, urine porphyrins, and skin biopsy.

217. **Sleep apnea:**
Pulmonary consult, polysomnography, neurology consult, endocrinology consult, and ENT consult.

218. **Sleep walking:**
Neurology consult, psychiatric consult, and wake and sleep EEG with nasopharyngeal electrodes.

219. **Sneezing:**
Nasal smear for eosinophils, radiograph of sinuses, ENT consult, nasopharyngoscopy, and trial of therapy.

220. **Snoring:**
Sleep diary, tape recording, polysomnography, ENT consult, pulmonary consult, and trial of continuous positive-airway pressure.

221. **Sore throat:**
Nasopharyngeal smear and culture, streptozyme test or ASO titer, Monospot test, culture for *Neisseria gonorrhoeae,* blood smear for atypical lymphocytes, culture for diphtheria bacilli, CBC, chemistry panel, ENT consult, sedimentation rate, and thyroid panel.

222. **Splenomegaly:**
A. CBC, platelet count, sedimentation rate, chemistry panel, febrile agglutinins, serum haptoglobin, ANA, Monospot test, serum protein electrophoresis, tuberculin test, chest radiograph, ECG, and flat plate of abdomen.
B. Hematology consult, hepatitis profile, red cell fragility test, blood smear for parasites, serial blood cultures, coagulation profile, and scan of liver and spleen.
C. CT scan of abdomen and pelvis, bone marrow examination, bone scan, GI workup for malignancy, splenoportogram, angiography, liver biopsy, and splenic aspiration.

223. **Steatorrhea:**
A. Stool for quantitative fat, sweat test, D-xylose absorption test, urine 5-HIAA, mucosal biopsy, serum $B_{12}$ and folic acid, stool for occult blood, ova, and parasites, and amylase and lipase.

B. GI consult, lactose tolerance test, hydrogen breath analysis, upper GI series and small bowel follow through, duodenal analysis, CT scan of abdomen, and therapeutic trial.

224. **Stress incontinence:**
Stress test, Q-Tip test, urology consult, and gynecology consult.

225. **Stretch marks:**
Serum cortisol, overnight dexamethasone-suppression test, endocrinology consult, and CT scan of abdomen and pelvis.

226. **Stridor:**
A. CBC, sedimentation rate, smear and culture of material from the nose, throat and sputum, radiograph of chest and sinuses, and ECG.
B. ENT consult, laryngoscopy, Tensilon test, thyroid profile, VDRL, and bronchoscopy.

227. **Stupor:**
A. CBC, sedimentation rate, urinalysis, chemistry panel, electrolytes, magnesium, drug screen, blood alcohol level, blood cultures, arterial blood gas analysis, carboxyhemoglobin determination, EEG, and CT scan of brain.
B. Neurology consult, CSF analysis, possibly MRI of brain, carotid duplex scan, and cerebral angiography.

228. **Syncope:**
A. Withholding of all drugs, alcohol, and caffeine, if possible, CBC, sedimentation rate, urinalysis, drug screen, chemistry panel, VDRL, thyroid profile, glucose tolerance test, C-peptide, ECG, chest radiograph, and several blood pressure recordings in recumbent and upright positions.
B. Cardiology or neurology consult, 24-hour Holter monitoring, EEG, 72-hour fast with glucose monitoring, echocardiography, carotid duplex scan, CT scan or MRI of brain, four-vessel cerebral angiography, 24-hour blood pressure monitoring, ambulatory EEG monitoring, and hospitalization for telemetry and video monitoring.

229. **Tachycardia:**
A. Withholding of all drugs, alcohol, and caf-

feine, if possible, CBC, sedimentation rate, urinalysis, drug screen, thyroid panel, ANA, VDRL, chest radiograph, ECG, and charting of temperature.

B. Cardiology consult, ASO titer, CRP, febrile agglutinins, serial blood cultures, arterial blood gas analysis, ventilation–perfusion scan, venous pressure and circulation time, pulmonary function studies, Holter monitoring, and hospitalization for telemetry and observation.

230. **Taste abnormalities:**
CBC, sedimentation rate, chemistry panel, urinalysis, drug screen, radiograph of sinuses, chest radiograph, oral surgeon consult, ENT consult, neurology consult, wake and sleep EEG with nasopharyngeal electrode placement, CT scan or MRI of brain, and psychiatric consult.

231. **Testicular atrophy:**
Urology consult, smear and culture of urethral or prostatic discharge, serum testosterone, FSH, urinalysis, urine gonadotropins, chromosome studies, liver function tests, serum iron and IBC, testicular biopsy, liver biopsy, and muscle biopsy.

232. **Testicular pain or swelling:**
A. CBC, sedimentation rate, urinalysis, urine culture, chemistry panel, VDRL, 24-hour urine gonadotropin, and smear and culture of urethral discharge before and after prostatic massage.

B. Urology consult, consultation with a general surgeon, testicular scan, ultrasonography of testicle, biopsy, and exploratory surgery.

233. **Thirst:**
A. CBC, sedimentation rate, urinalysis, chemistry panel, serum and urine osmolality, drug screen, blood alcohol level, and 24-hour urine calcium, sodium, and potassium.

B. Endocrinology consult, serum ADH, Hickey–Hare test, vasopressin injection test, PTH assay, CT scan of brain, and bone scan.

234. **Thyroid enlargement:**
A. CBC, sedimentation rate, urinalysis, thyroid

panel with TSH immunoassay, chemistry panel, chest radiograph, ECG, thyroid antibodies, and radiograph of neck.

B. Endocrinology consult, RAI uptake and scan, ultrasonography of thyroid, MRI, needle aspiration or biopsy, and surgical consult.

235. **Tinnitus:**

A. CBC, sedimentation rate, urinalysis, chemistry panel, thyroid panel, VDRL, audiometry, calories, radiographs of mastoids and petrous bones, and specialized audiometry (e.g., impedance audiometry, Békésy audiometry).

B. ENT or neurology consult, electronystagmography, CT scan or MRI of brain, CSF analysis, angiography, and glucose tolerance test.

236. **Tongue mass or swelling:**

A. Oral surgeon consult, ENT consult, CBC, sedimentation rate, urinalysis, chemistry panel, thyroid panel, VDRL, Tzanck test, ANA, coagulation profile, biopsy, and CT scan.

B. Therapeutic trial of vitamins, antibiotics, and antiviral agents or corticosteroids.

237. **Tongue pain and ulcers:**

Serum $B_{12}$ and folic acid, ANA, *Trichinella* antibody titer, upper GI series and esophagogram, CT scan, referral to a dentist or an oral surgeon, and therapeutic trial.

238. **Tooth and gum abnormalities:**

Radiographs of teeth and temporomandibular joints, heavy metal screen, drug screen, blood alcohol level, biopsy of gum, bone scan, and referral to a dentist or an oral surgeon.

239. **Tremor:**

Neurology consult, drug screen, blood alcohol level, serum copper and ceruloplasmin, CT scan or MRI of brain, EEG, CSF examination, liver function testing, and thyroid panel.

240. **Urethral discharge:**

Urethral smear and culture for *Neisseria gonorrhoeae* and *Chlamydia,* urinalysis and culture, PSA, prostatic examination, VDRL, and urology consult.

241. **Vaginal discharge:**
    A. Microscopic examination of saline and KOH preparations, endocervical smear and culture, search for clue cells, Pap smear, and culture for *Candida.*
    B. Gynecology consult, D&C, pelvic ultrasonography, VDRL, HIV antibody testing, and CT scan of pelvis.

242. **Varicose veins:**
    Liver profile, chest radiograph, flat plate of abdomen, CT scan of abdomen or chest, and exploratory surgery.

243. **Vulval or vaginal ulcerations:**
    CBC, sedimentation rate, urinalysis, VDRL, dark-field examination, smear and culture of exudate, Frei test, serologic test for lymphogranuloma venereum, biopsy, and gynecology consult.

244. **Weight loss:**
    A. CBC, sedimentation rate, urinalysis, chemistry panel, thyroid panel, serum amylase and lipase, febrile agglutinins, tuberculin test, ANA, serum protein electrophoresis, serum $B_{12}$ and folic acid, serum iron and IBC, chest radiograph, flat plate of abdomen, and HIV antibody titer.
    B. Gastroenterology consult, stool quantitative fat, stool trypsin, ova, and parasites, occult blood, upper GI series, small bowel series, barium enema, urine 5-HIAA, sigmoidoscopy, and CT scans of abdomen and pelvis.
    C. Endocrinology consult, plasma cortisol, rapid ACTH stimulation test, CT scan of brain, serum growth hormone, FSH, LH, RAI uptake and scan, and CSF analysis.
    D. Surgical consult, laparoscopy, and exploratory laparotomy.

245. **Wheezing:**
    CBC, sedimentation rate, chest radiograph, sputum analysis and culture, sputum for eosinophils, pulmonary function tests, bronchoscopy, and pulmonary consult.

# SECTION B

## SELECTION OF DIAGNOSTIC TESTS IN THE WORKUP OF DISEASES

**Acoustic neuroma:** Audiogram, calorie tests, CT scan, gadolinium-enhanced MRI, and combined CT scan and myelography.

**Acromegaly:** Growth hormone, FSH, LH, skull radiograph, CT scan, and MRI.

**Actinomycosis:** Smear for sulfur granules, culture of skin lesions, and chest radiograph.

**Addison's disease:** Plasma cortisol before and after ACTH, plasma ACTH, abdominal CT scan, and consultation with an endocrinologist.

**Adrenogenital syndrome:** Plasma 17-hydroxy-progesterone levels, urine 17- hydroxy and 17-ketogenic steroids, urine pregnanetriol, and CT scan of abdomen and pelvis.

**Agammaglobulinemia, congenital:** Serum electrophoresis and immunoelectrophoresis, blood type, and B-lymphocyte and T-lymphocyte counts.

**Agnogenic myeloid metaplasia:** CBC, blood smear, bone marrow biopsy, radiographs of bone, leukocyte alkaline phosphatase, and red cell survival time.

**Agranulocytosis, idiopathic:** CBC, platelet, bone marrow examination, and spleen scan.

**AIDS:** History and anti-HIV antibodies.

**Albright's syndrome**: Radiograph of long bones.

**Alcaptonuria:** Urinary homogentisic acid and radiograph of bones.

**Alcoholism:** Liver function tests, blood alcohol level, and liver biopsy.

**Aldosteronism, primary:** Serial electrolytes, 24-hour urine aldosterone, plasma renin, and CT scan of abdomen.

**Allergic rhinitis:** Nasal smear for eosinophils, serum IgE, RAST, and skin tests.

**Alpha$_1$-antitrypsin deficiency:** Serum protein electrophoresis.

**Alzheimer's disease:** CT scans and MRI.

**Amebiasis:** Stool for ova and parasites, hemagglutinin inhibition test, rectal biopsy, and therapeutic trial.

**Amyloidosis:** Congo red test, rectal biopsy, gingival biopsy, liver biopsy, kidney biopsy, and abdominal fat pad biopsy.

**Angina pectoris:** ECG, exercise tolerance test, thallium stress scan, coronary angiography, and therapeutic trial.

**Anthrax:** Smear and culture, biopsy of skin, and serologic tests.

**Aortic aneurysm:** Ultrasound, CT scan, sedimentation rate, VDRL, and aortography.

**Aplastic anemia:** Bone marrow examination and lymph node biopsy.

***Ascaris lumbricoides:*** Stool for ova and parasites, cathartic stool for ova and parasites, eosinophil count, and therapeutic trial.

**Asthma:** Sputum smear for eosinophils, pulmonary function tests before and after a $\beta$-adrenergic agonist, RAST test, and skin testing.

**Bacillary dysentery:** Stool smear, culture, and febrile agglutinins.

**Balantidiasis:** Stool for trophozoites or cyst.

**Basilar artery insufficiency:** MR angiography, four-vessel cerebral angiography, trial of anticoagulants, and consultation with a neurologist.

**Bell's palsy:** CT scan of mastoid and petrous bones, EMG, and consultation with a neurologist.

**Beriberi:** Erythrocyte transketolase activity, TPP test, thiamine-loading test, and therapeutic trial.

**Biliary cirrhosis, primary:** Liver function tests, antimitochondrial antibody titer, and open liver biopsy.

**Blastomycosis:** Skin test, sputum smear or culture, and culture of exudate.

**Boeck's sarcoid:** Kveim test, radiograph of chest and hands, scalene node biopsy, tuberculin skin test, transbronchial biopsy, and angiotensin-converting enzyme levels.

**Bornholm's disease:** Viral isolation from throat or stool and serologic tests.

**Botulism:** Demonstration of toxin in patient's serum, utilization of mice for bioassay, demonstration of toxin in stool or vomitus.

**Brachial plexus neuropathy:** EMG, NCV studies, somatosensory evoked potentials, and neurology consult.

**Brain tumor:** CT scan, MRI, and consultation with a neurosurgeon.

**Brill-Symmers disease:** Lymph node biopsy.

**Bronchial adenoma:** Bronchoscopy and biopsy.

**Bronchiectasis:** CT scan, bronchography, bronchoscopy, and sputum analysis.

**Bronchitis:** Chest radiograph and sputum smear and culture.

**Bronchopneumonia:** Chest radiograph, sputum

smear and culture, cold agglutinins, MG streptococci agglutinins, and complement-fixation test.

**Brucellosis:** Serologic tests, skin tests, and blood cultures.

**Bubonic plague:** Culture of bubo, blood or sputum, animal inoculation, and serologic tests.

**Buerger's disease:** Biopsy of affected vessels.

**Bursitis:** Clinical diagnosis, radiograph of joint, aspiration and therapeutic trial of corticosteroids, lidocaine injection, and consultation with an orthopedic surgeon.

**Cancer of the stomach:** Gastroscopy and biopsy and exploratory laparotomy.

**Carbon monoxide poisoning:** Blood carboxyhemoglobin level.

**Carbon tetrachloride poisoning:** Liver function tests, infrared spectrometry, and liver biopsy.

**Carbuncles and furuncles:** Smear and culture of exudate.

**Carcinoid syndrome:** Urinary 5-HIAA and exploratory laparotomy.

**Carcinoma of the ampulla of Vater:** ERCP and consultation with a gastroenterologist.

**Carcinoma of the breast:** Mammography, fine-needle aspiration, needle biopsy, and open biopsy.

**Carcinoma of the cervix:** Papanicolaou smears, cervical biopsy, colposcopy, and Schiller test.

**Carcinoma of the colon:** Colonoscopy and biopsy, exploratory laparotomy, and consultation with a gastroenterologist.

**Carcinoma of the endometrium:** Papanicolaou smear, D&C, and consultation with a gynecologist.

**Carcinoma of the esophagus:** Barium swallow, esophagoscopy and biopsy, ultrasonography, and scans to assess spread.

**Carcinoma of the lung:** Bronchoscopy and biopsy, needle biopsy, open resection, and consultation with a thoracic surgeon.

**Carcinoma of the ovary:** Ultrasonography, laparoscopy, serum CA-125, exploratory laparotomy, and consultations with a gynecologist and an oncologist.

**Carcinoma of the pancreas:** CT scan of abdomen, ERCP, liver function tests, and exploratory laparotomy.

**Cardiomyopathy:** ECG, echocardiography, cardiac catheterization, myocardial biopsy, and consultation with a cardiologist.

**Carpal tunnel syndrome:** NCV studies and neurology consult.

**Cat-scratch disease:** Skin test and lymph node biopsy.

**Cellulitis:** Smear and culture of exudates.

**Cerebellar ataxia:** Clinical diagnosis.

**Cerebral abscess (or cerebellar abscess):** CT scan, MRI, CSF examination and culture, exploratory surgery, and consultation with a neurosurgeon.

**Cerebral aneurysm:** CT scan, MR angiography, MRI, radiocontrast four-vessel cerebral angiography, spinal tap, and consultation with a neurosurgeon or neurologist.

**Cerebral embolism:** CT scan, MRI, angiography, spinal tap, and consultation with a neurologist.

**Cerebral hemorrhage:** CT scan, MRI, spinal tap, and neurology consult.

**Cerebral thrombosis:** CT scan, MRI, spinal tap, and consultation with a neurologist.

**Cervical spondylosis:** MRI, spinal tap, NCV study, EMG, dermatomal somatosensory-evoked potential study, and consultation with a neurologist for combined CT scan and myelography.

**Cervicitis:** Smear and culture or cervical biopsy and consultation with a gynecologist.

**Chagas' disease:** Blood smear and culture, CSF smear and culture, bone marrow or tissue biopsy, animal inoculation, and serologic tests.

**Chancroid:** Smear and culture or biopsy of lesion.

**Cholangiocarcinoma:** IV cholangiography, percutaneous transhepatic cholangiography, ERCP, CT scan, and GI consult.

**Cholangitis:** Liver function tests, CT scan, ultrasound, ERCP, percutaneous transhepatic cholangiography, and GI consult.

**Cholecystitis and cholelithiasis:** Ultrasonography, oral cholecystography, HIDA scan, and consultation with a surgeon.

**Choledocholithiasis:** Liver function tests, HIDA scan, ERCP, and percutaneous transhepatic cholangiography.

**Cholera:** Stool smear and culture for enteric pathogens.

**Choriocarcinoma:** Plasma $\beta$ subunit of hCG (pregnancy test) and consultation with a gynecologist.

**Cirrhosis:** Liver function tests and liver biopsy.

**Coarctation of the aorta:** Chest radiograph and aortogram.

**Coccidiomycosis:** Chest radiograph, serologic tests, skin tests, and consultation with a pulmonologist.

**Congenital heart disease:** ECG, echocardiography,

chest radiography, cardiac catheterization, angiocardiography.

**Conjunctivitis:** Gram or Giemsa stain of exudates and culture of exudates.

**Constipation:** Sigmoidoscopy, anoscopy, barium enema, colonoscopy, and consultation with a gastroenterologist.

**Coronary insufficiency:** ECG, exercise tolerance test, thallium stress scan, coronary angiography, consultation with a cardiologist, therapeutic trial, and echocardiography.

**Craniopharyngioma:** Skull radiograph, free $T_4$, TSH, FSH, LH, serum cortisol, CT scan, and MRI.

**Cretinism:** Radiographs for bone age, free $T_4$, and TSH.

**Creutzfeldt–Jakob disease:** EEG, CT scan, MRI, CSF protein, brain biopsy, and neurology consult.

**Cryptococcosis:** CSF examination, smear and culture, and sputum or blood culture.

**Cushing's syndrome:** Plasma cortisol, 24-hour urine free cortisol, plasma ACTH, dexamethasone-suppression test, high-dose dexamethasone-suppression test, metyrapone test, endocrinology consult, and CT scan of abdomen.

**Cutaneous larva migrans:** Clinical picture and skin biopsy.

**Cystic fibrosis:** Sweat test and consultation with a pulmonologist.

**Cysticercosis:** Biopsy of subcutaneous nodules for cysticerci, skull radiograph, CT scan, and indirect hemagglutination test or CSF complement-fixation test.

**Cystinosis:** Slit-lamp examination for crystals, urine

for cystine, and quantitative leukocyte or cultured fibroblast cystine content.

**Cystinuria:** Urinary nitroprusside test.

**Cytomegalovirus infection:** Viral isolation, fourfold rise or more in the titer of various serologic tests, and oncology consult.

**Dengue fever:** Hemagglutination inhibition or complement-fixation test.

**Depression:** Clinical picture and diagnostic tests to exclude endocrine and metabolic disorders.

**Dermatomyositis:** Muscle enzyme tests, RA factor, ANA, muscle biopsy, EMG, sedimentation rate, and consultation with a rheumatologist.

**Diabetes insipidus:** Hickey–Hare test, urine osmolality before and after vasopressin, and consultation with an endocrinologist.

**Diabetes mellitus:** FBS, glucose tolerance test, cortisone glucose tolerance test, and exclusion of other endocrine disorders.

**Diabetic coma:** Blood glucose, serum acetone, electrolytes, arterial blood gas analysis, and consultation with an endocrinologist.

**Digitalis intoxication:** Digoxin level, ECG, potassium infusion test, atropine test, and consultation with a cardiologist.

**Diphtheria:** History and physical examination and nose and throat culture on Loeffler's slant.

***Diphyllobothrium latum:*** Stool for ova and parasites and radiograph after barium enema.

**Diverticular disease:** Barium enema, colonoscopy, CT scan of abdomen and pelvis, gallium scan, and consultation with a gastroenterologist.

**Down's syndrome:** Clinical picture and chromosomal analysis.

**Dracunculiasis:** Eosinophil count, serum IgE, and antifilarial antibody titer.

**Dressler's syndrome:** CBC, sedimentation rate, ECG, and cardiology consult.

**Drug intoxication:** History, blood and urine tests for the drug, CBC, chemistry panel, and response to antidote.

**Drug reaction:** History, skin testing, RAST, and consultation with an allergist.

**Dubin–Johnson syndrome:** Liver function tests, cholecystogram, liver biopsy, and urine porphyrins.

**Eaton–Lambert syndrome:** EMG and search for carcinoma of the lung.

**Echinococcosis:** Chest radiograph, CT scans, ultrasonography, serologic tests, liver biopsy, Casoni intracutaneous test, and radiograph of long bones.

**Eclampsia:** Uric acid, renal function tests, renal biopsy, and urinalysis.

**Ectopic pregnancy:** Serum $\beta$-hCG, immunoassay, pelvic ultrasound, culdocentesis, peritoneal tap, and laparoscopy.

**Eczema:** Family history, skin testing, skin biopsy, RAST, and dermatology consult.

**Ehlers–Danlos syndrome:** Consultation with a rheumatologist, skin biopsy, and coagulation studies.

**Emphysema:** Chest radiograph, spirometry, and arterial blood gases.

**Empyema of the lung:** Chest radiograph, thoracentesis, and smear and culture of pleural fluid.

**Encephalitis, viral:** CSF examination, including search for herpes simplex virus, DNA in the fluid by PCR, CT scan and MRI of brain, neurology consult, viral isolation, and serologic tests.

**Encephalomyelitis:** Viral isolation from brain and CSF and serologic tests.

**Eosinophilic pneumonia:** Chest radiograph, sputum analysis, CBC, and tests to rule out parasites.

**Epididymitis:** Urethral smear and culture and ultra-sonography.

**Epidural abscess:** MRI or CT scan and culture of aspirated material.

**Epilepsy:** EEG, MRI, spinal tap, electrolytes, calcium, phosphorus, and neurology consult.

**Erysipelas:** Clinical picture, blood culture, culture of exudates, and surgical exploration.

**Erythema multiforme:** Clinical picture, dermatology consult, biopsy, and patch tests.

**Erythema nodosum:** CBC, sedimentation rate, skin tests, chest radiograph, dermatology consult, and biopsy.

**Erythroblastosis fetalis:** Bilirubin, CBC, direct Coombs' test on umbilical cord blood, type and cross match of infant's and mother's blood, and amniocentesis for bilirubin elevation.

**Esophageal varices:** Esophagoscopy, liver function tests, celiac and mesenteric angiography, and gastro-enterology consult.

**Essential hypertension:** Exclusion of renal and adrenal causes of hypertension, CBC, chemistry panel, plasma renin, 24-hour urine aldosterone, plasma cortisol, hypertensive IVP, renal angiography, and consultation with endocrinologist and urologist.

**Extradural hematoma:** CT scan, MRI, and neurosurgery consult.

**Fabry's disease:** Clinical picture, skin or renal biopsy, and ophthalmology or dermatology consult.

**Familial Mediterranean fever:** Family history and ethnic background.

**Familial periodic paralysis:** Family history, electrolyte determination during attacks, and response to treatment.

**Filariasis:** Blood, lymph, urine smears for microfilariae, *Dirofilaria* antigen intradermal test, complement-fixation test, and slit-lamp examination.

**Folic acid deficiency:** Serum folic acid and $B_{12}$, urinary formiminoglutamic acid, and tests for malabsorption syndrome (stool for quantitative fat, D-xylose absorption test, urine 5-HIAA, and mucosal biopsy).

**Friedreich's ataxia:** Clinical picture.

**Fungal infection of the skin:** KOH preparations, cultures, Wood's lamp examination, and dermatology consult.

**Galactosemia:** Red cell analysis of galactose-1-phosphate uridyl transferase, and elevated blood and urine galactose.

**Gas gangrene:** Clinical picture, smear and culture of exudates, radiograph of soft tissue, and frozen-section biopsy.

**Gastritis:** Gastroscopy and biopsy with urease testing to determine the presence of *Helicobacter pylori.*

**Gastroenteritis:** Stool smear for leukocytes, cultures, stool for ova and parasites, and *Giardia* antigen.

**Gilbert's disease:** Liver function tests and liver biopsy.

**Gingivitis:** Clinical picture, consultation with a dentist, and smear and cultures.

**Glanders:** Culture of exudates, skin tests, serologic tests, and animal inoculation.

**Glanzmann's disease:** Coagulation studies, CBC, platelet count, and clot retraction tests.

**Glaucoma:** Tonometry and ophthalmology consult.

**Glomerulonephritis:** Urinalysis, ASO titer, C3 complement levels, renal biopsy, and nephrology consult.

**Glycogen storage disease:** Chemistry panel, liver or muscle biopsy, and enzyme assay of tissue samples.

**Goiter, diffuse:** Free $T_4$, TSH, antithyroglobulin antibodies, RAI uptake and scan, and ultrasonography.

**Gonorrhea:** Urethral or vaginal smear and cultures, blood cultures, and ELISA.

**Goodpasture's disease:** Immunoassay of circulating antibodies to glycopeptide antigens related to basement membrane collagen, renal biopsy, and nephrology consult.

**Gout:** Blood uric acid levels, synovial fluid analysis, and response to colchicine.

**Granuloma inguinale:** Giemsa or Wright stain of scrapings from lesion and biopsy.

**Guillain–Barré syndrome:** CSF analysis, EMG, NCV studies, and neurology consult.

**Hamman–Rich syndrome:** Chest radiograph, pulmonary function tests, lung biopsy, and consultation with a pulmonologist.

**Hand–Schüller–Christian disease:** Radiograph of skull, bone biopsy, and bone marrow examination.

**Hartnup's disease:** Urinalysis for amino acids.

**Hashimoto's thyroiditis:** Free $T_4$, TSH, serum and antithyroglobulin antibodies.

**Hay fever:** Smears of nasal secretions for eosinophils, patch and intracutaneous skin tests, and therapeutic trial.

**Head injury:** Skull radiograph, CT scan, MRI, and neurology or neurosurgical consult.

**Heart failure:** ECG, chest radiograph, spirometry, venous pressure and circulation time, echocardiography, and cardiology consult.

**Heat-related disorders:** Clinical diagnosis.

**Hemangioblastoma:** CT scan, MRI, vertebral angiography, and neurosurgical consult.

**Hemifacial spasm:** Clinical diagnosis.

**Hemochromatosis:** Serum iron and iron-binding capacity, serum ferritin, liver or skin biopsy, and bone marrow biopsy.

**Hemolytic anemia, acquired:** CBC, red cell fragility test, direct and indirect Coombs' tests, and hematology consult.

**Hemophilia:** Coagulation time, prothrombin time, partial thromboplastin time, and assay of factors VIII, IX, and XI.

**Hemorrhagic fever:** Serologic tests and viral isolation.

**Hemorrhoids:** Digital examination, anoscopy, proctoscopy, and consultation with a proctologist.

**Hepatitis, toxic:** Liver function tests, toxicology screen, liver biopsy, and hepatitis profile.

**Hepatitis, viral:** Liver function tests, serologic tests for A, B, C, and D forms, liver biopsy, and consultation with a gastroenterologist.

**Hepatolenticular degeneration:** Serum and urine copper, serum ceruloplasmin level, liver biopsy, and slit-lamp examination of cornea.

**Hepatoma:** Liver function tests, alpha-fetoprotein, CT scans, liver biopsy, gastroenterology consult, and exploratory laparotomy.

**Hereditary ataxias:** Clinical diagnosis.

**Hereditary elliptocytosis:** CBC, blood sugar, serum haptoglobins, red cell survival time, and hematology consult.

**Hereditary spherocytosis:** CBC, blood sugar, red cell fragility, red cell survival time, and hematology consult.

**Herniated disc, cervical:** MRI, combined CT scan and myelography, EMG, dermatomal somatosensory-evoked potential study, and neurology consult.

**Herniated disc, lumbar:** MRI, CT scans, combined CT scan and myelography, EMG, and dermatomal somatosensory-evoked potential study.

**Herpangina:** Viral isolation and serologic tests.

**Herpes simplex:** Clinical picture, viral isolation, and serologic tests.

**Herpes zoster:** Tzanck test, serology, and animal inoculation.

**Hidradenitis suppurativa:** Clinical picture and cultures of exudates.

**Hirschsprung's disease:** Barium enema and surgical biopsy of the colon with the patient under general anesthesia.

**Histamine cephalalgia:** Histamine test and response to sumatriptan.

**Histiocytosis X:** Radiographs of skull, radiograph of long bones, bone scans, CT scans, and biopsy of the liver, spleen, or lymph nodes.

**Histoplasmosis:** Serologic tests, skin tests, sputum cultures, animal inoculation, and bone marrow smear and culture.

**Hookworm disease:** Stool for ova and parasites and eosinophil count.

**Huntington's chorea:** Clinical picture, family history, and neurology consult.

**Hurler's syndrome:** Urinary acid mucopolysaccharides, determination of alpha-L-iduronidase in cultured skin fibroblasts and leukocytes, and tissue biopsy.

**Hydrocephalus:** MRI, CT scan, lumbar isotope cisternography, and neurosurgical consult.

**Hypernephroma:** IVP, nephrotomography, ultrasonography, CT scan, and exploratory surgery.

**Hyperparathyroidism:** Serial serum calciums, parathyroid immunoassay, consultation with an endocrinologist, and radiograph of skull and long bones and mandible.

**Hypersensitivity pneumonitis:** Chest radiograph, spirometry, and immune response to offending agent.

**Hypersensitivity vasculitis:** CBC, ESR, and skin biopsy.

**Hypersplenism:** CBC, red cell survival, spleen-to-liver ratio, spleen scan, bone marrow, and epinephrine test.

**Hyperthyroidism:** Free $T_4$ and RAI uptake and scan.

**Hypoparathyroidism:** Serum calcium, phosphates, PTH assay, 24-hour urine calcium, magnesium, endocrinology consult, and therapeutic trial.

**Hypopituitarism:** Serum growth hormone, FSH, LH, TSH, free $T_4$, cortisol, Hickey–Hare test, ADH assay, skull radiograph, CT scan, and visual fields.

**Hypothyroidism:** Free $T_4$, TSH-sensitive assay, and therapeutic trial.

**Idiopathic postural hypotension:** Clinical picture and cardiology consult.

**Idiopathic pulmonary fibrosis:** Chest radiograph, CT

scan, spirometry, transbronchial or open lung biopsy, and pulmonology consult.

**Impetigo:** Smear and culture of exudates.

**Impingement syndrome:** MRI of shoulder, arthroscopy, and exploratory surgery.

**Infectious mononucleosis:** Blood smear, Monospot test, heterophil antibody titer, and repeat tests.

**Influenza:** Clinical picture, nose, throat, and sputum smears and cultures to rule out other pathogens, and chest radiograph.

**Insulinoma:** Frequent blood sugars during a 72-hour fast, plasma proinsulin, insulin, C-peptide levels, tolbutamide tolerance test, CT scan of pancreas to localize tumor, and endocrinology consult.

**Iron-deficiency anemia:** Serum iron and IBC, serum ferritin, and bone marrow for hemosiderin content.

**Irritable bowel syndrome:** Clinical evaluation and exclusion of other causes of diarrhea, constipation, and abdominal pain.

**Kala-azar:** Bone marrow or lymph node aspiration and biopsy, splenic aspiration, and serologic tests.

**Klinefelter's syndrome:** Buccal smear for sex chromatin, karyotype analysis, serum FSH, LH, testicular biopsy, and endocrinology consult.

**Korsakoff's syndrome:** History, blood alcohol levels, and response to thiamine.

**Lactose deficiency:** Lactose tolerance test, hydrogen breath test, measurement of lactose in a jejunal biopsy, and therapeutic trial.

**Langerhans' cell granulomatosis:** Lung or tissue biopsy.

**Laryngitis:** Nose and throat culture, throat washings

for viral isolation, laryngoscopy, lateral films of neck to exclude epiglottitis, and ENT consult.

**Lead intoxication:** Serum and urine lead level, urine for ALA, coproporphyrins, and free erythrocyte protoporphyrin.

**Legionnaires' disease:** Direct fluorescent antibody staining, cultures, and serologic tests.

**Leishmaniasis, cutaneous:** Smear and culture of aspirates or tissue, serologic tests, and skin test.

**Leprosy:** Wade's scraped incision procedure, culture of lesion, biopsy of skin, nerves, radiograph of hands and feet, histamine test, and lepromin test.

**Leptospirosis:** Blood, urine, CSF cultures, guinea pig inoculation, and serologic tests.

**Leriche's syndrome:** Aortography.

**Leukemia:** CBC, blood smear, bone marrow examination, and hematology consult.

**Lichen planus:** Skin biopsy.

**Lipoproteinemias:** Lipid profile, overnight plasma refrigeration, lipoprotein electrophoresis, and gel electrophoresis.

**Listeriosis:** CSF analysis, CSF culture, and blood and amniotic fluid culture.

**Liver abscess:** CT scan, MRI, ultrasonography, gallium or indium scan, serologic tests, and exploratory laparotomy.

**Lung abscess:** Sputum culture, chest radiograph, bronchoscopy, CT scan of chest, and needle aspiration.

**Lupus erythematosus:** ANA, double-strand DNA, anti-Smith antibodies, and tissue biopsy.

**Lyme disease:** Serologic tests.

**678**

**Lymphangitis:** Clinical diagnosis.

**Lymphogranuloma venereum:** Cultures of lesions, complement-fixation test, and Frei test.

**Lymphoma:** Radiographs, CT scans, biopsy, exploratory laparotomy, and bone marrow examination.

**Lysosomal storage disease:** Urinalysis, chemistry panel, radiographs, CT scans, biopsy, and culture of skin fibroblasts.

**Macroglobulinemia:** CBC, blood smear, serum protein electrophoresis, immunoelectrophoresis, and blood viscosity.

**Malabsorption syndrome:** Stool for quantitative fat, D-xylose absorption test, urine 5-HIAA, and mucosal biopsy.

**Malaria:** Giemsa stain of thick and thin blood smears and bone marrow examination.

**Mallory–Weiss tear:** Esophagoscopy.

**Marfan's syndrome:** Chest radiograph, slit-lamp examination, urine for homocystine, and ultrasonography of aorta.

**Mastoiditis:** Radiographs of mastoids, CT scan, and culture of aural discharge.

**McArdle's syndrome:** Muscle enzyme tests, myoglobin in urine, and muscle biopsy.

**McCune–Albright syndrome:** Radiographs of skull and long bones and bone scan.

**Meckel's diverticulum:** Small bowel series and exploratory laparotomy.

**Mediastinitis:** Chest radiograph, CT scan of chest, MRI, and mediastinoscopy.

**Melanoma:** Biopsy.

**Meniere's disease:** Audiograms, caloric testing, and electronystagmography ENT consult.

**Meningitis:** CSF analysis and culture, India ink preparation, blood cultures, and serologic tests.

**Meningococcemia:** Blood cultures, CSF analysis and cultures, petechial scrapings for smear and culture, and serologic tests.

**Menopause:** Serum FSH and estradiol, Pap smear for maturation index, and therapeutic trial.

**Mesenteric artery insufficiency, embolism, thrombosis:** Digital subtraction angiography, aortography, and selective mesenteric angiography.

**Methemoglobinemia and sulfhemoglobinemia:** No change in color of blood by exposure to air and spectrophotometry before and after adding cyanide.

**Migraine:** Histamine test and response to sumatriptan orally or subcutaneously.

**Milroy's disease:** Clinical diagnosis.

**Mitral valvular disease:** ECG, chest radiograph, echocardiography, MRI, and cardiac catheterization and angiocardiography.

**Mucormycosis:** Smear of crushed tissue, sputum smear and culture, and tissue biopsy.

**Multiple myeloma:** Serum protein electrophoresis, immunoelectrophoresis, bone marrow examination, and urine for Bence Jones protein.

**Multiple sclerosis:** MRI of brain and spinal cord, CSF for gamma globulin and myelin basic protein, and evoked potentials.

**Mumps:** Serologic tests, viral isolation, and skin test.

**Muscular dystrophy:** EMG and muscle biopsy.

**Myasthenia gravis:** Antiacetylcholine receptor antibody titer, Tensilon test, EMG, and search for thymoma.

**Myocardial infarction:** Serial ECGs, serial cardiac enzymes, and PYP resting heart scan.

**Myotonia atrophica:** EMG and muscle biopsy.

**Narcolepsy:** Wake and sleep EEG and sleep study.

**Nephrolithiasis:** 24-hour urine, chemistry panel, PTH, IVP, renal ultrasonography, and stone analysis.

**Nephrotic syndrome, idiopathic:** Serum protein electrophoresis, 24-hour urine protein, and renal biopsy.

**Neuroblastoma:** CT scan of abdomen, ultrasonography, urine homovanillic acid and catecholamines, and bone marrow examination.

**Neurofibromatosis:** Family history, tissue biopsy, urine catecholamines, and CT scan of brain.

**Neuroma, traumatic:** Nerve conduction studies and exploration and biopsy.

**Niemann–Pick disease:** Bone marrow examination and enzyme assay and culture of skin fibroblasts.

**Nocardiosis:** Acid-fast smears, fungal cultures, bronchoscopy, needle aspiration, and lung biopsy.

**Nutritional anemia:** CBC, blood smear for red cell morphology, serum iron and IBC, serum ferritin, serum $B_{12}$ and folic acid, and bone marrow examination.

**Obesity:** Free $T_4$, TSH, serum cortisol, 72-hour fast, serum C-peptide, tolbutamide tolerance test, and CT scan of brain.

**Optic neuritis:** Visual field examination, visual-evoked potential study, MRI, and consultation with ophthalmologist.

**Orchitis:** Careful exclusion of testicular torsion, ultrasonography, mumps serology and skin test, and urethral smear and culture after prostatic massage.

**Oroya fever:** CBC, red cell fragility tests, red cell survival time, and blood cultures.

**Osteoarthritis:** Radiographs of joints, bone scan, and exclusion of other forms of arthritis.

**Osteogenesis imperfecta:** Radiographs and clinical evaluation.

**Osteogenic sarcoma:** Radiographs of bones, bone scan, CT scan, and acid and alkaline phosphatase.

**Osteomalacia:** Chemistry panel, urine calcium, radiographs of bone, and serum vitamin D levels.

**Osteomyelitis:** Radiographs of bones, bone scan, MRI, cultures of exudates, blood cultures, and CT scans.

**Osteopetrosis:** Radiograph of skull and long bone.

**Osteoporosis:** Radiographs of bone, dual energy radiograph absorptiometry, and quantitative CT.

**Otitis externa:** Clinical evaluation and culture of discharge.

**Otitis media:** Clinical evaluation, tympanogram, and culture of transtympanic aspirate.

**Ovarian cancer:** Serum CA-125, pelvic and transvaginal ultrasonography, CT scan of abdomen, laparoscopy, and exploratory laparotomy.

**Paget's disease of bone:** Skeletal survey, bone scans, CT scans, biopsy, and alkaline phosphatase.

**Pancreatitis, acute:** Serum amylase and lipase, urine amylase, CT scan, MRI, and ultrasonography.

**Pancreatitis, chronic:** Serum lipase, stool for fat and trypsin, duodenal analysis, CT scan of abdomen, ultrasonography, and MRI.

**Panniculitis, acute:** Tissue biopsy.

**Paralysis agitans:** Clinical evaluation and exclusion of drug and manganese toxicity.

**Pellagra:** Urine *N*-methyl niacinamide, tests for deficiency of other vitamins, and response to niacin.

**Pemphigus vulgaris:** Skin biopsy.

**Peptic ulcer:** Upper GI series, serum gastrin, gastroscopy and duodenoscopy, and biopsy with urease testing or serology for *Helicobacter pylori*.

**Periarteritis nodosa:** Biopsy of involved tissue, angiography of involved arteries, and ANA.

**Pericarditis:** Chest radiograph, ECG, echocardiography, CT scan, and MRI.

**Perinephric abscess:** Plain abdominal films, ultrasonography, and CT scan.

**Peripheral neuropathy:** Nerve conduction studies, EMG, glucose tolerance test, heavy metal screen, ANA, and urine porphobilinogen.

**Peritonitis:** Peritoneal fluid analysis and culture, ultrasonography, CT scan of abdomen, and laparoscopy.

**Pernicious anemia:** Serum vitamin $B_{12}$ and folic acid, Schilling test, and bone marrow examination.

**Peroneal muscular atrophy:** Nerve conduction studies, EMG, and nerve biopsy.

**Peroneal neuropathy:** Nerve conduction studies and EMG.

**Pertussis:** Nasopharyngeal swab cultures and serologic tests.

**Peutz–Jeghers syndrome:** Small bowel series, barium enema, and colonoscopy.

**Peyronie's disease:** Clinical evaluation.

**Pharyngitis and tonsillitis:** Pharyngeal smears and cultures, rapid streptococcal tests, and serologic tests.

**Pharyngoconjunctival fever:** Cultures and serologic tests.

**Phenylpyruvic oligophrenia:** Plasma phenylalanine, serum tyrosine, and loading tests with phenylalanine.

**Pheochromocytoma:** 24-hour urine, VMA, catecholamines or metanephrines, CT of abdomen and chest, and aortography.

**Phlebotomus fever:** Clinical diagnosis.

**Pinealoma:** CT scans or MRI of brain.

**Pinworm disease:** Microscopic examination of cellulose acetate tape specimen, and therapeutic trial.

**Pituitary adenoma:** CT scan, MRI, prolactin, growth hormone, ACTH, TSH, FSH, LH, and target organ hormones.

**Pityriasis rosea:** Clinical evaluation and skin biopsy.

**Plague:** Culture of aspirated material from buboes, culture of blood and sputum, and serologic tests.

**Pneumoconiosis:** History of exposure to coal dust, silica or asbestosis, chest radiograph, pulmonary function tests, and open lung biopsy.

***Pneumocystis carinii* infection:** Sputum smear, fiberoptic bronchoscopy, and transbronchial biopsy.

**Pneumonia:** Sputum smear and cultures, cold agglutinins, serologic tests, and culture for *Legionella.*

**Pneumothorax:** Chest radiograph.

**Poliomyelitis:** Clinical examination and CSF analysis.

**684**

**Polycystic kidney disease:** IVP, ultrasonography, and CT scans.

**Polycystic ovary syndrome:** Elevated LH:FSH ratio, androstenedione, testosterone, and laparoscopy.

**Polycythemia vera:** CBC, red cell mass, ABG, thrombocytosis, leukocytosis, erythropoietin, serum $B_{12}$, and leukocyte alkaline phosphatase.

**Polymyalgia rheumatica:** Sedimentation rate and temporal artery biopsy.

**Porphyria:** Urine porphyrins, zinc protoporphyrin, urine porphobilinogen, $\delta$-aminolevulinic acid.

**Preeclampsia–eclampsia:** Clinical evaluation, proteinuria, and uric acid.

**Premenstrual tension syndrome:** Clinical evaluation.

**Prostatic carcinoma:** PSA, acid phosphatase, chemistry panel, transrectal ultrasonography, and needle biopsy.

**Prostatic hypertrophy:** Catheterization for residual urine, IVP, cystoscopy, ultrasonography, and prostatic biopsy.

**Prostatitis:** Urinalysis, urine cultures, smear of prostatic fluid, exclusion of gonorrhea, and MRI.

**Pseudogout:** Synovial analysis for calcium pyrophosphate crystals.

**Pseudohypoparathyroidism:** Family history, serum calcium, phosphorus levels, PTH, and response of blood and urine to exogenous PTH.

**Pseudopseudohypoparathyroidism:** Family history, serum calcium, phosphorus, PTH, and normal response of urinary cyclic AMP to exogenous PTH.

**Pseudotumor cerebri:** CT scan of the brain and lumbar puncture.

**Psittacosis:** Sputum or blood culture and serologic tests.

**Psoriasis:** Family history and skin biopsy.

**Pulmonary alveolar proteinosis:** Chest radiograph and lung biopsy.

**Pulmonary embolism:** Chest radiograph, arterial blood gas analysis, ventilation perfusion scan, and pulmonary angiography.

**Pyelonephritis:** Urinalysis, urine culture and colony count, IVP, and cystoscopy.

**Pyloric stenosis, congenital:** Clinical evaluation, electrolytes, and exploratory laparotomy.

**Pyridoxine deficiency:** Clinical evaluation, pyridoxal phosphate level, and therapeutic trial.

**Q fever:** Chest radiograph and serologic tests.

**Rabies:** Clinical evaluation, fluorescent antibody stain of tissue, serologic tests, and animal observation and autopsy.

**Rat-bite fever:** Dark-field examination, cultures of blood and infected tissue, and animal inoculation.

**Raynaud's disease:** Clinical observation, ice water test, and exclusion of other causes of Raynaud's syndrome.

**Reflex sympathetic dystrophy:** Radiographs of involved extremities, response to stellate ganglion or lumbar paravertebral block, and thermography.

**Reflux esophagitis:** Barium swallow, upper GI series, esophagoscopy and biopsy, and radionuclide reflux study.

**Refsum's disease:** Plasma phytanic acid and pipecolic acid.

**Regional enteritis:** Small bowel series, barium enema, colonoscopy and biopsy, and exploratory laparotomy.

**Reiter's syndrome:** Clinical evaluation and HLA–B27 antigen.

**Relapsing fever:** Staining of blood smears, culture, and serologic tests.

**Relapsing polychondritis:** Clinical evaluation and biopsy of cartilage.

**Renal failure, acute:** CBC, chemistry panel, urinalysis, serum and urine osmolality, electrolytes, and renal biopsy.

**Renal failure, chronic:** CBC, chemistry panel, urinalysis, serum and urine osmolality, and renal biopsy.

**Renal vein thrombosis:** Selective renal venography.

**Retinal artery occlusion:** Retinoscopy, ocular plethysmography, fluorescein angiography, and carotid angiography.

**Rheumatic fever:** ASO titer, CRP, sedimentation rate, and throat culture.

**Rheumatoid arthritis:** Sedimentation rate, RA titer, radiographs of joints, bone scan, and synovial fluid analysis.

**Rheumatoid spondylitis:** Radiographs of lumbar spine, bone scans, and HLA–B27 antigen.

**Riboflavin deficiency:** Clinical observation and therapeutic trial.

**Rickets:** Chemistry panel, skeletal survey, and serum vitamin D level.

**Rickettsialpox:** Weil–Felix reaction and serologic tests.

**Rocky Mountain spotted fever:** Weil–Felix reaction and serologic tests.

**Rubella:** Clinical picture and serologic tests.

**Rubeola:** Stains of nasal secretions, sputum and urine for multinucleated giant cells, and serologic tests.

**Salmonellosis:** Stool cultures and serologic tests.

**Salpingitis:** Vaginal or endocervical smear and culture (on special media), ultrasonography, endometrial biopsy, laparoscopy, and CT scan.

**Sarcoidosis:** Chest radiograph, scalene node biopsy, transbronchial biopsy, Kveim–Siltzbach skin test, and mediastinoscopy.

**Scabies:** Microscopic examination of scrapings and biopsy of papulovesicular lesions.

**Scarlet fever:** Rapid streptococcal tests, throat cultures, and Dick test.

**Schilder's disease:** MRI or CT scan of the brain, EEG, and CSF analysis.

**Schistosomiasis:** Stool, urine or tissue for ova and parasites, and ultrasonography of liver.

**Schizophrenia:** Clinical evaluation and psychometric testing.

**Scleroderma:** ANA, antinucleolar antibody titer, antiscleroderma antibody test, and skin biopsy.

**Scrub typhus:** Weil–Felix reaction and serologic tests.

**Scurvy:** Plasma ascorbic acid levels, platelet ascorbic acid level, and therapeutic trial.

**Seborrheic dermatitis:** Clinical picture and skin biopsy.

**Septic arthritis:** Synovial fluid analysis, smear and culture, and blood cultures.

**Septicemia:** Multiple blood cultures.

**Serum sickness:** Sedimentation rate and serum complement.

**Shigellosis:** Stool smear and culture and serologic tests.

**Shy–Drager syndrome:** Tilt-table test and fall in blood pressure of 30 mm Hg or more on rising.

**Sickle cell anemia:** Sickle cell preparation and hemoglobin electrophoresis.

**Sinusitis:** Transillumination, radiographs of sinuses, CT scan, and nose and throat cultures.

**Sjögren's syndrome:** ANA, RA test, ribonucleoprotein antibody test, and anti-SS-A/Ro antibody titer.

**Skin cancer:** Biopsy of lesion.

**Sleep apnea:** Polysomnography.

**Small intestinal tumors:** Small bowel series, CT scans with contrast, and exploratory laparotomy.

**Snake bite:** Clinical evaluation.

**Spasmodic torticollis:** Clinical evaluation.

**Spinal cord tumor:** MRI of spinal cord, combined CT scan and myelography, and CSF analysis.

**Sporotrichosis:** Culture of exudate or synovial fluid and sputum and skin biopsy.

**Sprains, common:** Clinical picture, radiographs of spine and joints, and MRI to rule out serious pathologic processes.

**Stasis dermatitis:** Clinical evaluation and venography.

**Strongyloidiasis:** Stool for ova and parasites, duodenal analysis, Entero-Test, string method, and serologic tests.

**Sturge–Weber syndrome:** CT scan of brain and skin biopsy.

**Subacute bacterial endocarditis:** Serial blood cultures, routine and transesophageal echocardiography, and CT scan or MRI.

**Subdiaphragmatic abscess:** Chest radiograph, abdominal plain films, ultrasonography, CT scans, MRI, and gallium scan.

**Subdural hematoma:** CT scan or MRI of brain.

**Syphilis:** Dark-field examination, direct fluorescent antibody identification test (DFA–TP), VDRL, and FTA–ABS test.

**Syringomyelia:** MRI of spinal cord and combined CT scan and myelography.

**Systemic mastocytosis:** 24-hour urine histamine, blood histamine level, and skin and bone marrow biopsy.

**Takayasu's disease:** Sedimentation rate, protein electrophoresis, and arteriography.

**Tapeworm disease:** Stool for ova and parasites, fluorescent antibody test, tissue biopsy, radiographs, and CT scans.

**Temporal arteritis:** Sedimentation rate and superficial temporal artery biopsy.

**Testicular tumors:** CT scan of abdomen and pelvis, chest radiograph, alpha-fetoprotein, and urine chorionic gonadotropin.

**Tetanus:** History of IV drug use and clinical picture.

**Thalassemia:** CBC, blood smears, and hemoglobin electrophoresis.

**Thoracic outlet syndrome:** Somatosensory-evoked potential study, digital subtraction angiography, and brachial angiography.

**Thromboangiitis obliterans:** Arteriography and excisional biopsy.

**Thrombocytopenic purpura, idiopathic:** CBC, platelet count, platelet antibody titer, platelet function tests, and bone marrow examination.

**Thrombophlebitis:** Duplex venous ultrasonography, impedance plethysmography, iodine-125 fibrinogen scan, and venography.

**Thrombotic thrombocytopenic purpura:** CBC, platelet count, blood smears, Coombs' test, and gingival and bone marrow biopsy.

**Thymoma:** Chest radiograph, CT scans of mediastinum, and MRI.

**Thyroiditis, subacute:** CBC, sedimentation rate, TSH, thyroid profile, and RAI uptake and scan.

**Tourette's syndrome:** Clinical picture.

**Toxoplasmosis:** Serologic tests and animal inoculation.

**Trachoma:** Giemsa staining of conjunctival smears, cell cultures, *Chlamydia,* PCR, and therapeutic trial.

**Transfusion reaction:** Repeat of type and cross match, direct and indirect Coombs' test, CBC, platelet count, prothrombin time, PTT, serum haptoglobin, fibrin split products, and fibrinogen.

**Transient ischemic attacks:** Carotid duplex scan, ocular plethysmography, echocardiography, and four-vessel cerebral angiography.

**Trichinosis:** Eosinophil count, muscle enzyme tests, serologic tests, skin test, and muscle biopsy.

**Trigeminal neuralgia:** Clinical diagnosis.

**Trypanosomiasis:** Giemsa-stain thick and thin blood smear for parasites, animal inoculation, blood cultures, and direct microscopic examination of fluid from chancre.

**Tuberculosis:** Chest radiograph, smear and culture for AFB, tuberculin test, serologic tests, animal inoculation, and biopsy.

**Tuberous sclerosis:** Family history, skin biopsy, and MRI of brain.

**Tularemia:** Serologic test.

**Turner's syndrome:** Serum FSH and LH, buccal smear for Barr body analysis, and chromosomal analysis.

**Typhoid fever:** Stool, urine, blood cultures, and Widal antibody test.

**Typhus, epidemic:** Weil–Felix reaction and complement-fixation tests.

**Ulcerative colitis:** Colonoscopy and biopsy and barium enema.

**Urinary tract infection:** Urinalysis, urine culture and colony count, and IVP and cystoscopy.

**Urticaria:** Clinical evaluation, RAST, skin test, and IgE.

**Uterine fibroids:** Ultrasonography, CT scans of pelvis, and laparoscopy.

**Vaginitis:** Microscopic examination of smears in saline and 10% KOH and cultures for *Candida* and *Trichomonas*.

**Varicella:** Tzanck smear and serologic tests.

**Varicose veins:** Venography.

**Variola:** Viral isolation from skin lesions, oropharynx, conjunctiva, and urine, and serologic tests.

**Venereal disease:** Smear, culture, dark-field examination, skin tests, biopsy, and serologic tests.

**Viral myelitis:** CSF analysis, viral isolation, and acute- and convalescent-phase fluid for viral serology.

**Visceral and ocular larva migrans:** ELISA for toxocaral antibodies.

**Von Willebrand's disease:** Prolonged bleeding time, plasma vWF concentration, ristocetin cofactor activity, and factor VIII assay.

**Warts:** Clinical evaluation and biopsy.

**Wegener's granulomatosis:** Lung biopsy, upper airway biopsy, renal biopsy, antineutrophil cytoplasmic antibody, ANA.

**Wernicke's encephalopathy:** Therapeutic trial of thiamine.

**Whipple's disease:** Small bowel biopsy.

**Yaws:** Dark-field examination, RPR, and FTA–ABS test.

**Yellow fever:** Viral isolation from blood and serologic tests.

**Zollinger–Ellison syndrome:** Serum gastrin, secretin injection test, and calcium infusion test.

# BIBLIOGRAPHY

Bakerman S. ABC's of interpretive laboratory data. 3rd ed. Myrtle Beach, SC: Interpretive Laboratory Data, 1994.

Chernecky CC, Krech RL, Berger BJ. Laboratory tests and diagnostic procedures. Philadelphia: WB Saunders, 1993.

Eisenberg RL, Margulis AR. Radiology pocket reference. Philadelphia: Lippincott-Raven, 1996.

Eng J. Manual of radiology. Philadelphia: Lippincott-Raven, 1997.

Fischbach F. A Manual of laboratory diagnostic tests. 2nd ed. Philadelphia: JB Lippincott, 1984.

Gomella LG. Clinician's pocket reference. 7th ed. Norwalk, CT: Appleton & Lange, 1993.

Griner PF, Panzer RJ, Greenland P. Clinical diagnosis and the laboratory. Chicago: Year Book, 1986.

Hall R. The ultrasound handbook. 2nd ed. Philadelphia: JB Lippincott, 1993.

Landberg GD. Using the clinical laboratory in medical decision-making. Chicago: American Society of Clinical Pathologists Press, 1983.

Mayne PD. Clinical chemistry in diagnosis and treatment. 6th ed. London: Arnold, 1994.

Nicoll D, McPhee SJ, Chou TM, et al. Pocket guide to diagnostic tests. 2nd ed. Stamford, CT: Appleton & Lange, 1997.

Ravel R. Clinical laboratory medicine. 4th ed. Chicago: Year Book, 1984.

Sox HC Jr, ed. Common diagnostic tests. Philadelphia: American College of Physicians, 1987.

Speicher CE. The right test. 2nd ed. Philadelphia: WB Saunders, 1993.

Tietz NW. Clinical guide to laboratory tests. 3rd ed. Philadelphia: WB Saunders, 1995.

Wallach J. Interpretation of diagnostic tests. Boston: Little, Brown, 1996.

Worthley LIG. Handbook of emergency laboratory tests. New York: Churchill Livingstone, 1996.

# INDEX

--Page numbers followed by an 'a' denote an algorithm--

Abdominal pain, acute, 617
Abdominal pain, chronic recurrent, 617
Abdominal plain films, 3, 4a
Abdominal swelling, focal, 617–618
Abdominal swelling, generalized, 618
Absent or diminished pulse, 618
Acetone, 5, 6a
Acetylcholine receptor antibody test, 7
Acid phosphatase, blood, 8, 9a
Acid phosphatase, vaginal, 10
Acoustic neuroma, 662
Acromegaly, 662
ACTH (Adrenocorticotropic hormone)
    infusion test, 13, 14a
    plasma, 11–12, 12a
Actinomycosis, 662
Activated partial thromboplastin time (APTT), 422, 423a
ADB (Streptococcal antibody test), 537
Addison's disease, 662
ADH (Antidiuretic hormone), 46–47, 47a
Adrenocorticotropic hormone (ACTH)
    infusion test, 13, 14a
    plasma, 11–12, 12a
Adrenogenital syndrome, 662
Agammaglobulinemia, congenital, 662
Agnogenic myeloid metaplasia, 662
Agnosia (see Aphasia)
Agranulocytosis, idiopathic, 662
AIDS, 662
Alanine aminotransferase (ALT) (SGPT), 68–69, 69a
Albright's syndrome, 662
Albumin, serum, 15–16, 16a
Alcaptonuria, 662
Alcoholism, 662
Aldolase, 17
Aldosterone, serum or urine, 18–19, 19a
Aldosteronism, primary, 663
Alkaline phosphatase, 20–21, 22a, 23b
Allergic rhinitis, 663
Alopecia, 618
Alpha$_1$-antitrypsin deficiency, 663
Alpha$_1$-antitrypsin test, 25, 26a
Alpha$_1$-fetoprotein, 27
ALT (Alanine aminotransferase), 68–69, 69a
Alzheimer's disease, 663
Amebiasis, 663
    antibody test, 28
Amenorrhea, 618
Amino acids, 29–30, 30a
$\delta$-Aminolevulinic acid, urinary, 31
Ammonia, 32

Amnesia, 618
Amniocentesis, 33
Amylase, serum, 34, 35a
Amyloidosis, 663
ANA (Antinuclear antibody test), 53, 54a
ANCA (Antineutrophil cytoplasmic antigen) antibodies, 52
Androstenedione, 36, 37a
Angina pectoris, 663
Angiocardiography, cardiac catheterization and, 131–132
Angiography, 38–39, 40a
    digital subtraction, 221
    fluorescein, 261
Angiotensin I-converting enzyme, 41
Animal inoculation, 42
Anion gap, 43
Ankle/brachial index, 44–45
Ankle clonus, 618–619
Anorexia, 619
Anoscopy, 516
Anosmia, 619
Anthrax, 663
Anti-DNA antibody test, 48
Anti-DNase-B, 49
Anti-GBM (Antiglomerular basement membrane antibody titer), 50
Anti-HCV (Hepatitis C antibody), 319, 320a
Anti-HDV (Hepatitis D antibody), 319, 320a
Anti-HEV (Hepatitis E antibody), 319, 320a
Anti-Smith antibody titer, 58
Antidiuretic hormone (ADH), 46–47, 47a
Antiglomerular basement membrane (anti-GBM) antibody titer, 50
Antimitochondrial antibody test, 51
Antineutrophil cytoplasmic antigen antibodies (ANCA), 52
Antinuclear antibody (ANA) test, 53, 54a
Antiparietal cell antibody, 55
Antiplatelet antibody, 56
Antisclerodermal antibody titer, 57
Antismooth muscle antibody test, 59
Antisperm antibody test, 60
Antistreptolysin O (ASO) titer, 61
Antithrombin III, 62
Anuria, 619
Anxiety, 619
Aortic aneurysm, 663
Aortic sonography, 63
Aortography, 64
Aphasia, 619
Aplastic anemia, 663
Apraxia (see Aphasia)
APTT (Activated partial thromboplastin time), 422, 423a
Arsenic, urine, 65
Arthrography, 66
Arthroscopy, 67
Ascaris lumbricoides, 663
Ascites, 619–620
ASO (Antistreptolysin O) titer, 61
Aspartate aminotransferase (AST) (SGOT), 68–69, 69a
Aspergillus antibody titer, 70
Asthma, 663
Ataxia, 620
    hereditary, 675
Athetosis, 620
Audiometry, screening, 71–72, 72a
Autohemolysis, 73

**696    Index**

Axillary masses, 620

Babinski's sign, 620
Bacillary dysentery, 663
Back pain, 620
Balantidiasis, 663
Barium enema, 74–75, 75a
Barr body analysis, 76
Bart's hemoglobin, 315
Basilar artery insufficiency, 664
Basophilic stippling, 77
Basophils, 78
Bell's palsy, 664
Bence Jones protein, urine, 79
Beriberi, 664
Bernstein test, 80
Bicarbonate, 81–82, 82a
Biliary cirrhosis, primary, 664
Bilirubin, serum, 83–84, 84a-85a
Bilirubin, urine, 86
Biopsy, 87
Blastomycosis, 664
    antibody test, 88
    skin test, 89
Bleeding gums, 621
Bleeding time, 90, 91a
Blindness, 621
Blood, culture of, 92
Blood, microscopic examination, 520
Blood chloride, 150–151, 151a
Blood smear for histiocytes, 321
Blood smear for morphology, 93–94, 95a
Blood typing, 96–97, 98a
Blood urea nitrogen (BUN), 99–100, 100a-101a
Blood volume studies, 102–103
Blurred vision, 621
Boeck's sarcoid, 664
Bone marrow
    examination, 104–105, 106a
    scan, 107, 108a
Bone mass or swelling, 621
Bone scan, 109
Bornholm's disease, 664
Botulism, 664
Brachial plexus neuropathy, 664
Bradycardia, 621
Brain scan, 110
Brain tumor, 664
Brainstem-evoked potential, 245
Breast discharge, 621
Breast mass, 621
Breast pain, 621
Breast ultrasonography, 111
Brill-Symmers disease, 664
Bronchial adenoma, 664
Bronchiectasis, 664
Bronchitis, 664
Bronchography, 112
Bronchopneumonia, 664–665
Bronchoscopy, 113
Brucella antibody test, 114
Brucellosis, 665
    skin test, 115

Bubonic plague, 665
Buerger's disease, 665
BUN (Blood urea nitrogen), 99–100, 100a-101a
Bursitis, 665


C-AMP (Cyclic adenosine monophosphate), renal, 208
C-peptide, 189, 190a
C-reactive protein (CRP), 191, 192a
Calcitonin, 116, 117a
Calcium, 118–119, 120a
   urine, 24-hour, 121–122
Cancer, ovarian, 682
Cancer, skin, 689
Cancer, stomach, 665
Capillary fragility test, 124, 125a
Carbon dioxide, 126–127, 127a
Carbon monoxide diffusing capacity (DLCO), 475
Carbon monoxide poisoning, 665
Carbon tetrachloride poisoning, 665
Carboxyhemoglobin, 128
Carbuncles, 665
Carcinoembryonic antigen (CEA), 129, 130a
Carcinoid syndrome, 665
Carcinoma
   of the ampulla of Vater, 665
   of the breast, 665
   of the cervix, 665
   of the colon, 665
   of the endometrium, 665
   of the esophagus, 666
   of the lung, 666
   of the ovary, 666
   of the pancreas, 666
Cardiac arrhythmia, 621–622
Cardiac catheterization and angiocardiography, 131–132
Cardiac murmurs, 622
Cardiac series, 133
Cardiomegaly, 622
Cardiomyopathy, 666
Carotene, 134, 135a
Carotid duplex scan, 136
Carpal tunnel syndrome, 666
Casts, 137–138, 138a
Cat-scratch disease, 666
Catecholamines, vanillylmandelic acid (VMA) and, 590
CD4 and T-Cell lymphocyte count, 139
CEA (Carcinoembryonic antigen), 129, 130a
Cell studies (see Cytologic studies)
Cellulitis, 666
Cerebellar ataxia, 666
Cerebral abscess (or cerebellar abscess), 666
Cerebral aneurysm, 666
Cerebral embolism, 666
Cerebral hemorrhage, 666
Cerebral thrombosis, 666
Cerebrospinal fluid (CSF), culture of, 203–204, 206
Cerebrospinal fluid (CSF), microscopic examination of, 523
Cerebrospinal fluid (CSF) pressure, 140–141, 141a
Cervical bruit, 641
Cervical spondylosis, 667
Cervicitis, 667
Chagas' disease, 667

**698      Index**

Chancroid, 667
  skin test, 142
Chest deformity, 622
Chest pain, 622
Chest radiography
  cardiac silhouette abnormalities, 144, 145, 147a
  lung abnormalities, 143–144, 145, 146a
  lung findings, 148a
  pleural effusion workup, 144–145, 149a
Chest tenderness, 622–623
Chills, 623
Choledocholithiasis, 667
Chloride, blood, 150–151, 151a
Cholangiocarcinoma, 667
Cholangiography, intravenous, 340
Cholangitis, 667
Cholecystitis, 667
Cholecystography, 152, 153a
Cholelithiasis, 667
Cholera, 667
Cholesterol, 154–155, 156a
Choreiform movements, 623
Choriocarcinoma, 667
Chromosome analysis, 157
Cirrhosis, 667
Cisternography, 158
*Clostridium difficile* toxin assay, 159
Clot retraction, 160, 161a
Clubbing of fingers, 623
CMV (Cytomegalovirus) antibodies, 217
CMV (Cytomegalovirus) infection, 669
Coagulant factors, 162–163, 163a
Coagulation time, 164, 165a
Coarctation of the aorta, 667
*Coccidioides* antibody test, 166
Coccidiomycosis, 667
  skin test, 167
Cold agglutinins, 168, 169a
Colonoscopy, 170
Color, urine, 171, 172a
Colposcopy, 173
Coma, 623
Complement C3, 174, 175a
Computed tomography (*see* CT-Computed tomography)
Congenital heart disease, 667–668
Conjunctival fluid culture, 205, 206
Conjunctivitis, 668
Constipation, 623–624, 668
Convulsions, 624
Coombs' test, direct and indirect, 184
Copper and ceruloplasmin, 185, 186a
Coronary insufficiency, 668
Cortisol, 187–188, 188a
Cough, 624
Cramps, menstrual, 624
Cramps, muscular, 624
Craniopharyngioma, 668
Creatine phosphokinase, 193, 194a
Creatinine, 195–196, 196a
  clearance, 197
Crepitus, 624
Cretinism, 668
Creutzfeldt-Jakob disease, 668

CRP (C-reactive protein), 191, 192a
Cryoglobulins, 198
Cryptococcosis, 668
*Cryptococcus* antigen titer, 199
Crystals, urine, 200, 200a
CSF (Cerebrospinal fluid), culture of, 203–204, 206
CSF (Cerebrospinal fluid), microscopic examination of, 523
CSF (Cerebrospinal fluid pressure), 140–141, 141a
CT (Computed tomography)
    abdomen, 176
    brain, 177
    chest, 178
    extremities and joints, 179
    head, 180
    neck, 181
    pelvis, 182
    spine, 183
Cultures of miscellaneous body fluids
    cerebrospinal fluid, 203–204, 206
    conjunctival fluid, 205, 206
    ear, 205–206
    nasal, 201, 206
    nasopharyngeal, 201, 206
    peritoneal fluid, 204–205, 206
    pleural fluid, 204, 206
    skin and wound, 201–202, 206
    stool, 203, 206
    urethral, 202, 206
    vaginal, 202–203, 206
Cushing's syndrome, 668
Cutaneous immunofluorescence biopsy, 207
Cutaneous larva migrans, 668
Cyanosis, 624
Cyclic adenosine monophosphate (C-AMP), renal, 208
Cystic fibrosis, 668
Cysticercosis, 668
Cystine, 209
Cystinosis, 668–669
Cystinuria, 669
Cystometric studies, 210
Cystoscopy, 211
Cytologic studies
    breast, 212
    cerebrospinal fluid, 212–213
    female genital tract (Papanicolaou smear), 213
    gastrointestinal tract, 213–214
    peritoneal effusion, 214
    pleural effusion, 214–215
    respiratory tract, 215
    urinary tract, 215–216
Cytomegalovirus (CMV) antibodies, 217
Cytomegalovirus (CMV) infection, 669

D-Xylose absorption, 613
Deafness, 625
Deformities, foot, 633
Dehydroepiandrosterone sulfate (DHEA-S), 218
Delayed puberty, 625
Delirium, 625
Delusions, 625
Dementia, 625
Dengue fever, 669
Depression, 625, 669

Dermatomal somatosensory-evoked potential (DSEP), 245
Dermatomyositis, 669
Dexamethasone-suppression test, 219–220, 220a
DHEA-S (Dehydroepiandrosterone sulfate), 218
Diabetes insipidus, 669
Diabetes mellitus, 669
Diabetic coma, 669
Diaphoresis, 625–626
Diarrhea, acute, 626
Diarrhea, chronic, 626
Difficulty in urinating, 626
Digital subtraction angiography, 221
Digitalis intoxication, 669
Diphtheria, 669
*Diphyllobothrium latum*, 669
Diplopia, 626
Diverticular disease, 669
Dizziness, 626–627
D$_{LCO}$ (Carbon monoxide diffusing capacity), 475
Down's syndrome, 669
Dracunculiasis, 670
Dressler's syndrome, 670
Drop attacks, 627
Drug intoxification, 670
Drug reaction, 670
Drug screen, serum or urine, 222
DSEP (Dermatomal somatosensory-evoked potential), 245
Dubin-Johnson syndrome, 670
Duodenal analysis, 223
Dwarfism, 627
Dysarthria, 627
Dysentery, bacillary, 663
Dysmenorrhea, 627
Dyspareunia, 627
Dysphagia, 627–628
Dyspnea, 628
Dysuria, 628

Ear discharge, 628
Ear fluid culture, 205–206
Earache, 628
Eaton-Lambert syndrome, 670
ECG (Electrocardiography), 227–228, 229a, 230a
Echinococcosis, 670
*Echinococcus* stain test, 224
Echocardiography, 225
Echoencephalography, 226
Eclampsia, 670
Ectopic pregnancy, 670
Eczema, 670
Edema, generalized, 628–629
Edema, localized, 629
EEG (Electroencephalography), 231–232, 232a
EGD (Esophagogastroduodenoscopy), 240
Ehlers-Danlos syndrome, 670
Electrocardiography (ECG), 227–228, 229a, 230a
Electroencephalography (EEG), 231–232, 232a
Electromyography (EMG), 233
Electrophoresis
    hemoglobin, 316–317, 317a
    lipoprotein, 366–367, 367a
    protein, 462–463, 464a, 465
Elliptocytosis, hereditary, 675

EMG (Electromyography), 233
Emphysema, 670
Empyema of the lungs, 670
Encephalitis, viral, 670
Encephalomyelitis, 671
Endocarditis, subacute bacterial, 690
Endoscopic retrograde cholangiopancreatography (ERCP), 234
Enlargement, forehead, 633
Enuresis, 629
Eosinophil count, 235
Eosinophilic pneumonia, 671
Epididymitis, 671
Epidural abscess, 671
Epilepsy, 671
Epiphora, 629
Epistaxis, 629
Epithelial cell casts, 137–138, 138a
Epstein-Barr antibody test, 236–237, 237a
ERCP (Endoscopic retrograde cholangiopancreatography), 234
Erysipelas, 671
Erythema, multiforme, 671
Erythema, nodosum, 671
Erythroblastosis fetalis, 671
Erythropoietin, 238–239, 239a
Esophageal regurgitation, 655
Esophageal varices, 671
Esophagogastroduodenoscopy (EGD), 240
Esophagogram, 577, 578a
Essential hypertension, 671
Estradiol, blood and urine, 241–242, 242a
Estriol, blood, 243
Estrogen and progesterone receptor proteins, 244
Euphoria, 629
Evoked potential studies, 245
Exercise tolerance testing, 246
Exophthalmos, 629
Extradural hematoma, 671
Extremity pain, 629
    upper extremity, 629–630
Eye pain, 630

Fabry's disease, 671
Face pain, 630
Facial flushing, 630
Facial mass, 630
Facial paralysis, 630
Facial swelling, 630
Factor VII-Factor XIII (see Coagulant factors)
Failure to thrive, 631
Familial periodic paralysis, 672
Fat bodies, oval, and fatty casts, 413
Fatigue, 631
Febrile agglutinins, 247–248
Femoral mass or swelling, 631
Fern test, 249
Ferritin, 250–251, 251a
Ferrokinetic studies, 252–253
Fetal hemoglobin in maternal blood, 254
Fever, of unknown origin, 631–632
Fever, relapsing, 687
Fibrin split products, 255, 256a
Fibrinogen, 257
Fibrinolysis/euglobulin lysis time, 258, 259a

Filariasis, 672
Fishberg concentration test, 260
Flank mass, 632
Flank pain, 632
Flatulence, 632–633
Flow volume loops (FV loops), 474
Fluorescein angiography, 261
Fluorescent treponemal antibody absorption test (FTA-ABS), 262
Flushing, facial, 630
Folic acid, 263, 264a
Folic acid deficiency, 672
Follicle-stimulating hormone (FSH), blood and urine, 265–266, 267a
Foot and toe pain, 633
Foot deformities, 633
Foot ulceration, 633
Forced vital capacity (FVC), 471–472, 478a
Forehead enlargement, 633
Free thyroxine index (FTI), 270
Free thyroxine (T4), 268–269, 269a
Free triiodothyronine (T3), 271, 272a
Frei test, 273
Frequency of urination, 633
Friedreich's ataxia, 672
Frigidity, 633–634
Fructosamine assay, 274
FSH (Follicle-stimulating hormone), blood and urine, 265–266, 267a
FTA-ABS (Fluorescent treponemal antibody absorption) test, 262
FTI (Free thyroxine index), 270
Functional residual capacity (FRC), 472
Fungal infection of the skin, 672
Furuncles, 665

γ-Glutamyltransferase, 296, 297a
Gait disturbances, 634
Galactose-1-phosphate uridyl transferase, 275
Galactosemia, 672
Gallbladder or hepatoiminodiacetic acid (HIDA) scan, 276
Gallbladder ultrasonography, 277
Gallium scan, 278
Gangrene, 634
Gas gangrene, 672
Gastrin, 279, 280a
Gastritis, 672
Gastroenteritis, 672
Gastrointestinal bleeding scan, 281
Gigantism, 634
Gilbert's disease, 672
Gingivitis, 672
Girdle pain, 634
Glanders, 672
Glanzmann's disease, 673
Glaucoma, 673
Gliadin antibody, 282
α₁-Globulin electrophoresis, 462–463, 464a
α₂-Globulin electrophoresis, 462–463, 464a
β-Globulin electrophoresis, 462–463, 464a
γ-Globulin electrophoresis, 462–463, 464a
Glomerulonephritis, 673
Glucagon, 283, 284a
Glucose
    blood, 285–286, 286a
    cerebrospinal fluid, 287, 288a
    urine, 289, 290a

Glucose-6-phosphate dehydrogenase (G6PD), 294, 295a
Glucose tolerance test, 291–292, 293a
Glycogen storage disease, 673
Glycosylated hemoglobin, 298
Goiter, diffuse, 673
Gonorrhea, 673
Goodpasture's disease, 673
Gout, 673
G6PD (Glucose-6-phosphate dehydrogenase), 294, 295a
Granular casts, 137–138, 138a
Granuloma inguinale, 673
Growth hormone, 299, 300a
Guillain-Barré syndrome, 673
Gum abnormalities, 660
Gums, bleeding, 621
Gynecomastia, 634

Halitosis, 634–635
Hallucinations, 635
Ham test, 301
Hamman-Rich syndrome, 673
Hand-Schller-Christian disease, 673
Haptoglobin, 302, 303a
Hartnup's disease, 673
Hashimoto's thyroiditis, 673
Hay fever, 673
HBsAg (Hepatitis surface antigen), 319, 320a
β-hCG assay (see Pregnancy test)
Head injury, 674
Head mass or swelling, 635
Headache, 635
Heart failure, 674
Heart shunt scan, 304
Heartburn, 635
Heat-related disorders, 674
Heavy metals
    arsenic, serum, urine, hair and toenails, 305–306, 307
    lead, blood, 305, 307
    mercury, urine, 306, 307
    urine screen, 305, 307
    zinc, blood, 306, 307
Heel pain, 635
Heinz bodies, 308
Hemangioblastoma, 674
Hematemesis, 635
Hematocrit, 309–310, 310a
Hematuria, 311–312, 312a, 635–636
Hemianopsia, 636
Hemifacial spasm, 674
Hemiparesis, 636
Hemiplegia, 636
Hemochromatosis, 674
Hemoglobin, 313–314, 314a
    Bart's, 315
Hemoglobin electrophoresis, 316–317, 317a
Hemoglobin F, 318
Hemolytic anemia, acquired, 674
Hemophilia, 674
Hemoptysis, 636
Hemorrhagic fever, 674
Hemorrhoids, 636, 674
Hepatitis, toxic, 674
Hepatitis, viral, 674

Hepatitis panel, 319, 320a
Hepatoiminodiacetic acid (HIDA) scan, 276
Hepatolenticular degeneration, 674
Hepatoma, 674
Hepatomegaly, 636–637
Herniated disc, cervical, 675
Herniated disc, lumbar, 675
Herpangina, 675
Herpes simplex, 675
Herpes zoster, 675
5-HIAA (5-Hydroxyindoleacetic acid), 330
Hiccups, 637
HIDA (Gallbladder or hepatoiminodiacetic acid) scan, 276
Hidradenitis suppurativa, 675
Hip pain, 637
Hirschsprung's disease, 675
Hirsutism, 637
Histamine cephalalgia, 675
Histiocyte smear, blood, 321
Histiocytosis X, 675
Histoplasmosis, 675
    antibody test, 322
    skin test, 323
HIV antibody tests, 324
HLA testing, 325
Hoarseness, 637
Holter monitoring, 326
Homogentisic acid, urine, 327
Homovanillic acid, urine, 328
Hookworm disease, 675
Horner's syndrome, 637–638
Huntington's chorea, 676
Hurler's syndrome, 676
Hyaline casts, 137–138, 138a
Hydrocephalus, 676
Hydrogen breath analysis, 329
25-Hydroxycalciferol (Vitamin D metabolites), 600, 601a
5-Hydroxyindoleacetic acid (5-HIAA), 330
Hydroxyproline, urine, 331, 332
Hyperactive reflexes, 638
Hyperkinesis, 638
Hypernephroma, 676
Hyperparathyroidism, 676
Hyperpigmentation, 638
Hypersensitivity pneumonitis, 676
Hypersensitivity vasculitis, 676
Hypersomnia, 638
Hypersplenism, 676
Hypertension, 638–639
Hyperthyroidism, 676
Hypoactive reflexes, 639
Hypochondriasis, 639
Hypoparathyroidism, 676
Hypopituitarism, 676
Hypotension, chronic, 639
Hypothermia, 639
Hypothyroidism, 676
Hysterosalpingography, 333

IBC, (Iron binding capacity, total), 345–346, 346a
Idiopathic postural hypotension, 676
Idiopathic pulmonary fibrosis, 676–677
IgM anti-HAV (Hepatitis A antibody), 319, 320a

IgM anti-HBc (Hepatitis B core antigen antibody), 319, 320a
Immunoelectrophoresis, IgA, IgE, IgG, IgM, 334–335, 336a
Impedance phlebography, 337
Impetigo, 677
Impingement syndrome, 677
Impotence, 639–640
Incontinence
    of feces, 640
    due to stress, 658
    of urine, 640
Indigestion, 640
Infectious mononucleosis, 677
Infertility, female, 640–641
Infertility, male, 641
Influenza, 677
Inguinal swelling, 641
Insomnia, 641
Insulin, 338, 339a
Insulinoma, 677
Intracranial bruit, 641
Intravenous cholangiography, 340
Iron, serum, 343, 344a
Iron-binding capacity (IBC), total, 345–346, 346a
Iron-deficiency anemia, 677
Irritable bowel syndrome, 677
IVP (Intravenous pyelography), 341–342, 342a

Jaundice, 641–642
Jaw pain, 642
Jaw swelling, 642
Joint pain, 642
Joint swelling, 642

Kala-azar, 677
17-Ketogenic steroids, urine, 347–348, 348a
17-Ketosteroids, urine, 347–348, 348a
Klinefelter's syndrome, 677
Korsakoff's syndrome, 677
Kyphosis, 642–643

Lactic acid, arterial blood, 349
Lactic acid dehydrogenase (LDH), 350, 351a
    cerebrospinal fluid, 352, 353a
    isozymes, 354, 355a
Lactase deficiency, 677
Lactose tolerance, 356
Langerhans' cell granulomatosis, 677
LAP (Leucine aminopeptidase), blood, urine, 360, 361a
Laparoscopy, 357
Larva migrans (see Visceral and ocular larva migrans)
Laryngitis, 677–678
LATS (Long-acting thyroid stimulator), 370
Lead intoxication, 678
Leg ulceration, 643
Legionella antibody, 358
Legionnaires' disease, 678
Leishmaniasis, cutaneous, 678
Leprosy, 678
Leptospirosis, 678
    antibody titer, 359
Leriche's syndrome, 678
Leucine aminopeptidase (LAP), blood, urine, 360, 361a
Leukemia, 678

Leukocyte alkaline phosphatase, 362, 363a
Lichen planus, 678
Lip pain, 643
Lip swelling, 643
Lipase, 364, 365a
Lipoprotein electrophoresis, 366–367, 367a
Lipoproteinemias, 678
Listeriosis, 678
Liver abscess, 678
Liver scan, 368
Liver ultrasonography, 369
Long-acting thyroid stimulator (LATS), 370
Lordosis, 643
Lung abscess, 678
Lupus erythematosus, 678
Lyme disease, 678
   antibody, 371
Lymphadenopathy, 643
Lymphangiography, 372
Lymphangitis, 679
Lymphogranuloma venereum, 679
Lymphoma, 679
Lysosomal storage disease, 679
Lysozyme, blood and urine, 373

Macroglobulinemia, 679
Magnesium, 374–375, 375a
Malabsorption syndrome, 679
Malaria, 679
Mallory-Weiss tear, 679
Mammography, 383
Marfan's syndrome, 679
Mastoiditis, 679
Maximum midexpiratory flow rate (MMFR), 476–477
Maximum voluntary ventilation (MVV), 477–478
McArdle's syndrome, 679
McCune-Albright syndrome, 679
Mean corpuscular hemoglobin concentration (MCHC), 386, 387a
Mean corpuscular hemoglobin (MCH), 384, 385a
Mean corpuscular volume (MCV), 388–389, 389a
Meckel's diverticulum, 679
Mediastinitis, 679
Mediastinoscopy, 391
Mediterranean fever, familial, 672
Melanin, urine, 390
Melanoma, 679
Melena, 643–644
Memory loss, 644
Meniere's disease, 680
Meningitis, 680
Meningococcemia, 680
Menopause, 680
Menorrhagia, 644
Mental retardation, 644
Mesenteric artery insufficiency, embolism, thrombosis, 680
Methemoglobin, 392, 393a
Methemoglobinemia, 680
Metrorrhagia, 644
Metyrapone test, 394, 395a
Microscopic examination of body fluids
   blood, 520
   cerebrospinal fluid, 523
   penile lesions, 522

   skin lesions, 522
   sputum, 519–520
   stool fluid, 523
   urethral, 521
   urine, 520–521
Migraine, 680
Milroy's disease, 680
Minimum inhibitory concentration (MIC), 396
Mitral valvular disease, 680
Monoplegia, 644–645
Monospot test, 397, 398a
Mouth pigmentation, 645
MRI (Magnetic resonance imaging)
   abdomen, 376
   brain, 377
   chest, 378
   joints, 379
   neck, 380
   pelvis, 381
   spine, 382
Mucopolysaccharide screen, urine, 399
Mucoproteins, 400, 401a
Mucormycosis, 680
Multiple myeloma, 680
Multiple sclerosis, 680
Mumps, 680
Muscular atrophy, 645
Muscular dystrophy, 680
Musculoskeletal pain, generalized, 645
Myasthenia gravis, 680–681
Myelin basic protein, cerebrospinal fluid, 402
Myelography, 403
Myocardial infarction, 681
Myoglobin, blood and urine, 404, 405a
Myotonia atrophica, 681

Nail abnormalities, 645–646
Narcolepsy, 681
Nasal discharge, 646
Nasal fluid culture, 201, 206
Nasal obstruction, 646
Nasopharyngeal fluid culture, 201, 206
Nausea and vomiting, 646
Neck pain, 646
Neck stiffness, 646–647
Neck swelling, 647
Nephrolithiasis, 681
Nephrotic syndrome, idiopathic, 681
Nerve conduction studies, 406, 407a
Neuroblastoma, 681
Neurofibromatosis, 681
Neuroma, traumatic, 681
Niemann-Pick disease, 681
Nightmares, 647
Nitrite test, 408
Nocardiosis, 681
Nocturia, 647
Nose, regurgitation of food through, 647
Nutritional anemia, 681
Nystagmus, 647–648

Obesity, 648, 681
Obstetric ultrasonography, 409

Odor, 648
Oliguria (*see* Anuria)
Opisthotonos, 648
Optic neuritis, 681
Orbital and ocular ultrasonography, 410
Orchitis, 681–682
Oroya fever, 682
Orthopnea (*see* Dyspnea)
Osmolality, serum, 411–412, 412a
Osteoarthritis, 682
Osteogenesis imperfecta, 682
Osteogenic sarcoma, 682
Osteomalacia, 682
Osteomyelitis, 682
Osteopetrosis, 682
Osteoporosis, 682
Otitis externa, 682
Otitis media, 682
Oval fat bodies and fatty casts, 413
Ovarian cancer, 682
Oxygen, arterial, 414–415, 415a

Paget's disease of bone, 682
Palpitations, 648
Pancreatic scan, 416
Pancreatic ultrasonography, 417
Pancreatitis, acute, 682
Pancreatitis, chronic, 682
Panniculitis, acute, 683
Papanicolaou smear, 213
Papilledema, 648
Paralysis
    agitans, 683
    facial, 630
    periodic, familial, 672
Paranasal sinus radiography, 418
Parathyroid hormone (PTH), 419, 420a
Parathyroid ultrasonography, 421
Paresthesias
    of the lower extremity, 648–649
    of the upper extremity, 649
Partial thromboplastin time (PTT), 422, 423a
Pathologic reflexes, 649
Peak expiratory flow rate (PEFR), 476
Peak inspiratory flow rate (PIFR), 475–476
Pellagra, 683
Pelvic mass, 649
Pelvic pain, 649–650
Pelvic ultrasonography, 424
Pelvimetry, 425
Pemphigus vulgaris, 683
Penile lesions, microscopic examination, 522
Penile pain, 650
Penile sores, 650
Peptic ulcer, 683
Periarteritis nodosa, 683
Pericarditis, 683
Perineal pain, 650
Perinephric abscess, 683
Periorbital edema, 650
Peripheral neuropathy, 683
Peristalsis, visible, 650

Peritoneal fluid analysis, 426, 427a
Peritoneal fluid culture, 204–205, 206
Peritonitis, 683
Pernicious anemia, 683
Peroneal muscular atrophy, 683
Peroneal neuropathy, 683
Pertussis, 683
Peutz-Jeghers syndrome, 683
Peyronie's disease, 684
pH, 428, 429a
   urine, 430, 431a
Pharyngeal smear, 432
Pharyngitis and tonsillitis, 684
Pharyngoconjuctival fever, 684
Phenylalanine, blood, 433
Phenylpyruvic oligophrenia, 684
Pheochromocytoma, 684
Phlebotomus fever, 684
Phonocardiography, 434
Phosphorus, 435–436, 437a
Photophobia, 650
PIFR (Peak inspiratory flow rate), 475–476
Pinealoma, 684
Pinworm disease, 684
Pituitary adenoma, 684
Pityriasis rosea, 684
Plague, 684
Platelet aggregation, 438
Platelet antibodies, 439
Platelet count, 440, 441a
Pleural fluid analysis, 442–443, 443a
Pleural fluid culture, 204, 206
Pneumoconiosis, 684
*Pneumocysitis carinii* infection, 684
Pneumonia, 684
Pneumothorax, 684
Poliomyelitis, 684
Polychondritis, relapsing, 687
Polycystic kidney disease, 685
Polycystic ovary syndrome, 685
Polycythemia vera, 685
Polydipsia, 650–651
Polymyalgia rheumatica, 685
Polyuria, 651
Popliteal swelling, 651
Porphyria, 685
Porphyrins, urine, 444, 445a
Potassium, 446–447, 447a
   urine 24-hour, 448–449, 449a
Precocious puberty, 651
Preeclampsia-eclampsia, 685
Pregnancy test, blood and urine, 450, 451a
Pregnanediol, urine, 452, 453a
Pregnanetriol, urine, 454
Premenstrual tension syndrome, 685
Priapism, 651
Prolactin, 455, 456
Prostate-specific antigen (PSA), 457
Prostatic carcinoma, 685
Prostatic hypertrophy, 685
Prostatitis, 685
Protein, cerebrospinal fluid, 458, 459a
Protein, urine, 460, 461a

Protein electrophoresis, 462–463, 464a
  cerebrospinal fluid, 465
Prothrombin consumption test, 466, 467a
Prothrombin time, 468, 469a
Pruritis
  ani, 652
  generalized, 651–652
  vulvae, 652
PSA (Prostate-specific antigen), 457
Pseudogout, 685
Pseudohypoparathyroidism, 685
Pseudopseudohypoparathyroidism, 685
Pseudotumor cerebri, 685
Psittacosis, 686
Psoriasis, 686
PTH (Parathyroid hormone), 419, 420a
Ptosis, 652
PTT (Partial thromboplastin time), 422, 423a
Ptyalism, 652
Pulmonary alveolar proteinosis, 686
Pulmonary capillary wedge pressure, 470
Pulmonary embolism, 686
Pulsatile swelling, 652
Pulse, absent or diminished, 618
Pulse, irregularity of, 652–653
Pulses, unequal, 653
Pupil abnormalities, 653
Purpura and abnormal bleeding, 653
Pyelography, intravenous (IVP), 341–342, 342a
Pyelography, retrograde, 502
Pyelonephritis, 686
Pyloric stenosis, congenital, 686
Pyridoxine deficiency, 686
Pyruvate kinase, 479

Q fever, 686

Rabies, 686
Radioactive iodine (RAI)
  fibrinogen venogram, 480
  total body scan, 481
  uptake and scan, 482, 483a
  uptake stimulation test, 484
Radioallergosorbent test (RAST), 485
Radiography, chest, 144–145, 146a–149a
Radiography, paranasal sinus, 418
Rales, 653
Rapid plasma reagin (RPR), 591
Rash, 654
RAST (Radioallergosorbent test), 485
Rat-bite fever, 686
Raynaud's disease, 686
Raynaud's phenomena, 654
Rectal bleeding, 654
Rectal discharge, 654
Rectal mass, 654
Rectal pain, 654–655
Red blood cell count (RBC), 486–487, 487a
Red cell casts, 137–138, 138a, 488, 489a
Red cell fragility, 490, 491a
Red cell size distribution width (RDW), 492
Red cell survival time, 493, 494a
Reflex sympathetic dystrophy, 686

Reflexes, hyperactive, 638
Reflexes, hypoactive, 639
Reflux esophagitis, 686
Refsum's disease, 686
Regional enteritis, 686–687
Regurgitation, esophageal, 655
Regurgitation, of food through nose, 647
Reiter's syndrome, 687
Relapsing fever, 687
Relapsing polychondritis, 687
Renal failure, acute, 687
Renal failure, chronic, 687
Renal ultrasonography, 495
Renal vein thrombosis, 687
Renin, 496, 497a
Renogram, 498
Residual volume (RV), 473–474
    urine, 499
Respiration abnormalities, 655
Restless leg syndrome, 655
Reticulocyte count, 500, 501a
Retinal artery occlusion, 687
Retrograde pyelography, 502
Retroperitoneal ultrasonography, 503
Rheumatic fever, 687
Rheumatoid arthritis, 687
Rheumatoid factor, 504, 505a
Rheumatoid spondylitis, 687
Riboflavin deficiency, 687
Rickets, 687
Rickettsialpox, 687
Rocky Mountain spotted fever, 687
    antibodies, 506
RPR (Rapid plasma reagin), 591
Rubella, 688
    antibody test, 507
Rubeola, 688

Salivary gland scan, 508
Salmonellosis, 688
Salpingitis, 688
Sarcoidosis, 688
Scabies, 688
Scalp tenderness, 655
Scarlet fever, 688
Schilder's disease, 688
Schilling test, 509, 510a
Schistosomiasis, 688
Schizophrenia, 688
Scleroderma, 688
Scoliosis, 655–656
Scotoma, 656
Scrotal swelling, 656
Scrub typhus, 688
Scurvy, 688
Seborrheic dermatitis, 688
Sedimentation rate, 511–512, 512a
Semen analysis, 513
Sensory loss, 656
Septic arthritis, 688
Septicemia, 688
Serum prothrombin time, 466, 467a
Serum sickness, 689

SGOT (aspartate aminotransferase, AST), 68–69, 69a
SGPT (alanine aminotransferase, ALT), 68–69, 69a
Shake test, 514
Shigellosis, 689
Shoulder pain, 656
Shy-Drager syndrome, 689
Sickle cell anemia, 689
Sickle cell test, 515
Sigmoidoscopy, 516
Sinusitis, 689
Sjögren's antibody test, 517
Sjögren's syndrome, 689
Skin and wound fluid culture, 201–202, 206
Skin cancer, 689
Skin lesions, microscopic examination, 522
Skin test
    blastomycosis, 89
    brucellosis, 115
    chancroid, 142
    coccidioidomycosis, 167
    histoplasmosis, 323
    toxoplasmosis, 569
    Trichinella, 570
Skin testing, allergy, 24
Skin thickening, 656–657
Sleep apnea, 657, 689
Sleep walking, 657
Small bowel series, 518
Small intestinal tumors, 689
Smear
    blood, 520
    cerebrospinal fluid, 523
    Papanicolaou, 213
    penile lesions, 522
    pharyngeal, 432
    skin lesions, 522
    sputum, 519–520
    stool fluid, 523
    urethral, 521
    urine, 520–521
Snake bite, 689
Sneezing, 657
Snoring, 657
Sodium, 524–525, 525a
    urine, 526–527, 527a
Somatomedin C, 528
Somatosensory-evoked potential, 245
Sonography, aortic, 63
Sore throat, 657
Spasmodic torticollis, 689
Specific gravity, urine, 520a, 529
Spherocytosis, hereditary, 675
Spinal cord tumor, 689
Spleen scan, 531
Spleen ultrasonography, 532
Splenomegaly, 657
Sporotrichosis, 689
Sprains, common, 689
Sputum, microscopic examination, 519–520
Sputum culture, routine, 533, 534a
Stasis dermatitis, 689
Steatorrhea, 657–658
Stomach cancer, 665

Stool analysis, 535–536, 536a
Stool fluid, microscopic examination, 523
Stool fluid culture, 203, 206
Streptococcal antibody tests (ASO, ADB, Streptozyme), 537
Streptozyme (Streptococcal antibody test), 537
Stress incontinence, 658
Stretch marks, 658
Stridor, 658
Strongyloidiasis, 689
Stupor, 658
Sturge-Weber syndrome, 690
Subacute bacterial endocarditis, 690
Subdiaphragmatic abscess, 690
Subdural hematoma, 690
Sulfhemoglobin, 538
Sulfhemoglobinemia, 680
Sweat test, 539
Syncope, 658
Synovial fluid analysis, 540, 541a
Syphilis, 690
Syringomyelia, 690
Systemic mastocytosis, 690

T4, free thyroxine, 268–269, 269a
T3, free triiodothyronine, 271, 272a
T and B lymphocytes, 542–543, 543a
T-Cell lymphocyte count, CD4 and, 139
T$_4$ (Total Thyroxine), 566, 567a
Tachycardia, 658–659
Takayasu's disease, 690
Tapeworm disease, 690
Taste abnormalities, 659
TBG (Thyroxine-binding globulin), 561, 562a
Technetium-99M resting heart scan, 544
Teichoic acid antibody titer, 545
Temporal arteritis, 690
Testicular atrophy, 659
Testicular pain or swelling, 659
Testicular tumors, 690
Testosterone, 546, 547a
Tetanus, 690
Thalassemia, 690
Thallium gated equlibrium heart scan, 548
Thallium stress scan, 549
Therapeutic drug monitoring, 550
Thirst, 659
Thoracic outlet syndrome, 690
Throat culture, routine, 551, 552a
Thrombin time, 553, 553a
Thromboangiitis obliterans, 691
Thrombocytopenic purpura, idiopathic, 691
Thrombophlebitis, 691
Thromboplastin time, activated partial (APTT), 422, 423a
Thrombotic thrombocytopenic purpura, 691
Thymoma, 691
Thyroglobulin, 554
Thyroid antibodies, 555
Thyroid enlargement, 659–660
Thyroid-stimulating hormone (TSH)-sensitive assay, 557, 558a
Thyroid ultrasonography, 556
Thyroiditis, subacute, 691
Thyrotropin-releasing hormone (TRH) stimulation test, 559, 560a
Thyroxine-binding globulin (TBG), 561, 562a

Tinnitus, 660
Tomography (*see* CT-Computed tomography)
Tongue mass or swelling, 660
Tongue pain and ulcers, 660
Tonsillitis and pharyngitis, 684
Tooth abnormalities, 660
Torch test, 563
Torticollis, spasmodic, 689
Total protein, 564–565, 565a
Total Thyroxine ($T_4$), 566, 567a
Tourette's syndrome, 691
Toxoplasmosis, 691
  antibody test, 568
  skin test, 569
Trachoma, 691
Transfusion reaction, 691
Transient ischemic attacks, 691
Tremor, 660
TRH (Thyrotropin-releasing hormone) stimulation test, 559, 560a
*Trichinella* skin test, 570
Trichinosis, 691
Trigeminal neuralgia, 691
Triglyceride, 571–572, 573a
Trypanosomiasis, 691
Trypsin, stool, 574
TSH (Thyroid-stimulating hormone)-sensitive assay, 557, 558a
Tuberculin test, 575
Tuberculosis, 692
Tuberous sclerosis, 692
Tularemia, 692
Typhoid fever, 692
Typhus, epidemic, 692
Typhus, scrub, 688
Tyrosine, urine, 576

Ulcerative colitis, 692
Ultrasonography
  breast, 111
  gallbladder, 277
  liver, 369
  obstetric, 409
  orbital and ocular, 410
  pancreatic, 417
  parathyroid, 421
  pelvic, 424
  renal, 495
  retroperitoneal, 503
  spleen, 532
  thyroid, 556
  urinary bladder, 583
Unusual odor (*see* Anosmia)
Upper gastrointestinal series, 577, 578a
Urethral discharge, 660
Urethral fluid, microscopic examination, 521
Urethral fluid culture, 202, 206
Uric acid, 579, 580a
  urine, 581, 582a
Urinary bladder ultrasonography, 583
Urinary tract infection, 692
Urinating, difficulty in, 626
Urination, frequency of, 633
Urine, microscopic examination, 520–521
Urine culture, 584–585, 585a

Urobilinogen, stool, 586, 587a
Urobilinogen, urine, 588, 589a
Urticaria, 692
Uterine fibroids, 692

Vaginal discharge, 661
Vaginal fluid culture, 202–203, 206
Vaginal ulcerations, 661
Vaginitis, 692
Vanillylmandelic acid (VMA) and catecholamines, 590
Varicella, 692
Varicose veins, 661, 692
Variola, 692
Veneral disease, 692
Venereal disease research laboratory (VDRL), 591
Venography, 592
Ventilation-perfusion scan, 593–594
Viral antibody tests, 595
Viral isolation tests, 595
Viral myelitis, 693
Visceral and ocular larva migrans, 693
Viscosity, blood, 596, 597a
Visual-evoked potential, 245
Vital capacity (VC), 472–473
Vitamin B$_{12}$, 598, 599a
Vitamin D metabolites (25-Hydroxycalciferol), 600, 601a
Vitamins, miscellaneous
    Vitamin A, blood, 602
    Vitamin B$_6$, blood, 602–603
    Vitamin C, plasma, 603
    Vitamin E, blood, 603–604
    Vitamin K, 604
VMA (Vanillylmandelic acid) and catecholamines, 590
Von Willebrand's disease, 693
Vulval ulcerations, 661

Warts, 693
Wegener's granulomatosis, 693
Weight loss, 661
Wernicke's encephalopathy, 693
Wheezing, 661
Whipple's disease, 693
White blood cell count (WBC)
    cerebrospinal fluid, 605, 606a
    differential, 607–608, 608a
    total, 609–610, 610a
    urine, 611, 612a
White cell casts, 137–138, 138a

Yaws, 693
Yellow fever, 693

Zinc protoporphyrins, 614
Zollinger-Ellison syndrome, 693

# *The quickest path from diagnosis to treatment.*

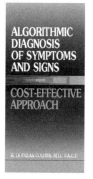

## Algorithmic Diagnosis of Symptoms and Signs: Cost-Effective Approach

R. Douglas Collins, MD, FACP

Start your search for the correct diagnosis with this fast-thinking guide that's organized by signs and symptoms, just like your patients. Each section opens with suggested questions that help you collect vital information. You then work through clear algorithms that highlight historic and clinical data that lead to the strongest diagnostic choice. Following the algorithms, guidelines direct you to the best tests for a diagnostic workup. Get ready for virtually any sign or symptom with 227 full-page algorithms that bring you a cost-effective approach to diagnosis.

1995/626 pages/0-89640-283-5

## Algorithmic Approach to Treatment

R. Douglas Collins, MD, FACP

Even after you reach a definitive diagnosis you still have to consider a number of possible treatment choices. This time-saving reference uses algorithms to present available therapies and divide patients according to the crucial factors that can influence your decision. You'll find 130 clear algorithms listed in alphabetical order by disease, covering both common and rare disorders. Order your copy for a logical, studied approach to treatment that leads you to the best results for your patients.

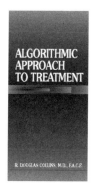

1997/640 pages/250 illustrations/0-683-30303-1

**We invite you to preview these texts for a full month** (US and Canada only).

Phone orders accepted 24 hours a day, 7 days a week (US only)
Prices subject to change without notice.

**From the US:**
Call: 1-800-638-0672
Fax: 1-800-447-8438

**From outside the US and Canada:**
Call: 410-528-4223
Fax: 410-528-8550

**From Canada:**
Call: 1-800-665-1148
Fax: 1-800-665-0103

**VISIT US ON THE INTERNET!**
E-mail: custserv@wwilkins.com
Home page:http://www.wwilkins.com

Printed in US 9 97     COLLBIA  >   S7B616